Ahead of the Curve

SHANE CROTTY

Ahead of the Curve

David Baltimore's Life in Science

UNIVERSITY OF CALIFORNIA PRESS
BERKELEY LOS ANGELES LONDON

University of California Press
Berkeley and Los Angeles, California

University of California Press, Ltd.
London, England

Library of Congress Cataloging-in-Publication

Crotty, Shane
    Ahead of the curve : David Baltimore's life in science /
Shane Crotty.
      p.   cm.
    Includes index
    ISBN 0-520-22557-0 (cloth : alk. paper)
      1. Baltimore, David.   2. Molecular biologists—
United States—Biography.   I. Title.
    QH506.C76   2001
    572.8'092—dc21   00-051170
    [B]

Manufactured in the United States of America

10   09   08   07   06   05   04   03   02   01
10   9   8   7   6   5   4   3   2   1

For my parents,
Mom and Dad

The people who are going to make the breakthroughs,
by analogy with history, are going to be young, well-trained
scientists working in unpredictable areas.

DAVID BALTIMORE

CONTENTS

PROLOGUE

*It has to do with the understanding I get from science. And some
of that understanding, I feel, leads me, has led me, to more activism
as a role. I mean, you can take a piece of information, and you can do
lots of things with it. You can try to publish it; you can try to develop
a practical aspect of it, like a therapy, or a machine; or you can look at
the implications in the public health arena, or the public policy arena.
I guess I've always considered those a kind of continuum of ways
that information becomes valuable, and ways that I take
information and then try and go further with it.*

DAVID BALTIMORE
January 20, 1995

ON A BLUSTERY AUTUMN day in 1986, the wind ripples across David Baltimore's trenchcoat and jostles his briefcase as he quickly crosses a courtyard in Cambridge, Massachusetts. His beard has a gray hair for every hundred times he has been asked when he will cure cancer. His navy blue suit is stylish; he dresses much better than he used to, back when biology wasn't lucrative and he was anticapitalist. His mind is actively planning, analyzing, and reviewing as he walks toward the Whitehead Institute for Biomedical Research, which he started four years earlier and where he has assembled perhaps the most brilliant and hardworking group of molecular biologists in the world. He knows that around the globe two hundred thousand people are succumbing to the stranglehold of AIDS. His newest project is to find a cure.

Baltimore has just spent two days in Washington, at the Institute of Medicine in the National Academy of Sciences, serving as cochair of the Committee on a National Strategy for AIDS. It has been five years since AIDS was identified, and the National Academy of Sciences is the first United States federal body attempting to deal with the epidemic. Congress and Ronald Reagan remain silent about AIDS. It is seen as the scourge of deviants, homosexuals, and heroin addicts. In Edmund White's words, "The AIDS epidemic has rolled back a big rotten log and revealed all the squirming life underneath it, since it involves, all at once, the main themes of our existence: sex, death, power, money, love, hate, disease, and panic." A world of turmoil is wrapped up in the tiny human immunodeficiency virus, and Baltimore is acutely aware of the complications. As director of the research half of the AIDS committee, he is charged with developing a national plan to create a cure and annihilate the AIDS epidemic.

On several counts he is the perfect choice. He is one of two men who discovered the protein heart of the retroviruses, a discovery that has allowed doctors and scientists to detect the elusive HIV virus. He is an experienced organizer, he is keenly attuned to problems with moral prerogatives, and he does not hesitate in a fight.

In other respects he is an unlikely candidate for this post. His lab did not even study AIDS in the early 1980s. But now, through his involvement with the AIDS committee, HIV has "intrigued" him, in much the same way that he was drawn into cancer research by the War on Cancer in the early 1970s. He currently has one graduate student studying HIV, although that project is basic research, not a directed search for a cure. Baltimore studies biology because he is curious, not because he wants to save the world. "My life is dedicated to increasing knowledge," he explains. "We need no more justification for scientific research than that." He wants a cure for AIDS, but his lab isn't looking for it.

At the same time, he knows the emotional toll of disease. Baltimore's mother, always a beacon for him, is succumbing to cancer. Each week he flies to New York to be with her. Her mind is deteriorating quickly, her health worsening slowly, and none of his discoveries can ease her suffering or prevent the inevitable. A few weeks ago he made a somber speech at Massachusetts General Hospital on the slow but steady pace of cancer research. "In my view," he said, "cancer is a problem that will be part of human life for a long time, if not forever . . . and I expect that therapy will be slow to come. Even when new therapeutics schemes come, the plasticity of tumor cells will make it very difficult to effect total cures. For those who hope for rapid progress, this is clearly a pessimistic view." But, disturbed by his own pessimism, he concluded: "But results *will* come, and we, as a nation, must maintain our commitment to finding everything we can about the disease and to try in every way possible to prevent or cure it. There is, of course, the real possibility that my whole analysis is wrong and that there lie out there magic bullets that will make a huge impact on cancer mortality rates in a relatively short time. To have judged so completely wrong would give me great pleasure."

Ever since Koch and Pasteur, society has placed heavy hopes on the ability of biologists to fight disease, but Baltimore entered biology research at a fairly benign time. By the time he graduated from college, the famous microbe hunters were all gone, smallpox was on its way to eradication, and a polio vaccine had been released. In the beginning his science had no medical importance. His fascination with animal viruses led him to research the mechanics of poliovirus, not because he was looking for a vaccine, but because there already was one, and thus poliovirus was safe to handle in the lab. Things changed when he and several colleagues revolutionized biology by creating the means to produce and use recombinant DNA, taking the fable of genetic engineering and making it a reality. Now the practical uses of his science keep drawing him into public life. He isn't interested in medicine, but medicine is interested in him. He did not volunteer for the AIDS committee role: his presence was requested. He was overwhelmed already with the Whitehead, his huge lab, and his mother's illness, but he felt he could not turn his back. With an estimated 25 million people infected by the year 2000, the war on AIDS will be a brutally pragmatic test of modern molecular biology, and Baltimore doesn't like it. Molecular biology is not poised to win a fight with HIV. Most viral vaccines take decades to develop, and no good retrovirus vaccine has ever been developed. He is not optimistic about a cure; HIV is a patient, methodical, spectral killer.

Inside the Whitehead Institute, Baltimore takes the elevator to the third floor. Stepping out, he is staring directly at a large, abstract, splattered acrylic painting on the wall. The rooms along the corridor to the right are all part of his laboratory. His office is to the left, next to a large picture window above a long, curving leather couch. Several token plants rest on the windowsill; they do not grow, and they have no viruses—they are silk. In his office there are no signs of his achievements, no evidence of his Nobel Prize or pictures of his wife and daughter. On a table, amid the piles of folders, papers, books, and magazines, are two neat stacks of documents. One consists of scientific discoveries to review for publication in *Science,* the other a similar stack for the *Journal of Virology.* On his desk, the galley proofs from his newest paper on immunological transcriptional regulation are in. Next to these are various memos about budgets and meetings at the Massachusetts Institute of Technology (the Whitehead's university affiliate). Baltimore enjoys the administrative work. There is a memo about the Imanishi-Kari/O'Toole conflict on the desk as well.

Leaving his office, Baltimore strides down the hall to the lab. A sign declares: "Laboratory Area—No unauthorized persons beyond this point. No food or drink allowed." The laboratory is bigger and busier than it has ever been before, with close to thirty people crammed into an area designed for fifteen. Graduate students and postdoctoral fellows work all hours, every day. Vacations and weekends are perceived as lost time. Some students come in at 7 A.M., while the kitchen staff are still bringing around clean glassware. Most students trickle in between 9 and 10 A.M., and a few don't show their faces until mid-afternoon. Completely nocturnal schedules are not uncommon. The work ethic draws from the motto of the Massachusetts Institute of Technology, *Mens et manus,* mind and hands. Students' motivations vary, but most are straightforward thinkers and tinkerers. They want to discover the multitudinous secrets of life—or at least one or two. Some work for Baltimore because his area of research fascinates them. Some are here because they have heard he is a great mentor. Some are here because they know Nobel mentors beget Nobel pupils. Their futures depend on their success here.

Latex-gloved students stride back and forth carrying plastic dishes filled with rich vermilion fluid growing mouse skin cells, large flasks full of artificial human saline, or photographs recording their most recent DNA concoctions. Baltimore himself has not done benchwork since 1975. Open doors expand into half a dozen laboratory areas on both sides of the hall that extend to the back of the institute. Researchers are crowded two to a bench. A few wear white lab coats; most are in casual clothes. Conversations are brimming with technical lingo. Even in the same lab, people working on different projects sometimes have difficulty understanding each other's vocabulary.

Two researchers stand at a chalkboard in the hall, exchanging scrawls and explanations. Their diagrams are scribbles of circles and lines and cryptic notations. Baltimore joins their discussion, which deals with designing a new NF-κB protein expression vector.

Students in the room to the right are studying poliovirus. The virus group is about the same size it has always been, but it now makes up a much smaller proportion of the lab. Nancy Andrews is studying the manufacture of the poliovirus replicase protein and the fundamental steps of poliovirus replication. Trillions of polioviruses are stored in filtered calf blood in the freezer. Peter Sarnow is studying poliovirus RNA synthesis. Karla Kirkegaard is analyzing the mechanism of RNA recombination, defining the flexibility and evolutionary potential of the virus. Vials full of poliovirus RNA, the living blueprint of the virus, sit in ice buckets while Kirkegaard works quickly to assemble the chemicals and proteins necessary to convert the RNA into more stable DNA.

A large group of students nearby is studying oncogenes, both viral and human: v-*abl*, v-*src*, c-*abl*, *myc*, c-*myc*, the *bcr-abl* hybrid, Ha-*ras*. These hieroglyphics are the names of cancer-causing genes discovered in humans and viruses. What is the Jekyll and Hyde connection between the normal function of human oncogenes and their cancer-causing mutants? Why do viruses like Abelson virus have cancer-causing oncogenes?

Students in the laboratory on the left are studying the immune system's production of antibodies in all of its trillion-cell complexity, teasing apart the plethora of messages and interactions that regulate even the mildest of immune responses. How are antibody genes regulated? What proteins are responsible? How do the parts of the immune system communicate with each other? What makes a B-cell a B-cell? In the tissue culture room, incubators hold flasks growing billions of human cells and mouse cells. Farther down the hall, some students are searching for genes, and others are adding and removing genes in mice. Racks of test tubes on benches swarm with bacteria full of mouse genes. Several students are constructing new genes, mixing pieces of DNA to match their designs. It is the heyday of molecular biology.

Baltimore revolutionized molecular biology with his codiscovery of reverse transcriptase, the enzyme that allows retroviruses like HIV to replicate. For this discovery he won the Nobel Prize at the age of thirty-seven. After that he became one of the foremost hunters of cancer-causing oncogenes and their cellular functions, and later his laboratory characterized crucial components of the immune system, including antibody diversity, NF-κB (a master control gene in immune responses), and the *rag* recombinase genes (which generate a large percentage of antibody diversity). Brilliant, eloquent, and personable, Baltimore is also a man whom even his closest friends refer to as arrogant and ruthless. One colleague at a cocktail party said of him, "He has the best killer instincts of any molecular biologist in the world." Another colleague remarked, "He's arrogant," and after a moment continued, "Why not? He's got every right to be." Perhaps the simplest gauge of his impact on biology is to ask biologists if they know Baltimore and his work; the answer will usually be yes. One colleague claims,

"Baltimore is the premier biomedical scientist of his time and has had a lasting impact on virtually every realm of modern biology." Another commented, "It is not an exaggeration to say that one could write a pretty decent history of the last 25 years in biology by reviewing Dr. Baltimore's contributions."

By the year 2000, at the age of sixty-two, Baltimore had published more than five hundred scientific papers. But his acclaim is by no means universal. Opinions of him are highly polarized, mostly because of the decade-long uproar over the scientific fraud case known as the Baltimore affair (or the Imanishi-Kari affair), which tore the research community into emotional factions. Baltimore went from a subject of awed conversation to a figure whose mention turned friends against each other and tainted conversations with a viciousness normally reserved for religion and politics. One fellow Nobel Prize winner swore venomously that Baltimore's Nobel Prize should be rescinded and his academic tenure revoked, and that he should be banned from scientific research for life.

Yet Baltimore's research has been among the best in the world for over thirty-five years, and his genius extends beyond the laboratory. He helped secure the future of genetic engineering in the recombinant DNA controversy, fought against chemical and biological warfare, organized the national AIDS research effort, founded the Whitehead Institute, served as the president of Rockefeller University, and is the current president of Caltech. On the flip side, he opposed the War on Cancer; became entangled in the nastiest, messiest and most publicized case of scientific fraud ever; and was forced to resign as the president of Rockefeller. He has never been afraid of a fight. "I know what I believe, and I stick by what I believe, and I'll defend what I believe. I understand that I could be wrong about things, but that's what I'm going to stay with. And I've paid a huge penalty for that." He has also reaped huge rewards from it.

One

No one has yet isolated the circumstances that help a child grow whole
and independent, but they were present.

JAMES GLEICK
Genius: The Life and Science of Richard Feynman

GREAT NECK WAS ONE of the many commutervilles lining the route of the
Long Island Railroad in the years following World War II. This sleepy little New York town had become famous up and down Long Island for its
excellent schools. Everyone at Great Neck High School was expected to go
to a four-year college; higher education was both imperative and assumed.
Here David Baltimore went to school. He was one of those students whom
everyone referred to as "gifted," and when his brother came through the
same classes four years later, the teachers still remembered David.

In school, David had no particular direction in mind, and biology classes
in the 1950s were unlikely to inspire budding scientists. David's biology class
consisted entirely of memorization. He learned the parts of a fern, the pieces
of a flower, how the five biological kingdoms were divided, the names of
all of the classes in the animal kingdom, the organs of a frog. The course
was descriptive; students were not encouraged to ask how or why, or to think
about how to solve a problem. And laboratory experiments were far beyond the capacity of the high school classroom in time, resources, and knowledge. The world of research remained foreign to him.

There are no child prodigies in biology. Future physicists may play with
radios or electronics, forcing electrons to flow along wire paths through light
bulbs or amplifiers, but there is no comparable pastime for biologists. Na-
ture-watching is no substitute. Simply looking at frogs is no more instruc-

tive than looking at a radio: the tinkering is the important component. Perhaps someday, when molecular biology has reached elementary and secondary schools, promising young biologists will play with molecular biology sets the way chemists and physicists play with chemistry sets and circuit boards. As it is, most young biologists do no experiments before college. Of the few who do, almost all experiment with chemistry sets, only to switch to biology in college when they learn about its experimental possibilities.

Experimentation is central to biology because, unlike the laws of physics and mathematics, the laws of biology cannot be derived from first principles. A mathematical genius sits down with a pencil and paper and derives the mathematical world. Theoretical physicists do the same; Einstein made three of his most profound discoveries before he was twenty-five without doing a single experiment. But you cannot derive the biological world from theory. Molecular biological systems have an untraceable history, stretching back through three to four billion years of evolution (scientists can find fossils of cells, but evidence of their molecular mechanics all disappeared long ago). And historical causes often completely undermine what seems logically intuitive. To illustrate this, biologists often compare the molecular biological world to a Rube Goldberg apparatus. Goldberg, a cartoonist, drew ludicrously complicated contraptions to accomplish simple tasks. For example, Rube Goldberg's Labor-Saving Potato Masher works by the following mechanism: A several-week-old hunk of cheese gets restless and moves down the incline it rests on, toward a duck. The duck is overcome by the fumes and falls over onto a see-saw, launching a spiked ball into the air. The spiked ball pops a balloon. A policeman hears the pop and thinks somebody has been shot, and so he pokes his head through the window, bumping his head on another lever, which tips over a pitcher of water. The water pours into a hopper and is forced out through a pipe, pushing an electric button, causing a motor to start cranking a music box. A Shimmy Bird starts dancing to the music, causing the platform it stands on to vibrate, which forces the potato masher to mash the potato sitting in a pot beneath the platform. Biological systems are analogous to a Rube Goldberg model: knowing the task to be performed does not allow a biologist, no matter how brilliant, to infer how that task is accomplished. Biological reality is a complex mix of historical and rational causes. Biological discoveries are made by experimenting, for which it takes training to develop the necessary skills and educated creativity.

David's introduction to experimental biology did not come from Great Neck High School, it came with a little help from his mother. He recalls having "a kind of knee-jerk reaction to premedical orientation, because that's what a successful Jewish boy did." David's younger brother, Bob, had the same reaction, and it eventually led him to become a professor of pediatrics at Yale University Medical School. Both sons held their mother in absolute respect. She was a working intellectual who had earned a master's degree in psychology from the New School for Social Research in New York during the 1940s and later became a tenured professor at Sarah Lawrence at the age of sixty-two. Even while she worked, she devoted herself to her sons' education. Early on she held David back in first grade for half a year, possibly to give him a social boost. She and her husband had moved from Queens to Great Neck when David was in the first grade because they wanted the best education for their two sons; they moved back to the city as soon as the kids went to college. She vested great faith in science and education, and, like many Jewish parents of the era, she and her husband hoped their sons would enter science or medicine. In David's junior year of high school, his mother nudged him into research by encouraging him to apply for a little-known summer research program at the Roscoe B. Jackson Memorial Laboratory in Bar Harbor, Maine. He was accepted, and in early summer his parents drove him up the coast to the remote mouse laboratory on Mount Desert Island.

JACKSON LAB

Maine. June, 1955. Sunlight fell through gaps in the gray clouds retreating over the north Atlantic, and sheets of light scattered across the waves, breached the shore, and brushed slowly over the rooftops of Bar Harbor. They skirted the oak- and beech-covered flanks of Cadillac Mountain in Acadia National Park and finally trickled through the lush green canopy surrounding Jackson Laboratory.

A future scientist's first exposure to experiments is of critical importance, and in David's case it was doubly so, because in those first days at Jackson Lab he met Howard Temin. As fate would have it, they would share the Nobel Prize exactly twenty years later for independently discovering reverse transcriptase, the enzyme that allows viruses such as HIV to replicate and reproduce. Jackson Lab scientists had trained Howard in the summer high school program five years earlier. Shortly thereafter, at age eighteen, he published his first scientific paper. In his Swarthmore College senior yearbook, his friends wrote: "Will be one of the future giants in experimental biology . . . could be a fine wrestler, but muscles too big for fascia." On the

Swarthmore wrestling team Howard fought with a quiet ferocity, tying opponents in knots with his gangly reach, but off the mat he maintained a mild-mannered decorum. Some of his friends called him Dean Howard. He had returned to Jackson Lab for the summer of 1955 to mentor the new students and to tinker with some genetics experiments of his own.

Baltimore, four years Temin's junior and distinctly smaller, readily engaged Howard. Their first impressions must have been positive. Howard knew that anyone accepted to the program had to be bright. For David, Howard was the first twenty-year-old he had ever met who was a real scientist. Years later David would fondly recall Howard as the summer "guru." The full group photo of the 1955 Jackson Lab whiz kids shows David displaying a certain adolescent awkwardness—the mundane sort, betraying clothes bought by mother and an uncertainty about the importance of attire. Temin has no such uncertainty, standing with arms akimbo and his jaw set in scientific seriousness.

The Jackson Lab geneticists structured their summer program around a core of daily lectures and three small research projects. The lab specialized in research on mouse genetics. In addition, Jackson was, and is, the largest supplier of lab mice in America. The Jackson Lab mouse library has the broadest, most scientifically potent, and most mind-boggling collection of mammalian genetic variations ever catalogued. In 1995, Jackson was shipping out two million mice a year. Thousands of mutant strains of scurrying mice rattled cages stacked from the floor to the ceiling in long warehouse buildings: black mice, white mice, sandy mice, spotted mice, mice with big ears, mice with pink eyes, fat mice, diabetic mice, mice that caught the flu, mice that shivered when they walked, bald mice, sick mice, mice that developed grotesque tumors. All of these mice lived, bred, and died for science.

Dr. Don Bailey supervised one of David's three small research projects, showing him the vagaries of mouse caretaking—feeding, cleaning, mating—and teaching him basic mouse genetics. The gene is the basic unit of heredity. A specific version of a specific gene is called an allele. For example, there is a gene for mouse hair color. There are many different alleles of that gene, such as white, tan, brown, and black. A complete set of genes, or the molecular instructions describing a complete mouse, is known as a genome. Mice, like almost all animals, have two copies of their genome. This redundancy allows animals to reproduce sexually (combining one copy from each mate), to have greater genetic complexity, and to have a backup copy of many of their genes. With these fundamentals covered, Bailey taught Baltimore how to set up matings that might yield novel traits and patterns.

The power of genetics is that it does not rely on knowing anything about the physical nature of the gene; the geneticist can study the inheritance pattern of hair color in mice, or certain cancers in humans, without any direct physical knowledge of what the gene actually is or does. The geneticist looks only at the gene's final effect. For example, using only genetics, scientists have determined that a certain gene can predispose mice to alcoholism. And in humans, using only genetics, scientists have determined that certain rare families have a predisposition for breast cancer.

For David's second project, Dr. Willys Silvers taught him techniques for examining how mouse skin pigment cells migrate through the body during the mouse's development from pup to adult. Silvers taught Baltimore the unexpected art of mouse dissection, flaying various layers of flesh with surgical precision, locating obscure muscles and tissue structures; and then he taught Baltimore how to examine tissue slices microscopically, searching for migrating pigment cells. Silvers knew the main stages of pigment cell migration, and he was attempting to determine which colors and migration patterns were dominant over others. To accomplish this, he cut patches of skin from one newborn mouse and grafted them onto another with a different skin color pattern. Months later, the mouse with the skin graft was sacrificed and sliced up like a loaf of bread to analyze what had happened to the cells in the skin graft.

Some people soon become desensitized to dropping mice in buckets of anesthetizing ice and then chopping their damp, furry heads off with razors and scissors. Others, plagued by dreams of bright-eyed mice pattering around on tiny pink feet, opt to experiment on something much less cute, something that doesn't bleed. David didn't like killing mice (even when he lived in a mouse-infested apartment years later, he threw washcloths over the mice caught in traps and waited for his roommate to throw them away), but at Jackson he managed.

Dr. Elizabeth Russell, known as Tibby around the lab, led Baltimore through his third project, examining blood cell formation. The cell is to biologists what the atom is to physicists. Though the specifics are lost in the haze of memory, David most likely bled a variety of mice—slicing off the tips of their tails to collect a few drops, or sliding a needle through the eye to extract large pools of blood—and analyzed the proportions of blood cell types present by observing them through a microscope. He had never seen cells before.

White blood cells, magnified five hundred times, floated beneath the lens like water balloons, swollen with grainy clumps of protein. Mature red blood cells appeared as swarms of dimpled discs, while rarer immature red blood cells drifted slowly, lugging their excess flying-saucer-shaped bulk. With different dyes David could identify neutrophils, basophils, and macrophages, each with specialized jobs in the immune system. David would sit at the microscope for hours, until someone reminded him that it was dinnertime. He made good progress on his projects and showed a promise for experimental science that surely did not go unnoticed by the faculty: he had patience, creativity, a meticulous lab manner, and a mind that was stuck in overdrive.

Biology fascinated David as it fascinated his new friends, including his summertime girlfriend and Howard Temin. Establishing an intellectual peer group must have been a vital part of Baltimore's positive experience with science at Jackson Lab; although studying cells and genetics can be intrinsically interesting, scientific benchwork can be as dull and repetitious as laying bricks. Tedious projects are often assigned to a summer student because no one else wants them. So, on days when perhaps David had been transferring mouse skin grafts every morning for a week or counting red blood cells through a microscope for eight hours, the other teenagers could tell him at dinner about the new techniques they had just learned, mouse strains they had seen, and what they thought of mating and killing mice.

Of all the people David met at Jackson Lab, Howard Temin was almost certainly the most influential. When Temin died of cancer in 1994 at the age of fifty-nine, Baltimore wrote a moving reflection titled "In Memoriam: Howard Temin, the Fierce Scholar." In it, he said that at Jackson Lab "[I] venerated him for his wide knowledge and deep commitment to science." At a historic gathering of cancer biologists in 1995, Baltimore lauded Howard Temin as a scientific hero. He encouraged young scientists in the audience to emulate Temin's scientific personality, much as David had as a young man.

Temin was a link for Baltimore between the unformed teenage summer interns like himself and the older, established faculty scientists. Before, David had presumed that real scientific research was far out of his reach, if he ever thought about it at all; but now a future in science didn't seem so impossible. Through his contact with Temin, Baltimore had the chance to ask, "Do I have what it takes to compare to Howard Temin?" Temin's accomplishments and rapid success set the bar for Baltimore; and, consciously or not, Baltimore would spend years working to match the skills of his first scientific role model. Little did he know the scope of that challenge.

After his experience at Jackson, David never wanted to do anything but experimental science. "That was it," he recalls, "It was fantastic, just fantastic. For a high school student it was unbelievable."

Because David was antsy to get out of Great Neck, there is no need to linger in his high school days, but there are a couple of memories worth saving from those years. The first, and more entertaining, is that David Baltimore and Francis Ford Coppola were the two-man tuba section of the Great Neck High School Marching Band—perhaps the most distinguished high school tuba section ever to oompah in America. Coppola recalled relying on Baltimore to count correctly, waiting for David to put his lips to the brass piece before doing so himself. They are friends to this day, and Baltimore occasionally visits Coppola at his vineyard in the Napa Valley.

The other notable aspect of David's high school life was his love of theater, which, as it turned out, dovetailed nicely with his political inclinations and those of his liberal mother. In his junior and senior years he led the thespian group, organizing all productions, and his favorite play was *The Madwoman of Chaillot.* Written by the French diplomat and playwright Jean Giraudoux when he was the French director of propaganda during World War II, and first produced on Broadway shortly after his death in 1944, *The Madwoman of Chaillot* was a blunt, satirical morality play about the evils of capitalism. David loved it. His personal philosophy and his family's political sympathies meshed well with those of Giraudoux. The Madwoman of Chaillot, who slips in and out of true lunacy, finds out about a plot of corporate villains to make millions by drilling for oil in the stately Chaillot district of Paris. With the help of the proletarian King of the Sewer Men, she convicts them in absentia of "the crime of worshipping money" and then convinces them to chase for oil down a bottomless staircase in her cellar, thereby ridding the world of greed. "They're greedy?" she remarks. "Ah, then, my friends, they're lost. If they're greedy, they're stupid." Giraudoux offers dark hyperbole about the merits of socialism and the sins of capitalism. The company president snivels: "I tell you, sir, the only safeguard of order and discipline in the modern world is a standardized worker with interchangeable parts. That would solve the entire problem of management. . . . Wherever the poor are happy, and the servants are proud, and the mad are respected, our power is at an end."

In the opposing camp, the ragpicker moans: "I remember well a time when a cabbage could sell itself just by being a cabbage. Nowadays it's no good being a cabbage—unless you have an agent and pay him a commission. . . . These days . . . every cabbage has its pimp."

David's senior year found him confused about where to go to college. He wanted to become an experimental biologist, but he wasn't in a hurry. Two factors pushed him toward the intellectual haven of Swarthmore College. The first was that Howard Temin had just graduated from Swarthmore, and he had liked it. The second was that David's mother favored Swarthmore. She knew some of the professors there from her years of studying for a psychology Ph.D. at the New School, which she never quite finished. Swarthmore was politically liberal, and David's mother and her parents had always sympathized with European socialist movements (though they never explicitly labeled themselves socialists or Communists), and that childhood influence shaped David's own liberal political philosophy. Swarthmore's academic reputation was undisputed: the *Saturday Evening Post* called it "the most scholarly" of American colleges and universities. For his mother, perhaps Swarthmore's most appealing quality was that it was close to home, so David could catch the train back to Great Neck for holidays. For David, the fact that his Jackson Lab girlfriend attended Swarthmore provided an extra incentive for him to take a good look at the college.

David visited Swarthmore in the spring. The entire campus is a nationally registered arboretum. When he visited, the rhododendrons were in bloom, the dogwoods were flowering, and early roses were budding. Even better, David stayed with his friends from Jackson Lab. He knew that Swarthmore wouldn't offer cutting-edge research, but it would provide an excellent liberal arts education, and he believed that trade-off was worthwhile for his undergraduate years. He enrolled at Swarthmore in the fall of 1956, planning to major in biology.

Two

Why else was the pause prolonged but that singing might issue thence?

COVER EPIGRAPH OF *HALCYON*
Swarthmore College yearbook, 1960

SWARTHMORE COLLEGE IS SNUGGLED in a quaint town outside Philadelphia. When Baltimore arrived, the streets were narrow and wooded, and the few small bridges were made of stone. The thousand students referred to the town beyond the college as "the Village" or simply "the Vil." The campus itself looked borrowed partly from the English countryside and partly from a Virginia plantation. It was the kind of place where, in the spring, once the chill left the air, professors sometimes held classes beneath a fragrant magnolia or near a patch of flowering lilacs. Parrish Hall, which housed the president's offices and the student center, sat at the top of a broad, gently sloping meadow, and the dormitories and academic halls radiated from Parrish to the wooded corners of the campus. Cold Crum Creek and a narrow forest created a natural borderland for the campus from north to west, and the Philadelphia commuter rail line and Swarthmore station sliced across the campus's southern edge. West of Parrish Hall was Scott Amphitheater, perhaps the campus's most famous landmark: an outdoor theater embraced by birch, oaks, and dogwoods. The grassy floor was perforated intermittently by white oaks standing like stone pillars, sprouting scores of leafy branches that wove themselves into a living canopy floating above the audience. At commencement, the dogwood trees and a thousand rhododendrons bloomed, carpeting the campus with red, cream, and pink petals.

Swarthmore was equally renowned for its politics. It was, and is, perhaps the most liberal college in America.* In 1996 the graffiti in the men's bathroom stalls was limited to magic marker peace signs and "Register to vote!" exhortations; the most vulgar epithet was "N.R.A., neurotics rave agitatedly." In 1956, during Baltimore's freshman year, a free-speech controversy raged over the cancellation of an appearance by Alger Hiss, six years after he was convicted of perjury after being tried for Communist espionage and treason. It was also one of the few places in America where people openly questioned the Korean War. In David's junior year, Swarthmore protested the National Defense Education Act because it required students to take a loyalty oath and sign an affidavit stating "that *he does not believe in* [emphasis added] and is not a member of and does not support any organization that believes in or teaches, the overthrow of the United States government by force or violence or by any illegal or unconstitutional methods." Swarthmore objected to the legislation of thought, and Swarthmore's president decried the Act as "un-American." Baltimore's liberalism was mainstream at Swarthmore.

David started out at Swarthmore in the male freshman dorm, Wharton Hall. Finding the rooms small and his roommate a bore, he set about obtaining better accommodations. No matter that freshmen were supposed to live in the freshman dorm, no matter that the Swarthmore administration frowned on attempts to change dorm rooms during the year. David soon discovered a huge room in the upperclass dorm Mary Lyons that was being vacated by a couple of students moving off campus. Mary Lyons was situated across the railroad tracks and about half a mile away from the main campus. The room was a double, so Baltimore needed a roommate. He had made a few friends on his hallway in Wharton, so he asked around to see if he could convince anyone to join him, and Detmar Finke leaped at the chance.

In January, David and Detmar moved into their new attic room, about twice the size of the freshman doubles. It had direct access to a fire escape, so that they could slip out without the dorm proctor seeing, and women could sneak up the three rickety flights into their room. One of the reasons Swarthmore enjoyed such popularity among students in the 1950s was that it was the only top college that was truly coeducational. Nevertheless, this was the mid-fifties, and women were not allowed in the Swarthmore men's dorm. Alcohol was also forbidden. The fire escape immediately became Det-

*Its rival, Reed College in Oregon, might contend that only a friendly game of ultimate Frisbee can settle the matter.

mar and David's window to freedom. As Detmar recalled, "Women were just as important in our lives as academics was—and so were friendships."

Detmar had a clear memory of that freshman year with David: "We didn't sit around in our rooms and study a lot, because we didn't have to. I don't want to sound vain, but in essence we were the top. So we didn't have to do as much work as everybody else had to do to get the same results." Swarthmore didn't expect students to study twenty-four hours a day. Gil Harman, a college friend of David's who later became a professor of philosophy at Princeton University, put it this way: "College in the fifties wasn't like college is today. The expectations were different. I majored in philosophy and mathematics, and the highest math course I took at college my daughter took in high school [in the 1990s]." And grades were less important. Baltimore got a C in organic chemistry in his freshman year, but it didn't keep him from taking honors organic chemistry two years later.

Detmar and David decorated the walls of their room, rearranged the furniture, and somehow became inspired to be morning disc jockeys for the campus FM radio station. They did a tag-team radio show, chattering back and forth, wondering if anybody was listening, and spinning their favorite vinyl: folk tunes and jazz.*

Not only did the two have a fire escape, they also had Detmar's illicit car. From Swarthmore's Quaker roots grew a series of college rules designed to maintain equality among students from different socioeconomic backgrounds. No students were allowed to have cars, and as late as the 1990s students weren't allowed to have their own telephones. Rules weren't of much interest to David and Detmar, however. They hid the car on side streets and alleyways so that they could use it to get to campus on freezing February mornings, and more important, they could take their dates and friends to jazz clubs and bars in Philadelphia on Saturday nights.

The most popular jazz clubs in Philadelphia were places like Pep's and Showboat near City Hall, and there were a few smaller clubs in the ghetto neighborhoods. Most of the patrons were black, and your average upper-middle class white college kid didn't go there. David, Detmar, and a couple of their friends were more adventurous than most, and those swinging bars became some of David's favorite weekend haunts.

*In his freshman year David also dabbled in the Little Theatre Club, orchestra, band, cross-country running, and junior varsity baseball, and ran for student council. By sophomore year he had faded out of most of those activities, except for being part of the Little Theatre Club lighting crew.

These were the years immediately following *Brown v. Board of Education,* when the civil rights movement was just starting to coalesce, and even liberal Swarthmore college had very few black students. Racial integration issues came up in political conversations regularly (though not nearly as regularly as the benefits of Communism) and David, Detmar, and Peter Temin (Howard's younger brother) were part of a loose-knit group of Swarthmore students who participated in occasional small civil rights protests: a sit-in at the Woolworth's in Chester or a public drive to integrate the Swarthmore town barber shops.

There was plenty of time to hang out with his friends. In his sophomore year, David's entire circle of friends lived in Mary Lyons: Peter Temin, Lannie Rubin, Gil Harman, and Detmar Finke, none of whom were biologists. They took over an entire floor, and they had a lot of fun together.

The *Halcyon* yearbook editor struggled to define the essence of Swarthmore: "The spirit of Swarthmore is not to be found in the football stands or in chorus; indeed, at times it seems to ignore the traditional 'togetherness' which a yearbook presumes to reflect. Rather it is felt individually as a persistent state of concentration." The idea of a "persistent state of concentration" was a perceptive one. That state, with all of its philosophical underpinnings, would become a way of life for Baltimore. Forty years later, both Gil Harman and Detmar Finke still remembered deeply intellectual conversations they had had with Baltimore. Life was full of situations to analyze, and these young intellectuals "would drive ideas into the ground" arguing with each other, according to Detmar. There were two conversations in particular that Detmar remembered; one was about love. David was dating a classmate by the name of Kay Senegas, and, as Detmar tells the story, "He came to me and he said, 'I have a real problem. I don't think that love exists.' This was a classic case of David being overintellectual—dividing an emotion to such a degree that it disappears. I mean, obviously he loved [Kay] and they had a relationship, but he had decided on the basis of analysis that love did not exist."

Detmar also remembered a running dialogue on great men and David's personal aspirations:

> David has always been arrogant, and so was I. That's how we ended up rooming together. . . . Right from the start, he was pointing toward something like a Nobel Prize. He was pointing toward very, very important stuff. And what bothered him was that the only people who get Nobel Prizes are those people who are very creative very early

in their career. "If you haven't made a really fantastic contribution in whatever area you're working in by the age of twenty-five, forget it." That was the way he used to put it. He saw this as one of the weird things about being a very talented scientist. All of your most creative work was done before you reached the age of thirty. This put quite a bit of pressure on him. But he came through, he did fine. But he was very conscious of that. . . . David was worried about having anything to do after he was thirty.

The two spent late nights arguing about a formula for success. Scientific accomplishments—any accomplishments—weren't enough, and they wrangled over the thorny issue of great men who were unscrupulous and cruel:

> There was a group of men who'd become Nobel Prize winners and important political leaders, but whom we didn't want to be like, because they hurt other people so much—they hurt the people they lived with, the people they worked with. It was very important to David to be a decent human being, not just a bright, high-powered human being. . . . When you are arrogant, you have to have a strong sense of morality or you get yourself in trouble. And David has that morality. That's why I think that he's not only an exceptional human being but a decent human being.

In addition to fostering long-winded philosophical and sociopolitical debates, from the nature of love to the true meaning of jazz, that sophomore year in Mary Lyons was a wonderful year for carousing; but one day Detmar got caught with his car on campus and the dean impounded it, taking the keys and banishing the car to a parking lot on the far side of Swarthmore. Without Detmar's car they couldn't make their weekend jaunts. The commuter rail line didn't make late-night Philadelphia runs.

There was only one way to get Detmar's car back: move off campus. Normally only seniors were allowed to do so. One way or another, the two sophomores managed to convince the dean to let them move off campus as soon as the summer came. In Detmar's opinion, the dean was probably happy to be rid of them.

MT. SINAI SUMMER, 1958

The previous summer (1957), David had been a waterfront counselor, lifeguarding and teaching swimming at the Children's Colony Camp, a summer camp in Connecticut attended largely by children of Jewish German refugees. It was a relaxing place where Baltimore read novels and watched the waves sweep across the lake. One of the other summer staff members, Bob Ledeen, worked in Mt. Sinai Hospital's research laboratories, and he eventually invited Baltimore to work for him at Mt. Sinai the following summer. Baltimore jumped at the opportunity to do some real science, and so he spent the summer after sophomore year analyzing a sea cucumber extract thought to possess an antitumor activity.

Sea cucumbers are simple, bottom-dwelling animals that look like colorful, rotten cucumbers, with a fleshy mouth at one end and little footpads on their underside. One approach to finding anticancer drugs has been to chemically synthesize molecules that might stop cancer ("lead compounds") and then synthesize and test related molecules for the ability to destroy tumors in mice. Such projects have kept chemists and biologists busy for a century. A related approach is to let nature do the organic chemical synthesis: to identify plants, animals, molds, or other organisms with potential anticancer properties. Scientists harvest the organism, grind it up, make extracts (concoctions in which chemicals have been separated into different groups), and look for those that cure tumors. Someone had detected a hint of antitumor activity in sea cucumber paste this way, and Ledeen was chasing it. Baltimore diced up sea cucumbers and made various extracts to try and isolate the putative cancer-fighting compound, distilling the chemical essence of a sea cucumber. Nothing ever came of Baltimore's work, but it was more stimulating than lifeguarding at the summer camp. He planned to return to Mt. Sinai the following year.

BLENDED HELIXES AND THE SECRET LIVES OF THE HUMAN COLON

For their junior year, David and Detmar had to find a place to live near Swarthmore. They didn't have much money, so they moved into a third-story dive in Chester, a blue-collar town about seven miles from Swarthmore. "It was sort of a dump," David recalled. Detmar's recollection was that "the second-floor apartment was always vacant because *no one* would live there."

They made good use of the place. Detmar mainly remembered the parties: "David and I used to have these parties, dinner parties. David would always cook flank steak. I made barbecued spare ribs, and he'd make flank steak, and we'd ferry people out to our apartment and throw a keg party."

Most of the old crew from Mary Lyons came by, though after college they would all go their separate ways. Baltimore enjoyed the social time, but he focused his energies more and more on biology.

Classes at Swarthmore weren't difficult for David, but when he began taking biology classes, he ran up against the legend of Howard Temin. Temin had become known as a scholar of herculean stature in the biology department even before he graduated, just a year before Baltimore's arrival. For the first time in his life, David was in the shadow of another student. In his 1994 memorial article on Temin, he wrote: "Temin's academic feats were central myths of the biology department. It was said that he had read every book in the biology library and the department purchased new ones by the month to satisfy his voracious appetite for knowledge." The quintessential Temin story, the one that Baltimore himself would retell for forty years, was the story of his honors exam. This ritual exam panicked seniors, because it was an oral exam covering every course the student had taken during the previous two years, and it was given by professors from other colleges. But it didn't faze Temin. As Baltimore later recalled, "Most students quiver, but Howard knew that examining his understanding of biological sciences was superfluous, so he sat astride a table and took the opportunity to engage the examiners in a dialogue about their work." As his brother Peter noted, "Howard was individual to the point of being cantankerous," and so when the examiners didn't award Howard a highest honors commendation, Swarthmore professors let it be known that Howard had "fought his examiners to a draw."

David Baltimore is a competitive man, and he saw Howard's fame as a challenge. Because Howard wasn't at Swarthmore any longer, this was a competition with a shadow, a myth, a sort of academic ideal, and it pushed David to try to be the greatest biology student the campus had ever seen.

Baltimore joined the honors program in the autumn of his junior year, along with nearly half his classmates. The Swarthmore honors program was unusual because it focused students' energies on two intensive seminars each semester. For David, however, the experience was unproductive. Because of his experience at Jackson and Mt. Sinai, Baltimore had been exposed to biochemistry, genetics, and molecular biology, but little of that biology had made its way into the Swarthmore curriculum. The biology courses focused on classical embryology, physiology, and cellular organization, none of which excited him. With a laugh, he later said, "At Swarthmore the teaching of biology was poor—at best. The courses were really generally *bad*." In one course, the professor stood in front of the class and read directly from the textbook. No classes focused his passion for molecular biology; the field was so new that no textbook was available. With only half a dozen professors in the department, Baltimore felt trapped.

Searching for knowledge in experimental biology and molecular biology, Baltimore took the train out to the libraries of nearby Haverford and Bryn Mawr on weekends. At a wooden table beside the science periodicals shelves, he read through a random selection of biology journals.

Because the intensely technical jargon of the journals was difficult to read, Baltimore soon sought out the more comprehensive, less esoteric review articles instead. Just as he started reading reviews, Joshua Lederberg, a young scientist at Columbia University, won the Nobel Prize in medicine and physiology, along with George Beadle at Caltech and Edward Tatum at the Rockefeller Institute, for establishing the connection between enzymes and genes.* The resulting publicity and scientific reviews showed Baltimore the promise of molecular biology.

Beadle and Tatum had carried out a long series of experiments using the fungus *Neurospora* to gather evidence for the theory that a single gene codes for a single enzyme. Enzymes are a large class of proteins that assist in metabolic reactions and other activities. For example, chymotrypsin is a digestive enzyme that breaks down proteins eaten as food. The protein enzyme alcohol dehydrogenase breaks down alcohol in the liver. Beta-galactosidase is a protein enzyme that cuts lactose, a sugar, into two pieces: glucose and galactose. By studying *Neurospora* mutants that were defective in the biosynthesis of various molecules (such as the amino acids arginine and tryptophan), Beadle and Tatum discovered that a given single specific gene codes for a single enzyme in *Neurospora*. For example, a *Neurospora* gene called *arg-3* codes for the enzyme that converts the molecule citrulline into the amino acid arginine, and this is the only enzyme that the *arg-3* gene codes for. The discovery was important for biologists because it gave a clear organization to the relationship between genes and enzymes.

Joshua Lederberg dedicated his considerable genius to developing *E. coli,* a bacterium that lives peacefully in the human colon, as a system for experimental genetics. Today, *E. coli* is the best-understood organism in the world. Lederberg made the extraordinary discovery of genetic transfer between bacteria. Two *E. coli* can come together, and one (the "male") can actually give genes to the other (the "female"). Lederberg then carried out a

---

*There is no Nobel Prize specifically for biology, so biologists are generally awarded the Nobel Prize in medicine and physiology, or sometimes the chemistry prize.

series of experiments that laid the foundation for bacterial genetics: he recapitulated Beadle and Tatum's "one gene, one enzyme" theory in *E. coli*. Lederberg isolated *E. coli* that were deficient in certain nutritional abilities. By carefully studying these bacteria and then mixing specific mutants and allowing them to exchange genes, Lederberg concluded that specific individual genes were indeed responsible for specific individual nutritional deficiencies in *E. coli*. Those nutritional deficiencies each resulted from the lack of a specific enzyme. Through extensive analysis he concluded that each gene in *E. coli* coded for one enzyme.

Through reviews on topics like Lederberg's study of bacterial genetics and enzymes and genes, Baltimore pieced together his own understanding. But it was isolated work, and during the winter it was unpleasant to trudge through the snow and down icy paths littered with holly berries to the Swarthmore train station. Unsatisfied with his solitary ventures, Baltimore joined the Swarthmore Biology Club and attended their weekly discussions. Through the club Baltimore learned about the origins of molecular biology. Watson and Crick's discovery of the DNA double helix in 1953, only four years earlier, was the breakthrough that clearly marked the beginning of the new field, but a number of important discoveries during the previous fifty years had contributed to its emergence. The discoveries came from a variety of experimental fields, which made it difficult for the Biology Club to follow the jumbled, stumbling procession toward the double helix. Fragments of research from genetics, biochemistry, microbiology, and immunology built up the techniques and knowledge that formed the framework of molecular biology.

Gregor Mendel discovered the basic laws of genetics in 1866, but no one paid much attention until they were rediscovered in the early 1900s. Thomas Hunt Morgan, probably the greatest geneticist of the early twentieth century, built on Mendel's ideas by using fruit flies *(Drosophila)* to study hereditary traits. Fruit flies gave quick results because of their short lifespan and rapid breeding: thus genetic experiments could be completed in two weeks instead of the months it took using Mendel's pea plants, or the years it took with Jackson Lab's mice. Huge numbers of flies could be stored in mason jars, and *Drosophila* had plenty of observable genetic traits to be explored, such as eye color, wing shape, and hair length. Admittedly, the fact that the average drosophila is the size of a sesame seed caused untold headaches and eyestrain among the geneticists who poked and probed flies for ten hours a day, but people made the sacrifice. One of Morgan's many discoveries using *Drosophila* was that chromosomes—certain visible structures within cells—contained all the genes. He and others discovered that chromosomes were linear and that genes were placed in a linear arrangement on chromosomes, as though a chromosome were a book and each gene a sentence. But what were chromosomes made of? Chemical analysis revealed a great deal of protein and a small amount of DNA (deoxyribonucleic acid). That discovery helped narrow the search but left the nature of hereditary material ambiguous. Was it protein or DNA?

Baltimore learned about this problem from his independent readings at Swarthmore. Most biologists from the 1920s to the 1940s believed proteins were the hereditary material, and their logic seemed solid. They reasoned that the hereditary material must have an enormous capacity for diversity and information storage, because it requires mind-boggling amounts of information to describe a living being and to provide for all the differences among the millions of species on the planet. It was well known that proteins had the potential to express far more diversity than DNA. DNA and proteins are both polymers made up of units (monomers) that link together to form a long chain. There are four different kinds of DNA monomers (nucleotides), which are distinguished by their different bases: adenine (A), thymine (T), cytosine (C), and guanine (G). In contrast, the monomers of proteins are amino acids, of which there are twenty different kinds, including glycine, methionine, glutamic acid, phenylalanine, and cysteine. For comparison, consider the musical scale, consisting of eight notes that, when arranged in long sequences, can express amazing complexity and information. In this analogy, DNA has a four-note scale and protein has a twenty-note scale. The larger the scale, the greater the number of possibilities that can be expressed. A protein that is twelve monomers long (or consisting of twelve "notes") has 100 million times more possible combinations than a polymer of DNA of the same length. Therefore it seemed obvious to most scientists that proteins should be the hereditary material. However, proving either case required experiments.

The secret lay with the "transforming principle," based on observations made by Frederick Griffith in the 1920s in *Streptococcus pneumoniae,* a bacterium that causes pneumonia. Griffith studied two types of pneumococcus bacteria, smooth and rough (referring to the appearance of the bacteria under a microscope). Injecting smooth pneumococcus bacteria into mice caused a lethal infection, but injecting rough bacteria did not. Additionally, Griffith showed that when he killed smooth bacteria (essentially by boiling) and injected them, the mixture did not kill the mice, which was not surprising. But when he mixed dead smooth bacteria with live rough bacteria, the mixture could kill the mice, and bacteria subsequently recovered from the dead mice were smooth. Somehow, the dead smooth bacteria had turned the rough bacteria into dangerous smooth bacteria! This change was caused by an unknown chemical or molecule, which they called "the transforming principle," that the rough bacteria acquired from the debris of the dead smooth bacteria.

The transforming principle molecule, whatever it was, must be the hereditary material. Oswald Avery, working at the Rockefeller Institute in the early 1940s, searched for it. Avery and his colleagues Colin MacLeod and MacLyn McCarty performed a series of experiments in 1943 and 1944 in which they took batches of killed smooth pneumococcus bacteria, which they knew contained the transforming principle molecule, and tried to purify different types of molecules from them. They showed that purified proteins, sugars, and fats did not transform the rough bacteria, but purified DNA did. Oswald Avery had proved that DNA was the hereditary material.

Unfortunately, proving a scientific fact is not the same thing as convincing other scientists that you have proved a scientific fact. As the 1940s wore on, few scientists were fully convinced by Avery's groundbreaking experiment. Some scientists thought his experiments might have been contaminated, and to others the result just did not make sense: how could a boring molecule like DNA contain all of the detailed genetic information necessary for life? In time, a different experiment, done by Albert Hershey using viruses, convinced the majority of biologists that DNA was the genetic material; and a third discovery, by Watson and Crick, beautifully demonstrated that DNA was a molecule "smart" enough to contain the hereditary information.

The foundation for Hershey's experiment was laid by Salvador Luria and Max Delbrück, who had assembled an informal group of scientists who became known as the Phage Group. They worked on the simplest possible biological system: viruses. Luria had emigrated from Italy and become a biologist at Indiana University. He knew everyone in virology, and everyone knew him. Delbrück, a boyish-looking German intellectual, was one of the first theoretical physicists to switch to biology. As a professor at Vanderbilt and later at Caltech, he had a driving creative energy that drew students to him and his viruses.

In essence, viruses are genetic material covered by a protein shell. Viruses that infect bacteria are known as bacteriophage, or simply phage. Luria and Delbrück were drawn to the possibilities of biology research using phage because of their amazing experimental possibilities. One milliliter of water can hold over a hundred billion phage. With those kinds of numbers, Luria and Delbrück could study genetic events that were extremely rare, conducting experiments that were simply impossible in *Drosophila* or mice. The virus experiments fascinated Baltimore.

Building on the Phage Group's experimental groundwork, Albert Hershey did a series of experiments with phage at the Cold Spring Harbor Laboratory on Long Island in 1952, with the help of his technician, Martha Chase. Phage geneticists knew that when a phage infected a bacterium, it injected only its genetic material into the bacterium and left its shell, or capsid, attached to the outside of the bacterium. Hershey and Chase labeled the virus DNA with ^{32}P (radioactive phosphorus) and the virus proteins with ^{35}S (radioactive sulfur). Then they let the viruses infect a swarm of bacteria and threw the bacterial culture into a Waring blender. The force of the blender was strong enough to strip viruses off the outside of the bacteria but not strong enough to rip apart the bacteria. Hershey and Chase then analyzed the bacteria to see what had been injected into them by the viruses. If protein was the hereditary material, the bacteria would be full of ^{35}S. If DNA was the hereditary material, the bacteria would be full of ^{32}P. The bacteria proved to be full of ^{32}P. The Hershey-Chase experiment convinced most biologists that DNA was the hereditary material. Whether because of the timing, the scientists involved, or the visceral appeal of the experimental design, the Hershey-Chase experiment was more convincing than Avery's experiment, and Albert Hershey later shared the Nobel Prize with Salvador Luria and Max Delbrück for their pioneering work using viruses to explore the nature of life.

The crowning achievement of the era was the deduction of the structure of DNA in 1953 by James Watson and Francis Crick at Cambridge University. Watson was a young American who was both cursed and blessed with the stereotypical physical characteristics of a brilliant scientist. He was almost ridiculously gangly, and Einstein himself would have been impressed with Watson's unruly coif. His research partner, Crick, was a fast-talking, hypercreative Brit. They analyzed X-ray diffraction images (a novel photographic technique for detecting repeated structures in molecules) of DNA that were taken by Maurice Wilkins and Rosalind Franklin of Kings College London. From those images, Watson and Crick predicted that DNA was a symmetrical double helix that could contain hereditary information coded in its linear sequence of As, Cs, Gs, and Ts (for instance, AGGGTCG-TACGTACGTACG). Their discovery showed the scientific community how DNA could be the hereditary material, the "blueprint of life." Crick, Watson, and Wilkins were later awarded the Nobel Prize in Medicine in 1962 for their discovery.* Watson and Crick were touted as the geniuses of molecular biology and lionized by the media. When a field is new, or newly fascinating in the public eye, a genius (or pair of geniuses) can become a lightning rod for the public's adulation; and molecular biology may never have another scientist who will attain the fame of Watson and Crick.

The prominence of Watson and Crick and the Phage Group made Baltimore all the more desperate to do some real experimental biology. During the spring of his junior year, Baltimore became president of the Biology Club and enrolled in a microbiology seminar that discussed the advances of Luria, Delbrück, Lederberg, and others. But he was sick of just talking about biology. He had understood very quickly that designing and completing experiments were the accomplishments that make a biologist; gathering an encyclopedic knowledge of facts simply makes a good student. "I was sick and tired of reading about bacteriophages and trying to understand the genetics of bacteriophages without having ever seen a bacteriophage plaque," he recalls. "I didn't know what a bacterial colony looked like, and I just had no idea what the manipulations people were talking about were." So he approached the professor in charge of the microbiology seminar. "If we can get some bacteriophage and bacteria," he asked, "could we just play around with it, just to see what it looks like?"

"Yeah."

"Well, where would I get it?"

"Cold Spring Harbor."

Baltimore knew of the Cold Spring Harbor Laboratory because of the Hershey-Chase experiment and his own childhood on Long Island. It was near the old Long Island Sound fish hatchery, thirty miles from his family's house in Great Neck. It would be easy to visit the labs while he was home for Easter vacation, and he hoped he could talk the scientists into giving him some phage samples.

EASTER VACATION

At Easter vacation, Baltimore took a train from Philadelphia out to Great Neck. He spent a couple of days at home relaxing with his family, and then he borrowed the family car one morning and sprinted to Cold Spring Har-

*Rosalind Franklin died of cancer in 1958. Nobel Prizes are not given posthumously, but neither is a prize given to more than three individuals, so there will always be debate about whether Franklin would have received the prize had she lived.

bor. The laboratories were quiet. Baltimore knew that Cold Spring Harbor was the summer mecca of the Phage Group, but he had no idea who was on the year-round staff. The only name he knew was Helen Gay; he had seen it on a *Drosophila* research paper that winter. He started wandering around, looking for someone who could give him directions. Plain buildings were scattered around a meadow that drifted down to a beach. The waters were calm in the cove off Long Island Sound. After a brief search, Baltimore found Helen Gay. Baltimore introduced himself, and they talked. Fortunately she was kind to him. When he asked about getting bacteria and bacteriophage, she took him to see George Streisinger.

One of the great experimenters of phage genetics, Streisinger had earned his doctorate under Luria and made scientific contributions to the study of phage proteins, genes, and chromosome structure. When Baltimore first saw him, Streisinger was standing next to a lab bench, wearing shorts and flip-flops and drinking Coca-Cola, pleasantly curious about the new arrival. Baltimore glanced around the lab and saw several laboratory workbenches, a few stools, a shelf full of bottled chemicals, and a couple of high windows. Gay introduced the two and left. Baltimore asked if Streisinger could possibly give him some bacteriophage and bacteria for his microbiology seminar. Streisinger said that he certainly could. Pleased by Baltimore's interest, Streisinger took some time to explain the basic techniques for handling bacteria and phage.

Scientists grow bacteria in Luria broth in large glass flasks. When it contains no bacteria, the broth is clear and golden, like beef bouillon. Inoculate a single bacterium into the broth, and overnight the mixture becomes thickly yellow with billions of progeny bacteria. Scientists mainly use the bacterial species *E. coli*. And since *E. coli* normally grows in the human colon, the optimal temperature for growth is 37° C, human body temperature. Streisinger's laboratory had several 37° C incubators.

Streisinger showed Baltimore how to grow bacterial colonies on a petri dish filled with agar, a gelatinous substance. First the bacteria must be diluted. If bacteria from a flask teeming with growth are poured onto an agar dish, the plate becomes a bacterial lawn, covered with growth. But for bacterial genetics experiments, individual bacterial clones are needed. So the bacterial culture is first diluted one million–fold, and then a small volume of culture, containing between ten and one hundred bacteria, is poured onto an agar dish. When each of those individual bacteria multiply over the next twenty-four hours in the incubator, they grow up into colonies on the agar surrounding the spots where each one started. When an individual bacterium grows into a colony (looking like a spot of mold on old bread), all of the bacteria in that colony are descended from that first bacterium. They have the same genetic makeup; they are clones. Once colonies of clones have developed, genetic experimentation can begin.

Phage experiments are similar. The biologist makes a bacterial lawn on an agar dish and then dilutes a phage sample and plates it over the lawn. An individual phage infects an *E. coli*, replicates within it, kills it, and releases a hundred new viruses, which infect the surrounding *E. coli*. After twelve hours, the viruses replicate to a point where they have killed all of the *E. coli* surrounding them, leaving a plaque—a vacant spot.

Streisinger saw something in Baltimore that he liked, and at the end of the brief tutorial he asked Baltimore whether he would like to come back to Cold Spring Harbor for the summer and work in Streisinger's laboratory. The question caught Baltimore off guard. Streisinger told him that he could probably get funding from a new National Science Foundation (NSF) summer program.

The NSF program at Cold Spring Harbor was known as the Undergraduate Research Participation Program (URPP), which is still active today. Cold Spring Harbor hadn't found student interns yet, so there was definitely space for Baltimore. David wasn't certain that he could come, because with Ledeen's help he had already arranged to work at the Haskins Laboratory in New York that summer. He promised to find out as soon as possible if he could get out of his commitment at Haskins. Before David left, they sat and talked for some time.

Back at home Baltimore checked with Haskins, and they agreed that David would do well to take advantage of the opportunity at Cold Spring Harbor. Baltimore wrote to Streisinger of the good news. He was coming to Cold Spring Harbor.

The spring term dragged on once Baltimore returned to college. Working with Streisinger would be great, but what would he do during his senior year? Desperately looking for ways to work in a laboratory, David switched his major to chemistry, without any intention of becoming a chemist. There was no research in the biology department, but in the chemistry department he could do a senior thesis. He ended up arranging to work with Philip George, a chemistry professor at the University of Pennsylvania, who was studying the chemistry of ATP, a biomolecule crucial for storing and using the energy of fat and sugar in cells.

From Philip George, Baltimore would learn biochemistry laboratory techniques, including protein purification. In the same way that geneticists were finding it powerful to study single genes, biochemists wanted to study individual proteins. To do so, they needed to purify their favorite protein from the thousands of others in an organism like *E. coli.* Using more sophisticated purification techniques than he had tried with the sea cucumber, David ground up batches of *E. coli* and flowed the batches through various "columns," which acted as thick filters to separate proteins according to their different properties, like size or electrical charge. Nothing much came of the data Baltimore collected, but what mattered most was creating the foundation for the skills he later used to make his Nobel Prize–winning discovery.

COLD SPRING HARBOR, 1959

After his junior year, Baltimore fled to Long Island. He lived at home and commuted to Cold Spring Harbor daily. He spent most of each day in the lab working on his summer project, which was nuts-and-bolts phage genetics. Streisinger had few scientific understudies, and so he worked with David extensively, teaching him bacteria and phage techniques. Streisinger showed Baltimore how to think about phage problems and design plausible experiments to test and prove ideas. Baltimore became convinced of the wisdom of Salvador Luria in working with phage, and of Lederberg's in the use of *E. coli.* These systems were simple enough to yield consistent results.

Every week Baltimore plated bacteria, harvested phage, and conducted experiments, but summertime at Cold Spring Harbor offered much more than lab space. It was the official summer watering hole for molecular biologists. Max Delbrück, James Watson, George Wald, Salvador Luria, and Albert Hershey were all there, and each either had won or would win a Nobel Prize. Dozens of other prominent scientists gathered to work, lecture, swim, barbecue, play tennis, and sunbathe. Cold Spring Harbor was designed as part campus, part resort, and part laboratory. Conversations were what made it such an invigorating place. People lounged on the ivy-covered terraces of the main buildings, talking for hours. James Watson, who later directed the Cold Spring Harbor Laboratory for many years, said: "I think during the summer, well, it is the most interesting place in the world, if you're interested in biology. Only place where you can be stimulated as much by what is going on, and by the people."

In addition, Cold Spring Harbor ran courses for researchers with lectures in the mornings and evenings. Baltimore, flushed with curiosity, attended some lectures. Researchers discussed the implications of a variety of major recent discoveries. In 1954, at Cambridge, Vernon Ingram had extended Beadle and Tatum's one gene, one enzyme theory when he showed that human sickle-cell anemia is caused by a difference of one amino acid between normal and sickle-cell hemoglobin enzyme. In 1956 Arthur Kornberg showed that DNA could replicate in a test tube with the proper enzymes added (a discovery for which he rapidly won the 1959 Nobel Prize). In 1957 Matthew Meselson and Frank Stahl proved how DNA replicates itself; and John Kendrew had just figured out the structure of the protein myoglobin, the first protein structure ever determined. It was obvious to Baltimore that modern biology was exploding, and Cold Spring Harbor was "the real world" of biology for him.

Streisinger was an important influence on Baltimore. He remembered Streisinger with fondness years later: "He was an extraordinary man. . . . He was one of the unknown men of the field [because he rarely published his research]. He just loved to work and think." And Streisinger's mentorship fueled Baltimore's determination to become an experimental biologist.

Toward the end of the summer, Baltimore had an opportunity to make his dream come true. Streisinger knew that Baltimore was talented, so he introduced him to Cyrus Levinthal and Salvador Luria. Levinthal was a trim young molecular biologist, a smoker with a cool James Dean look. By now Luria was the foremost virologist in the country, and he was also a wonderfully personable man. He had just moved to MIT along with Levinthal, and they were committed to building the department into a world-class research center. Streisinger highly recommended Baltimore. On that basis alone, Luria invited Baltimore to come to MIT as a graduate student the following year. The twenty-one-year-old Baltimore was elated.

That fall, Swarthmore felt small and isolated to Baltimore. Though the legend of Howard Temin still drove him, the Swarthmore biology department was fading into obsolescence. Graduating from Swarthmore College with a B.A. with high honors in chemistry and a minor in biology, Baltimore would always look back on Swarthmore as providing a terrible biology education (though he may have underestimated it) and an irreplaceable liberal arts experience. He became a lifelong devotee of classical music, art, photography, politics, and modern literature. In the spring of 1960 he graduated from the arboretum and headed off for the molecular world of MIT.

Three

Don't be afraid of being foolish.

PHILLIP SHARP
1993 Nobel laureate in medicine and physiology

THE EXPLOSIVE GROWTH OF molecular biology made the late 1950s both a great time and a chaotic time to become an apprentice molecular biologist. Baltimore could get involved in molecular biology immediately, but it was difficult to see how he could become a great scientist.

The MIT graduate program in biology was rigidly structured, requiring students to learn oceans of knowledge during their first year in a series of biological problem-solving classes. Students quickly developed a chalkboard understanding of experimentation, learning to wield a battery of biochemical and genetic approaches for solving biological problems: identifying a gene that gives fruit flies white eyes or isolating a protein responsible for gluing sugars together. Baltimore and his classmates virtually memorized heaps of scientific papers written by the masters of molecular biology. The rigid educational attitude of MIT was difficult to get used to after the more flexible structure of Swarthmore, but Baltimore adapted.

In classes, the professors lectured on mutation rates, phage genetics, or enzyme biochemistry, drawing models on the board and explaining experiments in confident tones—and Baltimore interrupted. He blurted out aggressive questions and challenged professors' interpretations of experiments. He refused to sit passively in a lecture hall and simply be indoctrinated. Science to him was not an immutable book of knowledge but a dynamic process, and if a professor mentioned a "scientific fact" in lecture that Baltimore thought was flaccid or simpleminded, he pointed out its weaknesses and besieged it. Baltimore quickly earned a reputation as a bombastic student. One professor thirty years later privately recalled Baltimore as one of the brightest and most troublesome students he ever had: "Baltimore was a pain in the ass."

His brilliant mind and blunt candor were a discomforting combination. He told one of his professors, "I can't attend your lectures, because they are terrible." Other professors privately agreed with him (and chortled behind closed doors), but his audacity shocked them. Yet although his manner could be abrasive and his arrogance was undeniable, his intelligence was difficult to ignore. In the words of Peter Medawar, winner of the 1960 Nobel Prize in medicine: "Humility is not a state of mind conducive to the advancement of learning."

The most important biological concept David learned at MIT was the "Central Dogma," the flow chart of genetic information. Whimsically named by Francis Crick, the great sage of molecular biology, this principle is emblazoned in the minds of all molecular biology students:

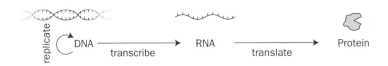

The Central Dogma of molecular biology.

The Central Dogma states, first, that all cells use DNA to store their genetic information. For example, in humans, genetic information is passed from generation to generation in the form of double-stranded DNA. Human DNA is three billion nucleotides long. Written out as a continuous string of letters, the information in DNA necessary to describe the entire genetic blueprint of a person would fill five thousand books. That entire three-billion-nucleotide string of DNA is crammed into every individual cell in the human body.

DNA is the genetic blueprint, but a blueprint by itself doesn't do anything. Human DNA is divided up into about fifty thousand genes. A simple way to think about this is to consider each gene a sentence in the code of life. It takes fifty thousand sentences to describe the human body plan.

The remainder of the Central Dogma addresses the question: How does the cell get the information out of a gene in the DNA for use in the cell? This is a two-step process. First, an enzyme called RNA polymerase synthesizes ("transcribes," in the scientific lexicon) RNA from the DNA. RNA is a polymer very similar to DNA, but less stable. Cells use RNA as the messenger molecule, a temporary replica of the gene. That RNA message of the gene is then "translated" into the protein, the final product, by molecular machines inside the cell, known as ribosomes, that read the RNA and synthesize the protein that the RNA contains instructions for.

Why does it have to be so complicated to get the information out of a gene and make a protein? (Some struggling biology students have been known to ask this question in more colorful language.) DNA is the genetic blueprint of a person, and a full copy of that blueprint is present in every cell in the human body. But you don't want all fifty thousand genes expressed in every cell in the body. Some genes are used only in the brain; some are specific to cells in the eye; some are used only by the immune system to fight viruses; and some are used in either women or men but not both. By analogy, every cell contains the blueprints for a thousand different types of houses, and it chooses one blueprint to follow (telegram from the architect inside a developing embryo: CELL #1547628 DEVELOP INTO A BRAIN CELL STOP). Once that blueprint is chosen, the appropriate pieces of the house are made: one gene codes for (determines the characteristics of) the front door, another gene codes for the doorbell, a third codes for a blue velvet loveseat with orange leopard spots. The body has evolved extraordinarily elaborate mechanisms to control gene expression so that a cell doesn't get its blueprints confused: brain genes don't make brain proteins in skin cells, and muscle genes don't make muscle proteins in the brain. The cell controls gene expression by regulating which genes are transcribed into RNA and translated into proteins, and every cell regulates how much of each gene is expressed so that there is no surplus or deficit of any protein.

A key part of the Central Dogma is that information does not transfer in the opposite direction; for example, from RNA to DNA. There is a hierarchy. DNA is the most stable information of the trinity; RNA and proteins survive in the cell only for a short while, with the RNA constantly driving more protein synthesis and the proteins cutting, welding, and torquing their way through the blue-collar work of the cell until they are destroyed. Their components are recycled as the cell changes its repertoire to adapt to the changing environment in the body. For example, as soon as the cells lining the small intestines detect food coming from the stomach, the RNA polymerase enzymes in each cell starts transcribing RNA from genes that are important for digestion. Those RNAs are translated into a carnival of specialized proteins (enzymes) that grab molecules of food from the gut—sugars, proteins, fats—and break them apart and convert them into useful building materials and energy supplies that can be passed through the blood to needy parts of the body. Once food stops coming from the stomach, the cells of the small intestines turn off all this molecular machinery.

Classes taught Baltimore the Central Dogma and the experimental strategies of biochemistry and genetics, but David wanted to do science, not listen to professors explain it. Science is the last great bastion of the apprentice system, and universities are its foundries. Baltimore needed a mentor. He liked the phage work done by Cyrus Levinthal, whom he had met at Cold Spring Harbor, and he decided that he wanted to work with Levinthal during his first year, even with the heavy courseload. Levinthal was happy to have him and set him up in a laboratory space on the fifth floor of the biology building, Building 16. This was an eight-story white box fused to the east side of the main MIT complex. From the laboratory Baltimore could see the Charles River and Boston's Back Bay.

MIT's central campus was a monumental neoclassical complex of interconnected limestone buildings, capped by a Pantheon-inspired Great Dome. Names of famous scientists were carved in foot-high letters along the parapets: Newton, Lavoisier, Pasteur, Faraday, Archimedes, Leonardo, Copernicus, Darwin. Inside this complex resided the world-famous departments of physics, mechanical engineering, and mathematics.

MIT's recent interest in biology, signaled by the recruitment of Salvador Luria and Cyrus Levinthal, had its roots in World War II. In the late 1930s, the university was receiving $100,000 a year in research funds. By the end of World War II, the university was flush with $40 million a year. Most of this money funneled into the Radiation Lab, which employed four thousand people who, among other accomplishments, developed 150 different types of radar to help win the war. (A number of historians have asserted that these people did more to influence the course of World War II than the developers of the atomic bomb.) The university has had strong military and government ties ever since. Virtually every U.S. naval ship built in the twentieth century was designed by an MIT alumnus. In 1957 James Killian, an MIT alumnus and former MIT president (who spent some time at 532 Beacon Street), became the first presidential science advisor, appointed by Eisenhower. When Baltimore arrived at MIT a few years later, after Sputnik and the start of the cold war, fifty million military research dollars were pouring into MIT annually. Most of that cash flowed to the electrical engineering and aeronautical engineering departments—which were developing missile guidance systems, magnetic core memory, avionics, atomic clocks, and digital computers—but some was used to extend MIT's reputation to the fields of economics, linguistics, and biology.

Reflecting its engineering focus, the intellectual atmosphere at MIT was, and always has been, intense, with a workaday, down-to-earth sensibility. Sometimes that mentality bordered on neurotic utilitarianism: all of the buildings were known by their numbers, like Building 16 and Building 2, and all of the majors were known by numbers instead of names: course 2 (mechanical engineering), course 18 (mathematics), course 7 (biology). Students meeting each other for the first time would say, "I'm course _____, I work in building _____." There was no use for names. Students worked uncommonly hard, submitting themselves to an education based on problem-solving and a humbling work ethic. Their humanities education and social lives were largely neglected.

Because of his heavy courseload, Baltimore wasn't able to spend much time in Levinthal's lab, but he did participate in one major project. Levinthal was running experiments to determine the character of a certain phage's genome. Specifically, he wanted to know if the phage's genome, the complete genetic identity of the virus, was entirely contained on one chromosome—one continuous length of DNA—or on many chromosomes. (The human genome consists of three billion nucleotides of DNA on twenty-three different chromosomes.) Underlying this question was the question of how much DNA—how much genetic information—it took to make a virus. No one knew how much DNA it took to make a living thing (the size of the enormous human genome was not determined until many years later). The phage viruses were the smallest beings on the planet, at once both breathtakingly simple and staggeringly complex.

Levinthal and other investigators had done sizing experiments numerous times before, but the results had always been uncertain. However, Alfred Hershey had recently shown that DNA was fragile to shearing forces. No one had imagined that the precious molecule of heredity could be so sensitive to physical abuse, but that explained the misleading results of the Levinthal lab's previous experiments: when they used syringes to handle the DNA, they broke the chromosomes into little pieces. This time around, Levinthal was committed to handling the DNA gently.

Quick results were imperative, because other labs were racing for the same goal, and modern biology is littered with stories of also-rans. Getting scooped on projects, often as not after years of work, is commonplace for biologists but no less painful on that account. Once a discovery is made, people race to build on that discovery, leading to more discoveries and more steeple-chases. Competition, coupled with curiosity, was and always will be biologists' fundamental motivator. Implicit in the process of discovery is the fact that one researcher must be first; for a brief moment that person must be the only one in the world who knows the result, otherwise the hunt is for nothing. Who wants to rediscover the wheel? Because the whole idea of competing for the truth appears unseemly, competition is often discounted as a minor part of the scientific process. But in the race for big answers, coming in first brings rewards of faculty jobs, prestige, and government research funds.

On the other hand, stories of successful collaborations also abound: Watson and Crick, Beadle and Tatum, Luria and Delbrück. Most scientists don't know much broad science; each specializes in a narrow subdiscipline. Both trapped and empowered by their specialty, researchers often have to solicit the help of other biologists' expertise. Biochemists need advice from geneticists on how to find a gene. Geneticists need advice from biochemists on how to study a protein.

A scientist also needs tools to construct experiments, and tools in molecular biology are precious. Sometimes scientists' careers are assured by the development of a single experimental tool. Often biologists have only a few of the many tools, or reagents—a virus, a protein, a drug, a mouse—needed for a set of experiments. To get the other reagents they have to ask their colleagues. A broad network of friends is often a scientist's greatest asset.

The ethics of competition in science are as complicated as the ethics of humanitarian aid to enemy nations. People hold scientists up to a high standard of ethics and morality; in a secular world, they are the truth-seekers. Of course, scientists come in all temperaments. As Peter Medawar has said, "Among scientists are collectors, classifiers and compulsive tidiers-up; many are detectives by temperament and many are explorers; some are artists and others artisans. There are poet-scientists and philosopher-scientists and even a few mystics." But even with their diversity, scientists as a group take these ethical standards seriously and do a fairly good job of upholding them. Truth always wins out; it is impossible to hide or obscure the scientific truth for long. But at the personal level, competition ranges from friendly rivalry to sabotage and backstabbing. Rules of etiquette strive to maintain honorable cooperative interaction among scientists, even those competing for Nobel

Prizes and multimillion-dollar grants. But the honor system sometimes breaks down as the prizes of prestige and financial gain soar.

One humorous story of scientific conduct, now a legend, involves a young molecular biologist who wanted to get a special phage stock, necessary for a certain experiment, from a competing scientist. The competitor had published a paper about this phage, and etiquette clearly required that he should provide the phage to other scientists. So the younger scientist wrote to ask for a sample. However, the phage discoverer didn't want to give his competitor the reagent that was making him famous. Scientists in this situation may take any number of evasive actions: they may send the wrong reagent, lie about it being lost in the mail, or stall, saying they are very busy. This particular competitor simply wrote a letter refusing to provide the reagent and apologized for any inconvenience. There were no "science police" to complain to, and so the young molecular biologist was left high and dry. However, scientists are a creative bunch. He cut the letter into little pieces and soaked them in a flask of bacterial medium. Then he added *E. coli* to the flask, incubated it, and grew up a stock of the phage! From the air in the lab enough viruses had stuck to the letter, like microscopic burrs, to generate a new stock. Versions of this legend differ as to whether the young scientist sent a thank-you note back. In other variations, the young molecular biologist invites the phage discoverer to give a lecture at his university and then scrapes samples of phage off the speaker's clothing or, even more mischievously, gives him a tour of a lab and then pulls the emergency shower handle, presumably flushing phage out of his hair and clothing and onto the laboratory floor.

Within this competitive environment, Levinthal's group scrambled for data. The phage chromosome-length experiment involved incorporating ^{32}P, radioactive phosphorus, into the phage DNA, much as Hershey had done in the original Waring blender experiment, and then counting how much radiation was emitted by a ^{32}P-labeled phage chromosome. The amount of radiation emitted by the DNA was directly proportional to the length of the DNA molecule. Baltimore and a number of other people spent mind-numbing hours tallying radiation counts for the experiment. Having learned from their past mistakes, this time they got the true answer: the phage possessed only one chromosome, and it was significantly longer than people had thought from the previous experiments.*

Apart from the "star experiment," as it came to be known (after the pat-

*The virus's DNA was about 50,000 nucleotides long, which is about 1/100,000 the length of human DNA.

tern radioactive decay makes on film), Baltimore tinkered around, plating phage and making stocks of phage, but for most of that first year he was busy with academic requirements. By late spring it was time to think about choosing a lab and getting started on a doctoral thesis project. There are many ways to choose a Ph.D. project. Some people choose a laboratory that explores a subject they love; others find that they have a particular experimental talent they should capitalize on; still others choose a laboratory based on the fame of the professor, the camaraderie of the lab members, or on how competitive a field is. And there are a few who look for a shortcut: a project that a professor says is guaranteed to work or will allow them to graduate quickly. Baltimore dreamed of important research, breaking open new areas of study, and so he chose an area based on a hunch about where greatness might hide.

Animal cells interested him, but they were too complicated to study directly. Luria, Levinthal, and the rest worked with viruses because of their simplicity. A bacteriophage has about ten to one hundred genes, whereas a human cell has about fifty thousand. Viruses, in essence, consist only of a protein shell encapsulating their genetic material (unlike cells, viruses can use either DNA or RNA as their genetic material). They have no metabolism, no protein synthesis machinery: they depend on the cells they infect to supply their metabolic needs. Without a cell, a virus is an inert chunk of information. Peter Medawar wrote, "A virus is a piece of bad news wrapped in protein."

How a bacteriophage virus invaded a bacterial cell and killed it was well known. The virus attached to the bacterium's cell surface and either injected its genetic material into the cell from the surface or entered the cell and then released its genetic material. In a cell a virus is a despotic, hyperactive micromanager. Its genetic material commandeers the cell's molecular machinery to furiously create more viruses. *Virus* is the Latin word for poison.

Baltimore had the notion that animal viruses could be the key to understanding the molecular mechanics of animal cells, in much the same way that bacteriophage research was revealing so much about bacteria. He decided that he wanted to skip the bacterial phase of molecular biology and start to work on animal systems, using animal viruses as his bridge. Animal viruses were a new field, but because they were viruses, Baltimore was confident that their molecular nature could be revealed. Thirty years later, while organizing a lecture for high school students, Baltimore reflected on his long love affair with viruses: "I love to teach about viruses, because they are the molecular biology stripped of all the proteins, right down to the

[RNA and DNA] nucleic acids. There's a wonderful logic to teaching about viruses. You can get your head around the whole organism."

There were three major complications with his hunch. First, most biologists were satisfied that the molecular biology of animal viruses would simply match that of the bacteriophage. Why shouldn't it? Biologists were rapidly determining the basic molecular biology of phage and bacteria, and they confidently assumed that the rules they were developing would hold true for higher organisms. Nevertheless, it would be necessary to study animal viruses and find out. Nature has a tendency to disprove biologists' gut feelings of how the world "should" be. The experimental scientist's canvas is damp with boldly colored brush strokes layered thick, sometimes building on previous vivid streaks, other times obliterating mistaken swaths and starting fresh. Many layers later, truth emerges.

The second complication was that Baltimore didn't know anything about animal viruses. Third, and most problematic, there was no one at MIT who did. Baltimore couldn't set out to study animal viruses alone; he needed a mentor. He and Cyrus Levinthal discussed whether he should research a thesis on phage with Levinthal and then move on to animal virology after graduate school, or start a thesis on animal viruses immediately. When Levinthal had no satisfactory answer, Baltimore went to talk to Luria. He felt a debt to Luria for bringing him to MIT; that was his first big break, and Baltimore has referred to Luria as "my angel." Both men had a passion for virology, literature, and socialism.

Luria had written *General Virology,* the preeminent book on virology, and he knew everyone who studied viruses. He arranged for Baltimore to work on animal viruses with Philip Marcus at the Albert Einstein School of Medicine in the Bronx for the month of June. Then Baltimore would go to Cold Spring Harbor and take their new summer laboratory course in animal virology. Normally these CSH classes were filled by older researchers, but in 1961 few people were interested in animal virology, and so Baltimore would be able to squeeze in. By the end of the summer a new professor studying animal viruses, Jim Darnell, would have arrived at MIT, and Luria suggested that Baltimore could join his lab.

Marcus, at Albert Einstein, was one of the few animal virologists in 1961 who grasped the promise of molecular biology, and he also knew the importance of quantitative science. The two fundamentals for starting research into a new area are an experimental vehicle, like Luria's phage or Morgan's fruit flies, and a method for quantifying the experimental conditions and results. Marcus introduced Baltimore to animal viruses, showing him day-to-day strategies for handling the viruses and carrying out experiments. Baltimore saw enough during this brief internship to be reassured that animal viruses were a viable experimental system, but he needed a much more substantial introduction to the techniques and scientific questions in animal virology. Cold Spring Harbor was the answer to his needs.

Cold Spring Harbor courses were, and still are, crammed into three neuron-scrambling weeks. The animal virology class was designed to start scientists making discoveries about viruses right away. Half of the class time was filled with demonstrations by the instructors, highlighting the core questions in virology; the other half was devoted to hands-on experiments. The two course professors, Richard Franklin and Ed Simon, walked around the laboratory benches daily, discussing the viruses. The questions people were asking fascinated Baltimore: How do animal viruses get into cells? How do they take over the cell? How do they replicate? The course was a revelation. Within a fortnight he had been mesmerized by the enormous possibilities of animal virology: "I was convinced that *is* what I wanted to do."

At Cold Spring Harbor Baltimore ran into Jim Darnell, who was attending one of the summer conferences. Baltimore introduced himself and asked to join Darnell's MIT laboratory in the fall. Darnell hesitated. He was a young scientist, and this professorship at MIT would be his first experience of running a lab. He didn't know Baltimore, and he was already bringing someone else to work with him. Darnell didn't think he could use Baltimore, so he turned him down. Baltimore was mortified. Darnell's rejection meant that he couldn't do animal virology at MIT.

Fortunately, Richard Franklin was interested by Baltimore's curiosity and intelligence from their daily interactions at the lab bench. The two hit it off, and Franklin told Baltimore that he could join his animal virology lab at the Rockefeller Institute in Manhattan. "That's all I really wanted to do," recalled Baltimore later, "and Richard was perfect."

When Baltimore returned to MIT in August he told Luria all that had transpired; he wanted to transfer to Rockefeller. Luria saw Baltimore's newfound love of animal viruses and agreed. He wrote a letter of recommendation for Baltimore to Detlev Bronk, the president of Rockefeller. Bronk interviewed and accepted Baltimore. In early September, 1961, Baltimore moved from Cambridge to New York and was ready to begin his lifelong cat-and-mouse game with animal viruses.

As with most history, another reality existed within and parallel to this one: Darnell's. That day at Cold Spring Harbor, two conversations happened simultaneously and contradictorily between Darnell and Baltimore. Darnell heard himself suggest that he needed the summer to set up his lab and get settled, but that Baltimore could join the lab once autumn rolled around. Baltimore heard Darnell politely turn him down. Darnell recalls with a wistful smile, "So I lost my chance to have David as a graduate student." Acknowledging the myth of a singular history, neither man harbored hard feelings, and David would join Darnell's lab soon enough.

ROCKEFELLER

Baltimore loved New York City. His childhood on Long Island's north shore was the kind that survives as memories of sunshine, bicycles, and stickball. He had always enjoyed trips into the city. And the fabled Rockefeller Institute was a good place to be. At the time, the institute was still in its the boom years. Its incredible microbiology advances in the first two decades of the twentieth century and the molecular biology discoveries made there through the 1940s propelled Rockefeller to the forefront of biology research. As a result, the institute had recently decided to expand and become Rockefeller University. Baltimore was in one of the Rockefeller Institute's first classes of graduate students (it still hadn't quite changed its name). When Baltimore arrived, there were forty Rockefeller graduate students, and the institution spared no expense to provide an opulent home for them. Its amenities attracted the crème de la crème of young biologists.

Thoughts of the "fabulous" graduate student life at Rockefeller still brought a warm smile to Baltimore's face thirty years after he graduated. A maid cleaned his spacious single in the graduate dorm; breakfast and dinner were served in elegant Abbey Aldrich Rockefeller Hall (known as the Abbey by the regulars); candlelit dinners were graced by a large Franz Kline oil painting hanging on the blue velvet walls. A coat-and-tie affair, dinner always pleased. A group of students known as "the last of the big spenders" ate steak every night for an extra dollar. Lunches were even better, held in a huge, austere dining hall whose floor was lined with rows of long wooden tables in the English college tradition. Only graduate students, postdoctoral fellows, and professors were admitted, and dress was formal. They sat anywhere, without regard to seniority. Baltimore routinely sat next to Peyton Rous, winner of the 1966 Nobel Prize for his work on cancer, or Fritz Lipmann, winner of the 1953 Nobel Prize for his biochemical elucidation of basic metabolism. They gabbed about science over roast turkey and broccoli. The graduate program would be stripped of its luxury in the early 1970s because of its exorbitant costs, but during Baltimore's stay, lavishness reigned.

The pampering made Rockefeller a wonderful place to immerse oneself in research. Baltimore worked twelve to sixteen hours a day, without the worries of cooking, cleaning, or transportation. "All you had to do was work, didn't have to think about a thing. It was fabulous." Baltimore even took his laundry home by bus on weekends because his parents lived right across town. "I'd go to the movies occasionally, had some love affairs and things, but—I did an awful lot of lab work. I loved it! I mean, you know, that's all I really wanted to do."

Baltimore considered science a guilty pleasure. He anxiously wondered whether becoming a scientist was socially responsible. "Did I have the right to indulge my newfound passion?" He was happily surprised by the answer. "The only way to do research was on government money: could I really make a life spending the government's money to indulge my habit? As I looked to the feedback coming from the outside world in the early 1960s, the answer was a resounding yes. . . . My private passion was a public good."

Franklin's laboratory consisted of Franklin himself, a technician, and Baltimore, all carefully pulling viruses apart, handling up to a trillion viruses a day. Officially, Franklin worked for Igor Tamm, the full professor who ran the animal virology laboratory. Rockefeller was arranged like a European university, with a full professor overseeing the work of a group of junior professors. Almost all other American universities allowed junior professors to run their own laboratories freely.

Franklin worked hard, but it was Baltimore who spent nights working alone, one of a few scientists in the dark high-rise, tending to cells and protein extracts with stubborn vigilance. Beyond the Franklin lab, Baltimore found Rockefeller to be a wonderful community where he could wander around to other labs to get help. Everything seemed free and grand.

Arrowsmith, Sinclair Lewis's novel of medical and biological research, was heavily based on the Rockefeller Institute and its scientists in the 1910s. In one of the novel's most famous passages, Lewis describes Martin Arrowsmith's reaction on settling into his first laboratory:

> When he had closed the door and let his spirit flow out and fill that minute apartment with his own essence, he felt secure. . . . He would be free to work. . . .
> He looked out of the broad window above his bench. . . . Shut in to a joy of precision, he would nevertheless not be walled out from flowering life. He had, to the north, not the Woolworth Tower alone but the Singer Tower. . . . To the west, tall ships were riding, tugs were bustling, all the world went by. Below his cliff, the streets were feverish. Suddenly he loved humanity as he loved the decent, clean rows of test-tubes, and he prayed then the prayer of the scientist:

God give me unclouded eyes and freedom from haste. God give me a quiet and relentless anger against all pretense and all pretentious work and all work left slack and unfinished. God give me the restlessness whereby I may neither sleep nor accept praise till my observed results equal my calculated results or in pious glee I discover and assault my error. God give me the strength not to trust to God!

Baltimore's own words, formulated almost exactly thirty years after his arrival at Rockefeller, express a similar view: "That epiphanal time was to me a realization of what I was meant to do. Not being religious, I do not mean that I was meant by God to do research, but I do suspect that I was meant by my genetic inheritance to do research. Coming to that realization was like putting on a calfskin glove that fits perfectly: it was a warm, enveloping experience." Again, in his own words, his scientific life was "sanctioned self-indulgence."

Baltimore worked first on the replication of influenza virus and Newcastle disease (a bird virus), both of which were popular RNA viruses to study. (RNA viruses are viruses that use RNA instead of DNA as their genetic material.) The work went reasonably well, but a previous result from the lab kept nagging Baltimore. One of Franklin's summer interns, Jon Rosner, had radioactively labeled the RNA in cells infected with mengovirus, a mouse virus. Radioactive labeling did not damage the mengovirus RNA genome; it simply made the RNA detectable with a radiation counter (like a Geiger counter) or on X-ray film. By following the radioactively labeled mengovirus RNA, Rosner saw that normal RNA synthesis in the cell nucleus was shut down, and shortly thereafter RNA synthesis was detectable in the cytoplasm (the cellular material outside the nucleus). The nucleus is generally considered the "brain" of the animal cell because that is where the DNA is stored. The information in the DNA is read and transcribed (synthesized) into RNA inside the nucleus. RNA synthesis normally wasn't observed outside the nucleus, because there was no DNA in the cytoplasm. The experiment suggested to Baltimore that mengovirus was taking over RNA synthesis in the cell, shutting down the cell's normal RNA synthesis and restarting it from the mengovirus's genetic material in the cytoplasm. Mengo, which was easy to work with, quickly became the model virus for Baltimore.

Beginning in the winter of 1962, Baltimore followed two research trails to determine the fundamental biology of mengo, and perhaps the fundamental characteristics of all similar animal viruses. Mengovirus had to do at least two things to replicate: it had to commandeer the protein and RNA synthesis machinery of the cell, and it had to replicate its own genetic material.

All of Baltimore's experiments depended on a scientific development that underpinned all the new animal virology research: the technique of animal cell culture. Before this development in the 1950s, all animal virology work had to be done in whole animals, which was difficult work and impossibly slow. But now cells could be grown, or cultured, by the millions and billions in the laboratory. Certain animal viruses were capable of infecting cultured animal cells, and animal virologists like Franklin and Baltimore were just learning to use molecular and genetic techniques (similar to the ones used by Luria, Levinthal, and the Phage Group to study virus infections of bacteria) to study animal virus infections of animal cells.

Baltimore's weekly work involved growing dozens of flasks full of cultured L-cells, a type of cancerous mouse cell related to skin fibroblasts. Fibroblasts are the cells in the layers between muscle and outer skin. Baltimore grew cancerous L-cells in a layer so thin as to be nearly transparent to the naked eye. At maximum density, about fifty million cells grew in a single layer on the bottom of a dish the size of a paperback book. Magnified one hundred times under a microscope, each amoeba-shaped cell stretched out flat on the surface of the dish, with a tiny dark hump in the middle that was the nucleus. Human cells looked the same.

The cells absorbed their nutrients from a liquid made by mixing a variety of salts, amino acid supplements, and serum from newborn calf blood—a growth medium. Although it contained no red blood cells, the broth was tinted with a pH indicator, phenol red, that made the medium look like thinned blood. Baltimore grew the cells in incubators heated to body temperature and fed them a fresh batch of medium every other day. The cultures had an irritating tendency to get contaminated with airborne bacteria and fungi that landed in the fluid and overgrew the animal cells like mold devouring a loaf of bread. Contamination problems forced Baltimore and every other scientist growing animal cells to use sterile techniques, such as baking their equipment, scrubbing their hands, developing a paranoia of their invisible microbial enemies, and working under hoods that effectively enclosed the benchtops and circulated purified air.

L-cells and other animal cell lines are a fantastic phenomenon. In the 1950s a researcher cut out a chunk of tissue from a mouse and left the tissue mass in cell culture medium for a week. At the end of the week, some cells had pushed their way out of the hard knot of flesh and migrated onto the surface of the flask. A few of the cells began to divide, and they covered the flask in a matter of weeks. The scientist then scraped the L-cells off the flask and split them up into to five new flasks, which were coated with the new replicating L-cells within days. The aggressive cells were passed into more and more flasks, and some samples were frozen. Under appropriate conditions, it is routinely possible to take animal cells, concentrate them into a solid yellow blob (by spinning them in a centrifuge), put them in a plastic vial, and freeze them in liquid nitrogen (at −210° C), after which they can be stored for a decade or more and then thawed and grown again. (Scientists in the 1990s have grown cells from people who died in the 1950s.) The developer of L-cells froze vials and sent them out to friends in various labs; from these cultures, the L-cells became the most promiscuous mouse cells in the world. Eerily, these cells are as much a species as any other unicellular organism bred in labs, although no one classifies them that way. They thrive in their new environment, independent of the body they once inhabited, sucking nutrients from the filtered calf blood.

Though normal human cells grow for only fifty generations (a few months of continuous replication), tumor cells can go through a nearly infinite number of generations. They have been freed from the aging process. The best-known human tumor cell line, HeLa cells, isolated from a tumor in a woman fifty years ago, have been grown so successfully and widely that their progeny have long since surpassed the number of stars in the universe.

Once Baltimore grew enough L-cells to run experiments, he tried some trial infections with his mengovirus stocks. Mengo was a minor virus of rodents and cattle isolated some years previously, and it was interesting only because it was easy to study in the lab and because it was related to the rhinoviruses (largely responsible for the common cold) and poliovirus (the cause of paralytic poliomyelitis, or polio). Very few animal viruses would infect laboratory-cultured cells. This was an early problem with studying poliovirus and would be a problem, much later, with HIV. Mengo had no such qualms and happily infected L-cells, resulting in tens of thousands of new mengoviruses bursting from each cell after one day.

Using a technique developed by Renato Dulbecco of Caltech, it was possible to infect a monolayer of millions of cells with only a couple of dozen viruses, resulting in bare patches in the monolayer of cells where a virus had infected one cell, multiplied, killed the cell, and then infected and killed its neighbors. This was the animal virus plaque-making technique, similar to the bacteriophage plaque-making technique Baltimore learned from

George Streisinger. After running through a few plaque experiments to measure how much virus was present, Baltimore infected a series of flasks of L-cells with millions of mengoviruses. Every cell in the flask was dead in twenty hours. The virus stocks were good.

Baltimore planned to observe how mengovirus shut down cellular RNA synthesis and began its own RNA synthesis, confirming and extending Rosner's observations. The way to see how the cellular RNA synthesis was shut down was to look at the cellular RNA polymerase activity. To do that, he first had to extract the RNA polymerase from the cells. He ran two preparations in parallel: the experiment and the control. The control was just a flask of regular L-cells to which the experimental results would be compared. The experiment contained a series of flasks of L-cells that had been infected with mengovirus for between zero and nine hours. Baltimore followed a fairly standard protocol for crudely extracting RNA polymerase. He took each of the flasks independently, poured the cells into test tubes, and centrifuged them, which concentrated the cells into tight pellets. He washed each pellet several times to clean off any excess medium and debris. Then he added thousands of small glass beads to each tube and put the tubes in a homogenizer, a machine similar in function to a paint can shaker, which pulverized the cells by violently shaking the glass beads. Though this treatment disrupted the cell membrane, it left the nucleus of each cell intact. To tear open the nuclei and free the RNA polymerase, he centrifuged this slurry at six hundred times the force of gravity, or 600 Gs, for eight minutes. Then he sucked the excess liquid and debris away from the pellet of nuclei, washed the nuclei with a sugary solution to remove more debris, centrifuged the result, and repeated the process.

When he had a clean pellet of mouse cell nuclei at the bottom of each tube, he added a small amount of almost pure water to each tube. Animal cells and nuclei don't like pure water; they are designed to survive in the salty environment of the body. Osmosis caused the nuclei to explode as the water rushed in and the nuclear membranes couldn't withstand the pressure. Now the RNA polymerase should be free; but, just to make sure, Baltimore exposed each tube to a short burst of ultrasonic energy waves, causing the nuclei to vibrate so violently that they ripped apart, like an opera singer breaking a million tiny champagne glasses. To the resulting slurry, Baltimore then added a strong salt solution. The salt caused the DNA, RNA, and a variety of associated proteins to fall (or precipitate) out of the solution in a stringy white tangle. Baltimore watched the ghostly threads settle and then slid the tubes into a metal bench rack. Grabbing a long, rapier-thin glass rod, he passed it through the flame of a Bunsen burner, twisting the end of the rod into a red-hot hook. After quenching the rod with a quick dip in the water bath, he reached it into the first tube and twirled up the cottony precipitate. As he pulled it out of the tube, he could see clear, unprecipitated, gloopy DNA and protein hanging from the rod as well. That was fine. The DNA from one mouse cell would stretch two feet if laid out end to end (the DNA from the human body would stretch to the moon and back with length to spare), so the DNA from a flask full of cells made quite a tangle; various proteins were caught up in that tangle, including RNA polymerase. Slipping the mass into a new tube labeled "Control aggregate-enzyme 1," he had his RNA polymerase, somewhere in that gloop.

First he tried the uninfected control. He washed the aggregate-enzyme several times to clean it up again and change its salt concentration and pH. Now it was time to test for RNA polymerase activity. The recipe du jour was this:

> 50 micromoles Tris, pH 7.9
> 1.5 micromoles $MnCl_2$ (manganese chloride)
> 10 micromoles NaF (sodium fluoride)
> 2.5 micromoles β-mercaptoethanol
> Radioactive-hydrogen-labeled adenosine triphosphate
>   nucleotide (ATP)
> 60 micrograms each GTP, CTP, UTP
> 0.05 ml cold-saturated ammonium sulfate
> 0.2 ml "aggregate-enzyme"

Mix well and incubate at 37° C (human body temperature) for twenty minutes.

During the incubation, the RNA polymerase invisibly went to work, synthesizing new RNA that was radioactively labeled. After the incubation, Baltimore shoved the tubes into a bucket of ice for ten minutes to stop the polymerase action; enzymes from warm-blooded animals work only near body temperature. Then he precipitated the mixture again with a dense salt solution and centrifuged the ivory strings of DNA and RNA into a tight white pellet to separate the desired RNA polymers from the loose radioactive nucleotide monomers, like sifting long pearl necklaces away from loose pearls. He resuspended the pellet in a new solution and placed the pellet of RNA in the liquid scintillation radioactivity counter, a high-tech relative of a Geiger counter that told Baltimore how much radioactive RNA the RNA polymerase had synthesized.

The results were low. Very low. A different lab had published a paper on this technique and reported much higher radioactive nucleotide incorporation into RNA polymers. Disappointed, he knew that he had probably just made a mistake. Failure is part of daily laboratory life, and Baltimore would have to troubleshoot the problem and repeat the experiment.

What could have gone wrong? Just about anything. He sat at his desk and thought the experiment through again, step by step. Any one of those different reagents could be of the wrong concentration, or contaminated, or both. Or Baltimore could have made a mistake when he measured out the minuscule quantities of liquid. Was the radioactive reagent bad? He checked pure stock in the radiation counter. No, the radioactivity was fine. Were the cells poorly pulverized? Maybe. Had he lost his pellet in one of the washes? Maybe. Perhaps the procedure took too long and his RNA polymerase went bad. The only thing to do was repeat the experiment.

The experiment failed again, and again. But after a few more tries, normal RNA polymerase activity showed up like a radioactive flare in the scintillation counter. Success! The next day he ran the same experiment on the extracts from mengovirus-infected cells.

Success in biology often depends heavily on the Edison philosophy of 99 percent perspiration and 1 percent inspiration. For some, like Baltimore, research is an addiction. He was addicted to the hunt for results. What was the answer? How should he interpret the data? Would he figure out the experimental kinks? What did it all mean? Some people are so addicted they can't wait to see their newest results. Like kids opening Christmas presents the night before, they stop their experiments early, desperate to know the results—and lead a miserable existence repeating ruined or ambiguous experiments. Baltimore was patient and foresighted enough to stifle urges that would shortchange his experimental results. Still, the lab work was so addictive that he had difficulty tearing himself away to eat. Often he worked himself into a euphoric exhaustion before wandering back to his dorm room, leaving the lab only to avoid making careless mistakes.

Within months, Baltimore and Franklin optimized the RNA polymerase experiments and made substantial findings on how mengovirus commandeered the cell. In the RNA synthesis comparison between infected L-cells and uninfected L-cells, Baltimore saw that mengovirus reduced the RNA synthesis activity in cells to a scant 10 percent of normal: mengo inhibited the L-cells' ability to express their own genes, preventing information transfer from DNA to RNA. The virus had taken control of the cell's metabolism. Baltimore had made his first discovery.

By the end of his first academic year at Rockefeller, Baltimore had sent off his first scientific paper on mengovirus for publication in a scientific journal. It was time for the annual pilgrimage out to Long Island. This year at Cold Spring Harbor was particularly important to him, because the 1962 Symposium of Quantitative Biology was dedicated to animal viruses, and this was Baltimore's first conference as an official participant. The symposium, Cold Spring Harbor's biggest affair of the summer, was chaired by Renato Dulbecco from Caltech. If Salvador Luria was the godfather of bacterial virology, Baltimore saw Dulbecco as "one of the great godfathers of animal virology." Dulbecco was yet another pupil of Luria's and had shared a bench with James Watson for a time. Currently Dulbecco was researching cancer-causing animal viruses.

The major players in animal virology were all in attendance, Howard Temin, Ed Simon, and Jim Darnell among them. The major sessions focused on the geometric shape of viruses, how viruses replicated, and how some viruses caused cancer. Darnell lectured on poliovirus replication and continuously referred to Baltimore and Franklin's mengovirus work showing the devastating effects of mengovirus on RNA synthesis in infected cells. Franklin gave a lecture as well. Darnell's and Franklin's presentations were the centerpieces of the viral replication session and the basis of excited discussions throughout the week. Dulbecco was so fascinated by the work that he spent half of his concluding remarks on it.

A confusing array of viruses was discussed: poliovirus, mengovirus, a *Drosophila* virus, a chicken cancer-causing virus, rabbitpox, cowpox, influenza, Newcastle disease virus, and others. This variety of subjects was making the early days of animal virology much less organized than those of phage studies. Early on, the phage group had established an informal "treaty" whereby only two types of bacteriophage were chosen for study. However, out of this animal virus free-for-all, fascinating patterns were emerging: animal viruses were profoundly different from bacteriophages and from one another. They were so diverse that the participants were hardly able to agree on a vocabulary or a way to group the viruses into families.

Down at the Cold Spring Harbor beach, some scientists swam in Long Island Sound, and others sat on the rocks talking about poxviruses, cancerous transformation, and isometric viral shells. Back up the hill, other scientists drank beer and argued about viral replication strategies. For most of the week the scientists basked in sunny, warm days. They held picnics on the lawn or ate on the terrace overlooking the shore. Baltimore was perhaps the youngest person in attendance. He sported a black mustache to make himself look older. He wore the standard scientific attire: khaki pants and a white long-sleeved shirt. He was always in a conversation, talking science with everybody. The conversations were intense, but there was a lot of experimental space in animal virology, so the atmosphere was one of intellectual curiosity rather than competition.

Baltimore made a big impression on the other scientists. People could see the hunger in his eyes and hear it in his voice. On uncontroversial topics he was a gracious conversationalist with a pleasant sense of humor, an affable dinner companion. But when the talk turned to virology, Baltimore became a person to reckon with. At heart, David Baltimore is a passionate debater: he aims to be right. Backed up by his sharp mind and encyclopedic knowledge, his argumentative personality makes him stand out even in scientific discourse; he simply doesn't give up. There are few biologists more competitive. Paul Berg, later an important friend and ally of Baltimore's who met him for the first time at a similar conference, said, "It was clear that this was a guy who was very smart, and was not shy. Not shy at all. I mean, he certainly engaged everybody. Anybody who picked at him on his data or conclusions, he fought them tooth and nail. He was pretty aggressive. And so he sort of acquired a bit of a reputation as an enfant terrible."

Before the conference, Franklin had accepted a faculty position at Colorado Medical School in Denver and planned to leave Rockefeller the following spring. Baltimore hadn't said anything about going with Franklin yet, and Darnell noticed. One mild evening, Darnell asked Baltimore what his plans were after Franklin left Rockefeller. Baltimore said that he had been wondering that himself. In that case, Darnell suggested, Baltimore might come back to MIT. It was a reasonable plan, and Baltimore agreed to think about it. More than that, he started planning to work with Darnell.

Back at Rockefeller, Baltimore and Franklin were trying to find out how RNA viruses replicate. It was a big question, because no living organism used RNA as its genetic material. There was something unique about these viruses. Biologists were comfortable with the clean schema of DNA to RNA to protein, the Central Dogma. DNA stores the genetic blueprint. DNA

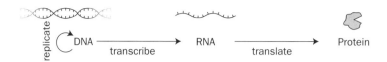

DNA $\xrightarrow[\text{transcribe}]{}$ RNA $\xrightarrow[\text{translate}]{}$ Protein

replicate

The Central Dogma.

replicates to make more DNA, using an enzyme called DNA polymerase, the molecular analog to those medieval monks who copied entire books letter by letter. From the information in DNA (the genes), RNA is transcribed by the RNA polymerase. The information on these RNA messages is then translated by the ribosomes (construction workers of the cell) to synthesize the appropriate proteins. But the existence of RNA viruses clearly put a kink in this elegant, simple scheme, because only DNA, and not RNA, was supposed to be able to replicate. But the RNA viruses clearly replicated *somehow.* The RNA virus had two logical possibilities. It could make DNA from its viral RNA genetic material, and then transcribe the DNA information back to RNA for protein synthesis and replication; or it could make RNA from the RNA and not use DNA at all. Both options were beyond the scope of the Central Dogma.

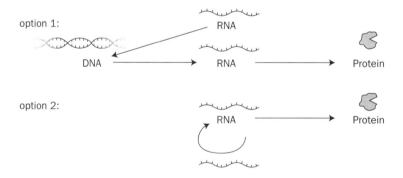

The two options for RNA virus replication that Baltimore and Franklin could diagram on the laboratory chalkboard.

What was the truth about RNA virus replication? Ed Simon, co-instructor of the Cold Spring Harbor animal virus course, showed that poliovirus replicated in human cells even when the cells were infused with drugs that destroyed DNA synthesis, a test something like pouring sugar in a car's gas tank to prove that the radio still works even though the motor won't run. DNA wasn't involved. That conclusion left everyone inferring that the RNA copied itself. A new rule was postulated: "RNA can beget RNA." But no one had proved it yet. Baltimore wanted to be the man to do it.

He had competition on three sides: poliovirus scientists, tobacco mosaic virus scientists, and RNA phage scientists. Tobacco mosaic virus, a plant RNA virus, had been studied by scientists for fifty years, and preliminary results about its replication cycle were finally coming in. But it looked as though the toughest competitors would be the RNA phage labs.

The first RNA bacteriophage was discovered in 1961 by Tim Loeb, a graduate student working for Norton Zinder at Rockefeller, with initial inspiration from Maurice Fox. More RNA phages might have been discovered earlier, but the "Phage Treaty" had limited the research. At Cold Spring Harbor one summer Fox had suggested that Loeb look for new phage, which was a disgusting job. The place to find *E. coli* phage was in human sewage. Since the Cold Spring Harbor area sewage would be overrun by the two types of phage all the scientists studied and washed down the drain, Fox suggested Loeb try Manhattan sewage. Loeb agreed and left to begin filtering phage from sewage samples. Loeb's uptown Manhattan phage was soon identified as having RNA as its genetic material. This was an important discovery, because hundreds of virologists knew how to gather molecular information about phage, whereas biochemical and genetic work with plant viruses and animal viruses moved comparatively slowly.

Baltimore rapidly hunted for evidence of a mengovirus RNA polymerase that could replicate the mengovirus RNA genetic material—the heart of the virus. How could he isolate this enzyme from the thousands of other cellular enzymes? One of his tools was the drug actinomycin, which kills cells by destroying RNA synthesis: it binds to DNA and prevents the cell's RNA polymerase from reading the DNA and synthesizing RNA. Such drugs have proved crucial to modern cell biology research in much the same way that mutations (also called alleles in the scientists' lexicon) provided the foundation for genetics experiments. A number of these drugs caused specific damage inside cells, which allowed biologists to study the workings of a cell in much the same way that someone might try to figure out how a car works by selectively disabling parts of the engine by disconnecting hoses or taking off the fan belt. Baltimore reached his hands into the molecular engine of the cells and started ripping out wires. Break it and figure out what went wrong; then break something else and keep looking.

Baltimore and Franklin found that in cells infected by mengovirus, actinomycin stopped the cellular RNA synthesis (in the nucleus), but not mengovirus RNA synthesis (in the cytoplasm). They reasoned that the mengovirus was using not the cell's RNA polymerase but some other RNA synthesis system, an independent system created by the virus. It must be an RNA polymerase that replicated RNA. This was the first direct evidence of an RNA-replicating RNA polymerase (a name soon simplified to RNA replicase) and it provided a new enzymatic twist to the Central Dogma.

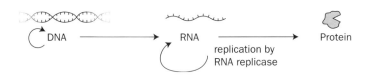

The discovery of RNA replication modified the Central Dogma.

Their data were good, but an even better proof would be to show that the enzyme activity had the full characteristics of an RNA polymerase. If they were lucky, they could isolate the mengovirus RNA replicase enzyme from all the other proteins in the cell and show that it had RNA polymerase activity. It was the difference between being able to deduce that a murderer had used a gun and actually catching the murderer holding the gun.

To handle this new biochemical aspect of the project and to ferret out the rogue viral enzyme, Baltimore learned new techniques from members of Fritz Lipmann's lab. Lipmann had won the Nobel Prize ten years earlier for his brilliant biochemical research, but by the early 1960s he was hardly ever around. Nevertheless, his Rockefeller laboratory was full of excellent scientists, and the expertise of one young biochemist in particular, Dan Nathans—a future Nobel winner—proved to be a boon for Baltimore. After learning some clever techniques from Nathans and discussing some strategies with Franklin, Baltimore set up a series of experiments to illustrate conclusively that the activity was an RNA polymerase. Data kept flowing in, but his efforts to isolate the mengovirus polymerase were failing.

Baltimore and Franklin were scared they'd be beaten to the punch in announcing the first RNA replicase by one of the RNA phage groups. With their preliminary data, the two quickly wrote a paper in late September and sent it off for publication while they finished up experiments for a more complete paper. The first paper was published late in 1962. Baltimore's instincts were good. Only a few months later, a lab at New York University, led by the Nobelist Severo Ochoa, showed the same activity in an RNA phage and published their results, but Baltimore's paper was first, and the NYU group duly noted that "Baltimore and Franklin have recently reported on the occurrence of a similar enzyme in L-cells infected with the RNA-containing mengovirus." Baltimore and Franklin's definitive paper on the RNA replicase came out several months after the NYU group's paper. Baltimore and Franklin proved that an RNA replicase was present, but neither they nor anyone else would manage to isolate the mengovirus enzyme for fifteen years; Baltimore's experiment remained one of the only proofs of the RNA replicase's existence.

The rapidity of the discoveries exhilarated Baltimore. His experiments with Franklin were clean, quick, and flexible and generated solid data, and few other groups had touched animal virus replication. Baltimore was young enough to maintain an exhausting laboratory schedule, and he stayed keenly aware of the need to publish papers quickly. There was a lot of data overlap in his early papers, and he also published a series of short letters and preliminary reports and made a series of presentations at Cold Spring Harbor and other meetings to stay ahead of the competition. "The way to do significant science is to be ahead of the curve," he has observed. "There is no other advice to give a budding scientist who wants to reach the top." That advice summarizes his personal philosophy, both in his relentless competitiveness and in his restless search for innovative projects.

As Baltimore cranked out data on the mengovirus replicase, he was already looking to expand his horizons. He hadn't purified the RNA replicase, but that was starting to look like a long-term project, and the most interesting part was over. He wanted to move on. What else was interesting? How about poliovirus?

CHOSEN PET

Igor Tamm ran the other animal virology laboratory at Rockefeller, and the Franklin and Tamm Labs held joint group meetings, in which every week people presented their findings and problems. Tamm's lab worked on a variety of animal viruses, and one of his postdoctoral fellows, H. J. Eggers, worked on poliovirus. Between Darnell and Tamm, Baltimore quickly became interested in poliovirus, the highly contagious cause of infantile paralysis. It can claw its way into human nerves and muscle tissue, and in the most severe cases it causes lifelong paralysis or death. In 1952, a polio epidemic in the United States infected 50,000 people, killing 3,300 and paralyzing roughly 10,000 more. That same year, Jonas Salk developed the first polio vaccine, using poliovirus cell culture techniques developed by John Enders, Frederick Robbins, and Thomas Weller of Harvard Medical School, who took home the 1954 Nobel Prize.

Poliovirus has an extraordinary ability to replicate. A single poliovirus that infects a human cell generates ten thousand progeny that rip the cell apart in only eight hours. Protected by Salk vaccinations, virologists like Darnell and Eggers cultured enough poliovirus on their lab benches to paralyze an entire city. For Baltimore, poliovirus was simply a more popular virus to work with than mengo. Instead of cancerous mouse L-cells, cancerous human HeLa cells were used as the viral hosts. Also, poliovirus studies at Rockefeller could segue conveniently into his future work with Darnell. Baltimore decided to pick up poliovirus work that summer. That work provided the evidence that his polio and mengovirus studies were compatible: he identified the poliovirus RNA replicase activity quickly enough to add it as a brief note to his mengovirus polymerase paper before it was published. Baltimore delved into the molecular brains of mengo and polio, splitting his time between two laboratories.

The RNA replicase experiments, isolating the active enzyme, were in vitro experiments: test-tube experiments. But a test tube is not a living cell. Now he wanted to do in vivo experiments to observe what happened in living cells infected by the virus.

Baltimore's poliovirus experiments always started with human HeLa cells growing on the bottom of a dish. Baltimore sucked out the pink media with a pipette (a glass straw) and replaced it with a swarm of poliovirus. He then returned the dish to the body-temperature incubator for fifteen minutes, allowing the polioviruses to slip inside the HeLa cells while he gathered together the remaining reagents he needed, thawing frozen stocks and mixing up pH-buffered solutions (often just called "buffers"). After scrubbing his hands again, he pulled out the infected dish and moved it to the sterile workspace, where he sucked off the polioviruses that hadn't entered the cells, disposing of them in a test tube full of bleach. Next he added ³H-leucine, a radioactively labeled amino acid, and placed the dish back in the incubator for fifteen minutes. Meanwhile he patiently read the newest issue of whatever scientific magazine was around. In the incubator, the HeLa cells were absorbing the leucine and incorporating it into the proteins they were continuously producing. At the end of fifteen minutes, Baltimore flooded the dish with an ice-cold vinegar and alcohol mixture, killing the cells and stopping their metabolic activity, as though taking a physical photograph of the cells' state. After another ten minutes he removed the vinegar solution and replaced it with a 70 percent ethanol solution, further preserving, or "fixing," the cells. To complete the fixing process, a fifteen-minute incubation in cold perchloric acid was followed by four washes with water. Then Baltimore dehydrated the cells with alcohol-ether and pure ether, turning them into protein-RNA-DNA shells, like microscopic radioactive crispy pastry balls. Next he placed the dehydrated cells in the radiation counter and determined how much protein the cells had made during their fifteen minutes in ^{3}H-leucine. By doing this experiment at a variety of time points, in uninfected and infected cells, and with various drugs, he determined that poliovirus sucked the life out of human cells by strangling their cellular protein synthesis and replacing it with poliovirus protein synthesis.

He published three papers with Tamm and Eggers demonstrating poliovirus's dictatorial effects on protein synthesis inside human cells. Looking back fifteen years later, he saw these years at Rockefeller as a time where he did some of his best research: "Everything started breaking. I walked into lab each day and made a discovery. It was unbelievable! . . . I found some methods that were particularly effective and ended up publishing a lot of papers," he paused and smiled, "and finding some pretty important things." By the end of 1963, Baltimore had ten scientific papers to his name, a huge number for a graduate student; even more remarkably, he was lead author on all but one of them.

The contents of these papers revealed some of the fundamental mechanics of the animal virus lifecycle. An excellent gauge of the significance of Baltimore's graduate work is a simple tally of how many times other scientists referenced Baltimore's work in their own papers. Three of his graduate school papers, the most complete ones, were cited 250 times in scientific papers before 1970. That was a rate of almost one per week, an extraordinary count even in the active microcosm of virology.

However, much of the credit for graduate students' work often goes to the supervising professors. Conflicts often arise from this policy, given the independence of many junior researchers and their years of hard labor. An often-cited example is the discovery of pulsars in space. In 1967, a Cambridge University graduate student, Jocelyn Bell, noticed "a bit of scruff" on the radiotelescope data chart. Remembering having seen a similar bit of scruff earlier, she checked through the charts and determined that it was a periodic signal from an extraterrestrial source. After further analysis with her professor, Andrew Hewish, they published a paper announcing the discovery of a new phenomenon, pulsars. Seven years later Hewish won a Nobel Prize for the discovery, and people cried foul at Bell's nonrecognition, although Bell herself, and others, asserted that as a graduate student she received adequate recognition. Such are the merits and spoils of the apprentice system.

Richard Franklin said farewell to Rockefeller in March 1963 and headed for the cool heights of Colorado. Baltimore prepared to follow suit and take up his paid postdoctoral position at MIT. He had only been at Rockefeller for eighteen months, but in that time he had completed more than enough work for a thesis. The easy path to a Ph.D. was to write up the mengovirus work. If there had been photocopiers in 1963, Baltimore probably would have xeroxed his papers, stapled them together, typed a cover page labeling it as "David Baltimore's Thesis," and dropped it off at the dean's office on his way to MIT. As it was, he called it "The Diversion of Macromolecular Synthesis in L-Cells towards Ends Dictated by Mengovirus."

The Rockefeller Institute, however, was not prepared to give Baltimore a Ph.D. for a scant eighteen months of work. Three to four years of lab work was the norm. They did not reckon on Baltimore's determination. He simply informed the Rockefeller that he was done and was leaving for MIT. Flabbergasted, but left without many options, the Rockefeller administration declared it a "domestic year abroad" and submissively suggested that Baltimore write his thesis slowly. Though no one keeps records of these kinds of feats, he was almost certainly the fastest Ph.D. student in the history of Rockefeller, and one of the fastest ever in molecular biology.

Baltimore wanted to stay in the area for the Cold Spring Harbor symposium, so he hung around the Tamm lab cleaning up some poliovirus experiments for publication with Eggers. Baltimore and Franklin again presented a paper at the Cold Spring Harbor meeting, and Baltimore again impressed the major players in virology. Then, with the heat of midsummer stifling Manhattan, Baltimore sped north.

POSTDOCTORAL DAYS

Cambridge hadn't changed much in the two years he was gone, and Baltimore settled right back in. Darnell's lab was, above all else, a comfortable place. Marc Girard from Paris joined the Darnell Lab as a postdoc shortly after Baltimore did, and his first Monday morning in an American lab was a memorable one. As befitted a French scientist of the 1960s, he showed up at 9 A.M. sharp, dressed in his best suit and a crisp blue tie. No one was there. The Darnell lab was dark and the shades were pulled closed, but the door was unlocked. So Girard went inside, sat on one of the bench stools and waited, listening to the hum of the freezers and refrigerators. Forty-five minutes later, a lab technician showed up and offered him coffee. They talked for a couple of minutes, and then the tech went off to take care of his daily chores. A little after ten, Darnell phoned to say that he'd be in around 1 P.M. Then, around 10:30 or so, a ratty-looking, unshaven guy in blue jeans and a dirty T-shirt walked in and said, "Ah! You must be Marc Girard. I'm David Baltimore."

Girard was shocked. "*Baltimore?* Of Baltimore and Franklin?"

"Yes, why?"

Girard was speechless, because in the feudal European system of science, the professor's name was always listed first on publications, and Girard didn't know that it was different in the United States: generally the person who did most of the work is first on the list, and the professor's name comes last. And so here was someone Girard thought was a famous professor, renowned for his discoveries over the past couple of years, dressed like a bum and only about twenty-five years old.

Darnell's lab was a place where Baltimore could relax a little after his long days at the Rockefeller. He worked a fairly regular, not too grueling schedule. Darnell noted, "No more than a couple of nights a week would people work [long hours], and David worked at that pace." He spent the rest of his time with his current girlfriend, reading, or hanging out with friends.

One of the big factors in the comfortable lab atmosphere was Darnell's fairness as a mentor. When Baltimore arrived at MIT, he was in the midst of experiments that showed directly that the RNA made by the polio RNA replicase was specifically poliovirus RNA and not HeLa cell RNA. This was a key confirmation that Baltimore had discovered the poliovirus replicase. Darnell not only encouraged Baltimore to see that project through but also allowed Baltimore to publish the results as the sole author. Darnell refrained from putting his name on work he didn't help do, and several students, Baltimore included, benefited from that graciousness. In that kind of nurturing environment, Baltimore's independence and creativity flourished. Darnell helped Baltimore to begin thinking as an independent researcher, learning to analyze problems and conceive clear experiments. In addition, as Baltimore recalled, "I thought it would be the perfect place—and it was the perfect place—to become more immersed in other technical ways of handling these problems." Baltimore learned the techniques well. Darnell recalled that "David was by no means the most technically adept [person] that's ever been in the lab—neither was I—but he was good. The data he collected he *devoutly* believed in. Usually for good reasons." From this training with Darnell came David's first publication in the topnotch journal *Science,* coauthored with Darnell, reporting observations on an unusually large, double-stranded poliovirus RNA that might be the key to understanding how the RNA replicase enzyme replicated the poliovirus genome.

Darnell and Baltimore became very good friends. They talked almost daily about the complexities of cells and viruses and theorized about the molecular clockwork of life. Baltimore also became good friends with Marc Girard. Girard was in a new country where he knew no one besides his wife, and Baltimore was a friendly guy who was happy to befriend a new labmate. For the two of them, research amounted to a molecular game of hide and seek.

Poliovirus bursts from cells as a tightly packed ball of proteins slotted together to wrap and protect the RNA genome from the outside world. But how were new viruses made inside cells? How were the virus proteins and the RNA genome assembled into this elegant structure? To generate ten thousand little viruses in one cell in less than eight hours seemed magical. The problem excited Baltimore, and he and Girard worked to gather clues about poliovirus assembly. It was like a Lego puzzle, except that each poliovirus was one-millionth the size of a Lego block.

But how important was poliovirus assembly to the outside world? How important was the science that Baltimore, Darnell, and Girard were doing? These are difficult questions to answer, and they are questions that scientists spend a lot of time avoiding, as though they were in poor taste. At some level, scientists profess that all basic research is equal, because it all increases humanity's knowledge of the known universe. But some discoveries are more equal than others. The value of Baltimore's poliovirus assembly project depended on one's perspective. Other scientists had already spent twenty years studying the assembly and structure of bacterial viruses, and they had generated an impressive understanding of how new viruses were slotted together from a bunch of proteins and strands of DNA or RNA. Other virologists had analyzed the structure of tobacco mosaic virus, a plant virus, for decades. But did that knowledge allow scientists to understand the assembly and structure of animal viruses like polio? Many scientists thought it did, but Baltimore didn't.

The value of a research project can also be judged by its possible value in applied science, such as drug development or clinical medicine. Baltimore didn't spend much time justifying the medical value of his research, because he didn't care about it. He studied viruses because they fascinated him, not because he wanted to cure anyone of anything. But since he was studying a human virus, it could be argued (and certainly was by the agency funding the project) that the knowledge could help cure viral diseases in the future.

Scientific research projects are further judged by pure aesthetics, which is often a powerful influence. Most of the known viruses had beautifully ordered, symmetrical structures. And it had been proposed that poliovirus was a nearly perfect icosahedron of proteins (a theory later proven true). The assembly of that polio icosahedron possessed a certain seductive quality.

In the big picture of scientific importance, then, the poliovirus assembly project might produce knowledge that would be generalizable to other viruses; it might be medically useful; and it was aesthetically pleasing. So the research fell somewhere in the featureless Great Plains of scientific work; it was interesting to animal virologists like Baltimore, but not to the vast majority of biologists and not to the public.

EINSTEIN

Within six months of Baltimore's return to MIT, Darnell accepted a professorship at the Albert Einstein College of Medicine. He planned to leave MIT during the summer of 1964. David was becoming a scientific nomad. Of course, Darnell offered to take Baltimore with him to Einstein, but David didn't accept the offer immediately. One evening Baltimore sat in his apartment weighing the science he knew versus the skills he needed to know. Darnell's science was good, but Baltimore had the impression that he had learned all he would from Darnell. David decided that this was an opportunity to move on. In the back of his mind, he was still bothered by his failure to isolate the purified polio replicase enzyme, so he decided that it would be best to apprentice himself to an enzymologist—a protein chemist—who might be able to teach him how to purify and analyze proteins more adeptly. And he thought it could be important to go to an enzymology lab to learn about other ways of thinking about biological problems. At the same time, however, he wanted to stay in touch with Darnell and Girard and finish the poliovirus assembly experiments. That would require his taking a postdoc position at Einstein. Baltimore arranged to work for two years with the enzymologist Jerry Hurwitz.

While he was packing up to move for the second time in a year, his Rockefeller diploma arrived in the mail. He was officially Dr. Baltimore. He happily tossed it in a box with everything else.

Back in New York, at the sixteen-acre Albert Einstein campus in the Bronx, Baltimore was yet again near enough to his parents' house to do his laundry there. By July 1964, he was appointed as a postdoctoral research fellow in both the Department of Biochemistry and the Department of Molecular Biology. Fixated on replication, Baltimore told Hurwitz he wanted to work on DNA polymerase. Hurwitz told him that would be fine and suggested that Baltimore work on the DNA synthesis initiation problem. It was unclear under what conditions DNA polymerase started its synthesis of DNA. The conditions for cellular RNA polymerase synthesis of RNA were known, at least in a minimal sense, and from there Baltimore might be able to reason his way to the necessary conditions for DNA polymerase.

Long days slipped into long weeks as his manipulations failed. Day after day he got nothing, and nothing again. That was okay; experiments fail. The secret to good science is to guess which variables to tinker with. He changed the temperature: maybe the enzyme liked to be warmer, maybe cooler. He got nothing but nucleotide monomer soup. Baltimore fought with the experiment, trying higher nucleotide concentrations, lower nucleotide concentrations, different pH levels. Maybe the polymerase was damaged in purification. Trying a gentler purification method took Baltimore a month and still resulted in no DNA synthesis. The invisible enzyme wholly rejected his methods.

Periodically retreating, Baltimore sought refuge in Darnell's poliovirus dissection, a more familiar and tractable project that yielded publications. Back in Hurwitz's lab, Baltimore scoured the literature for signposts that might lead to success. Comments about RNA polymerase in one paper keyed him to a novel experiment, something tangential to his bogged-down DNA polymerase work.

People knew that RNA polymerase synthesized RNA in vitro, given the right conditions, but details of the initiation still required explanation. Baltimore was sick of the DNA polymerase work, and he dropped it for a few days so that he could try his hands at RNA polymerase initiation. But he would need some reagents.

Baltimore borrowed RNA polymerase from one person in Hurwitz's lab and a radioactive nucleotide triphosphate (a batch of RNA monomer) from another. Then he carried out an experiment, optimized it a little, and proved that RNA polymerase uses nucleotide triphosphate to initiate synthesis of

RNA. This was his quickest discovery yet, and it was significant because RNA polymerase initiation was a basic reaction necessary to all cells.

The people he borrowed the reagents from were not amused. President Harry Truman once said, "It is amazing what you can accomplish if you do not care who gets the credit." But credit is often the only thing scientists work for, and they'll fight hard for it. Both the other lab members claimed that they were planning to do that same experiment soon, and that Baltimore was trespassing. Baltimore figured that since he had actually done the experiment, opportunistic as it was, he deserved the credit. Besides, he was fairly sure that neither of the people he borrowed the reagents from would have done the experiment, because they refused to share reagents with each other. Nevertheless, Baltimore backed down. Though he would always consider the discovery his own, Baltimore was relegated to the subordinate status of third author.

During David's free time at Einstein he met and, in a whirlwind romance, married Sandra Woodward, a young painter and sixties rebel from Swarthmore. The marriage wouldn't last.

Renato Dulbecco came through New York in the fall of 1964, when Baltimore was just getting started with his Hurwitz apprenticeship. Through Luria, Dulbecco had stayed informed about Baltimore's work. Dulbecco was moving his lab from Caltech to the Salk Institute of Biological Studies, a new research institute in La Jolla, California, financed and directed by Jonas Salk, inventor of the polio vaccine. He was recruiting people to join him, so he stopped by Hurwitz's lab and talked with Baltimore. Dulbecco told Baltimore that he would love to offer Baltimore a research position in his lab, but admitted that he wasn't sure the new Salk Institute was going to hold together. Unexpected bureaucratic problems were plaguing the Salk, and Dulbecco didn't want Baltimore caught in an administrative war zone. But, he said, if he decided the institute was stable, he would offer Baltimore an independent research position. Baltimore was certainly interested, and they kept in touch throughout the year. In February 1965, Dulbecco called Baltimore and offered him a five-year position as a Salk Institute research associate.

Baltimore was enchanted with the idea. California seemed wonderfully romantic, and quite a change from New York. Sandra was excited to go as well. There was one hitch: Baltimore's prior commitment to Hurwitz. But Baltimore continued to fail miserably at the DNA polymerase initiation experiment. It was later shown that DNA polymerase could not start without a primer, a short stretch of double-stranded DNA, a requirement Baltimore never thought of. His enzymatic mixtures were impotent. For Baltimore, the temptation of the Golden State and an independent position at a new institute, working with Renato Dulbecco, was too much to resist. Baltimore left Albert Einstein abruptly at the end of the academic year, yet again abandoning a position early, and headed for his own California poliovirus lab.

Baltimore's undergraduate, graduate, and postgraduate education was unusual because of the number of labs he worked in. Most undergraduates had no lab experience. Most graduate students worked in one lab and then might go on to a postdoctoral position in another. Baltimore worked in two different labs as an undergraduate, four as a grad student, and another two as a postdoc.* His mobility certainly strained the continuity of any given line of research, but it also indoctrinated him in the experimental techniques of multiple fields. What was Baltimore becoming? Virologist, molecular biologist, cell biologist, microbiologist, biochemist, enzymologist. The fields in biology were overlapping so much that titles had more to do with personal preference than real delineations. For Baltimore, the hat of choice was animal virologist.

---

*Graduate students now frequently "rotate" through several laboratories during their first year in graduate school to provide them with a variety of training and help them decide which laboratory to join. It is also much more common now for undergraduates to work in laboratories.

Four

SALK INSTITUTE

DAVID AND SANDRA DROVE out to California in his white Valiant. Spring 1965 was the height of the popularity of the Beach Boys and surfing in southern California. La Jolla, home of the Salk Institute, was a wealthy town on the coast, full of Mercedes Benzes, jewelry stores, and art galleries. It has only one season—spring. The Salk was a mile north of town, near the University of California at San Diego, about eighteen miles outside San Diego proper. David and Sandra rented a house in Solana Beach, two towns up the coast from La Jolla. It was a small town nestled along the shoreline, surrounded by avocado orchards and family vineyards. Mornings found Baltimore cruising down the coast to Salk.

The institute's postmodern main complex was still under construction, so David and everyone else worked in temporary labs in a cluster of wooden shotgun houses near a cliff overlooking the Pacific. Dulbecco kept his word and gave Baltimore complete independence. He was comfortably supplied with money and laboratory space. The position was comparable in salary to that of an assistant professor, but the only obligation was research: no teaching or administrative duties. Baltimore, like many research scientists, was thrilled that someone would pay him $13,000 a year to puzzle out the secrets of biology.

Baltimore's experiments and techniques flowed from the style he developed in Franklin's and Darnell's labs. He had invited Marc Girard to come

65

with him to the Salk. Girard's wife objected because she was anxious to return to France, but Girard convinced her that California would be a wonderful place to live for a couple of years. Having Marc around allowed David to double the number of experiments he was running. And, outside the lab, it was nice for David and Sandra to have a couple of good friends they could invite over for dinner on weekends. But Girard wasn't very fond of Sandra: "She was very *messy*. Not a messy artist, I mean she was," with a shake of his head, "she was not a housewife. Things turned sour after a while." Girard tended to avoid her, but he always enjoyed hanging out with David. Together they made a good research team. They dropped their work on the assembly of poliovirus particles because it wasn't moving along as quickly as Baltimore wanted, but in the two years that Girard stayed at the Salk, they published a series of four papers describing the steps of poliovirus RNA replication.

Before Girard left, he helped recruit two new scientists to the Baltimore lab: Michael Jacobson and Alice Huang. Jacobson was Baltimore's first graduate student, and Baltimore set him to work on poliovirus protein synthesis. Postdoctoral fellow Alice Huang was born in Nanchang in Kiangshi, China. As a grad student she had worked on vesicular stomatitis virus (VSV), a debilitating cattle disease, with Robert Wagner at Johns Hopkins University. Huang's postdoctoral project focused on the interactions between poliovirus and infected cells. Together they formed the polio group, and the three of them grew trillions of polioviruses.

The presence of live poliovirus scared some of the other Salk scientists. Everyone knew someone from childhood who had been crippled by polio. Baltimore found himself defending his lab's safety to neighboring scientists as often as he discussed his scientific results. "I . . . found a kind of know-nothing-ism among a lot of people working with phages and bacteria and biochemistry who didn't have anything to do with animal virology, who were just on me all the time." Everyone had swallowed polio vaccinations, so they were protected from the virus. If they still felt nervous, they could take a booster dose of the vaccine. Nevertheless, a bad batch of Sabin polio vaccine had caused a polio outbreak in 1962, just three years earlier, making people nervous about vaccination. Normally, however, the vaccine was highly effective. Even without the vaccine, fewer than 1 percent of people infected with poliovirus contracted poliomyelitis; the remaining 99 percent developed a poliovirus infection that resembled the common cold. Baltimore was comfortably certain that no vaccinated person was in danger. Historically, however, a number of scientists have died from working with bacteria, viruses, or chemicals more dangerous than they had thought. And before the polio vaccine was invented, several polio researchers had been crippled by the virus. So some of Baltimore's colleagues remained fearful and distrusting. "Those guys are crazy," they would comment in their own labs. Biohazard issues would haunt David Baltimore for a long time.

Meanwhile, Jacobson and Baltimore discovered that protein synthesis in poliovirus generated one huge protein that was later cut into the ten individual smaller poliovirus proteins. This was a biological strategy never observed before: manufacturing a polyprotein. Baltimore was ecstatic and very proud of the result because it significantly restructured the model of viral replication. By analogy, it was as if everyone knew that chocolate bars were always made one bar at a time, and then one day someone discovered that they could pour ten bars in a row all at once, as one long chocolate bar, and then cut it into ten individual chocolate bars afterwards. The polyprotein's novelty helped to establish Baltimore as an expert in animal virology, and he began receiving invitations to talk at symposia, conferences, and universities.

Along with his reputation as an excellent experimental biologist, Baltimore was ascribed "the Touch," the intuitive ability to know what to research and which experiments to try. His mentors—Richard Franklin, George Streisinger, and Dan Nathans—were all reputed to have the same ability. Baltimore understood that science was the art of the solvable; he also understood that staying competitive in important fields meant pushing the limits of his intuition. "Any pursuit so far beyond present knowledge to be pathfinding is not a logical progression from the established order. That, in fact, is the dirty secret of high science—it is not logical. At best it is analogical, and often one is driven by a simple hunch."

Within academia, Baltimore could enjoy the lifestyle he wanted without participating in the capitalist society he disdained. He had always sympathized with leftists and socialists, much as his parents and grandparents had done. His time at Swarthmore, Rockefeller, and MIT had not altered his views. His opinion was blunt: "I really was an anticapitalist." Though not an anticapitalism activist, Baltimore did engage in political activism. He joined antiwar groups, and he took time away from the lab to speak at rallies in San Diego and La Jolla protesting the Vietnam War. In the antiwar movement, he was just another vocal, angry young American protesting the imperialism of the U.S. government.

Sandra spent most of her time painting, but she too hated the war, and she involved herself heavily in the San Diego Coordinating Council for Social Action (SDCCSA). She and some friends published the *Gadfly,* an antiwar newsletter for the SDCCSA. She was its editor for about a year. The newsletter came out intermittently, but the volunteer staff tried to publish it monthly. It consisted of about eight pages of articles describing antiwar activities in San Diego County, announcing protest events and rallies, denouncing the federal government, and encouraging people to rebel against U.S. involvement in Vietnam. In addition, she was chair of the "Open Letter Committee," which raised $1,500 in a week to publish a five-column tirade in the *San Diego Union* expressing opposition to the president's policies and U.S. involvement in Vietnam.

Other colleagues were also involved in the antiwar movement. At MIT, Salvador Luria and several friends organized a nationwide antiwar media campaign by university faculty. Their group, named the Boston Area Faculty Committee on Public Issues (BAFCOPI), published full-page protest advertisements in national newspapers and magazines, often under the moniker of the "Ad Hoc Faculty Committee on Vietnam." Their statements were signed by renowned scientists and professors around the country. On January 15 and 22, 1967, two consecutive Sundays, the Ad Hoc Faculty Committee on Vietnam published full-page ads with the signatures of three thousand faculty from around the United States, including David Baltimore's. In the middle of the page, in inch-high bold type, was the command:

Mr. President:
STOP
the
BOMBING

In February, they published a more lengthy pronouncement in *Newsweek* with four thousand signatures:

> On January 29 in Boston five men, including the Chaplain of Yale University and the best-known pediatrician in our land, will be arraigned in Federal Court accused of a political crime: participation in overt resistance to the draft. . . . On campuses, from pulpits, and in the halls of the United States Congress itself, a profound opposition to the war in Vietnam has been voiced.
>
> Our Government's pursuit of this cruel and unjust war is depriving our country of the moral claim to the allegiance of decent and responsible men.

The war in Vietnam has passed all tolerable bounds of policy. . . . We place ourselves morally beside the defendants in the Boston indictment. They have acted in a just cause, that of putting an end to a war which endangers our national life by weakening the web of commonly held beliefs and values on which it rests.

THE PATH OF RESISTANCE CHOSEN BY THE BOSTON DEFENDANTS IS ONLY ONE OF MANY FORMS OF DISSENT THROUGH WHICH FREE MEN CAN OPPOSE THE ILLEGITIMATE USE OF LEGITIMATE POWER. SUCH DISSENT IS WITHIN THE TRADITION OF OUR NATIONAL HISTORY SINCE THE AMERICAN REVOLUTION AND THE FIGHT AGAINST SLAVERY. . . . A NATION CANNOT DO WITHOUT SUCH MEN IF IT IS TO PRESERVE ITS MORAL INTEGRITY.

IN THE NAME OF THAT TRADITION, WE URGE THE MORAL INNO-CENCE OF THE DEFENDANTS. AS CITIZENS, WE DEMAND HONEST ACTION BY OUR GOVERNMENT TO END THE WAR NOW.

In addition to participating in antiwar politics, Baltimore involved himself in Salk Institute politics, though no more efficaciously. His position as research associate included no administrative responsibilities. The senior faculty, the seven fellows, controlled everything at the institute. Baltimore's lack of influence grated on him whenever the fellows made decisions that he opposed. "In terms of my power over an institution, or my ability to deal with an institution, Salk was small enough that if I was going to be there and be a major publisher and doer of science, then I ought to have some say in the place," he felt. He wanted a more egalitarian power structure, and he griped with the other junior faculty members about their second-class status.

Near the end of 1966, everyone moved into the elegant white buildings sitting back away from the cliffs. The complex was gorgeous. The entrance to the Salk's courtyard followed a shimmering conduit of water flowing across the marble plaza to a gushing fountain, framed against the ocean. Later its beauty and status would attract a number of the great figures of molecular biology, including Francis Crick.

At the Salk, Baltimore grew to feel established as a molecular biologist, and he was confident in his ability to do good work. He was beginning to develop a molecular description of the poliovirus lifecycle. Poliovirus slowly developed into a classic experimental virus, and poliovirus replication became a classic model in animal virology.

In early 1967, reflecting the status he was earning among molecular biologists, a potential job offer from Harvard University arrived. As was usual, Baltimore was invited to give a seminar to the department. After the seminar he would interview with Bernard Davis, the department head. While Baltimore was in Boston, he stopped by MIT to visit Salvador Luria, still a good friend and colleague. Luria told him, "Well, look, if you're talking to them, let us give you an offer. Just put it in your desk." When Baltimore visited Harvard, he didn't get along with Davis: "I went there and I talked to him, and he didn't like me, and I didn't like him; he never gave me an offer."

Shortly after that, Baltimore helped organize an art show at the Salk for Sandra and another artist. As Baltimore recalled the show, the other artist was totally apolitical; he just liked symbols. But one of the symbols he manipulated, grotesquely, was the American flag. "I can't remember what he did with it, but there was something terrible about what he did to an American flag." The art disturbed various faculty members and the president, and they closed down the show. Baltimore was furious with the oligarchic Salk administration: "That was enough for me." At the same time, his marriage was breaking up, and he was frustrated by the impotence of the antiwar effort. His life outside the lab fell apart. He and Sandra divorced. One night, at the beginning of a beautiful California spring, crushed by personal crises and wearied of the Salk, he called Luria and told him he wanted to come back to MIT. An offer from the head of the department, Irwin Sizer, was mailed from MIT on April 17, 1967, welcoming Baltimore to the MIT biology department as an associate professor.

Sizer offered the position for the following fall, but he noted that if Baltimore needed more time, they could arrange for him to start in January. If he wanted to come earlier, he would simply need to let Sizer know, and MIT would arrange for appropriate financial support. Baltimore accepted the offer two weeks after he received the letter, taking Sizer up on the option to come in January. Immediately, he began to organize his things, tie up his research, and pull himself together.

Jim Darnell and his wife came to the Salk for the summer of 1967 and provided Baltimore with some much-needed stability. Baltimore found them a rental house in La Jolla not too far from his new apartment, and Darnell, his wife Jane, Alice Huang, and Baltimore played bridge and drank together almost every night that summer, talking about everything but Baltimore's troubles. Every few nights, instead of meeting at the Darnells' house, they would go down to Marty Weigert's house just up from the beach. Weigert was a good friend of Baltimore's at the Salk. Marty and his wife had a couple of young daughters, and the Darnells had three young boys. So the kids played together, and the six adults relaxed playing bridge. For Baltimore, it was a time to forget about the recent painful months. "I live in the future, not in the past," he later said. And Alice was there, becoming his closest companion. Come January, she would accompany him to MIT.

Five

MIT

Landing back on the east coast was a relief to Baltimore. He felt he was there to stay. He and Alice went apartment hunting together in the snowy Cambridge neighborhoods around Inman Square, Central Square, and Harvard Square. They picked a small flat on Soden Street, not too far from the MIT campus, and settled in together. Eight months later, they were married in a quiet ceremony inside the nearly invisible MIT chapel, with virtually no one in attendance. It was a private moment.

A photo of Associate Professor Baltimore taken during his first few weeks back in Cambridge shows him awash in the trappings of the 1960s. He wears a cream pinstriped jacket over a striped shirt that bounces off a kaleidoscopic tie. A single fat pen hangs in the lapel pocket. His hairline has receded, and his straight brown hair is draped over his ears. His beard has evolved into a dark mustache and a thick, pointed goatee. His eyes are as bright and striking as ever, though shaded by his boxy, black-framed glasses, popular among the serious thinkers of the era. His belt is clasped by a silver buckle adorned with a Santa Fe roadrunner etching.

Luria welcomed his prodigal son back to MIT, this time as a professor instead of a student, with a laboratory near Luria's in Building 16. For Baltimore, those early months as a new professor were a time to settle in and think about what direction his scientific work would take. After all, his thirtieth birthday was two months away, and only a few years earlier at Swarthmore he had predicted that his most creative work would be finished by now. In the intervening years he had obviously decided not to accept this landmark as the intellectual catastrophe he once feared. Nevertheless, the question "Where to now?" pestered him, as it always would.

He loved working with poliovirus, but a single virus couldn't captivate him for long. He became anxious to diversify. As he looked for a new virus his thoughts wandered to VSV, an RNA virus related to rabies that causes a mouth-blistering disease in cattle. VSV was very different from poliovirus, and Baltimore expected it to present a whole new range of intellectual possibilities. "I thought it would be fun to work on something other than polio. . . . And I was very enamored with the vesicular stomatitis virus that [Alice] had worked with. So I said, why don't you teach me, and we'll have a joint program for a while, on your virus instead of my virus. . . . It grew very fast, so it was easy to do experiments; made high-titer [i.e., high-concentration] virus stocks; it was very stable; and it had some interesting properties." One of VSV's "interesting properties" would lead him to a problem important enough to win the Nobel Prize.

As Baltimore began to explore the biochemistry of VSV, the campus political environment intruded. Whereas Baltimore's antiwar activities at Salk had been distinctly separate from the institute, MIT was immersed in social unrest. The tension in America was almost unbearable. Martin Luther King Jr. was shot to death in Memphis in April 1968. Turmoil rocked universities across the country as student disillusionment and angst led to wild attempts to overhaul the educational institutions. Like many other MIT professors, Baltimore joined a slew of political groups that protested everything from biological warfare agents to CIA agents. He belonged to the MIT chapter of the Union of Concerned Scientists (UCS) and participated in the New University Conference Group (NUC), one of many loosely organized, radical political organizations on campus. NUC produced a fourteen-page manifesto on radical campus unrest:

> We support the new student movement, for we believe it is the main hope for creating a movement for social change in America and within the universities. The society in which the student movement is growing is in need of radical change; it is in this context that we must understand the controversies now raging about the American University.
>
> The student movement includes . . . the struggle by humanist and radical white youth to end the complicity of the university with war and imperialism, with racism and domestic suppression of black and other minorities, with bureaucratic values and corporate interests. . . .

We share with student activists the aim of constructing a grass-roots movement in this country that can have real effect in stopping American efforts to dominate other people, that can win a fundamental reordering of priorities in this country so that genuine equality can become a realistic hope, . . . [and] that can find new modes of political and social organization which will permit our vast resources to be shared for the benefit of all men and provide the basis for personal liberation.

Baltimore tried to focus his anger on the war: "Different people had different views of the protests of that time. Some people saw it narrowly in terms of the war, and other people tried to bring in a whole range of ancillary issues, everything from socialism to student rights to university reform. I think what was going on . . . was that the war had activated people to think more deeply about the world around them, and they tended to lump all of their thoughts and complaints together. It led to some fragmentation. I was much more of the opinion that the issue was the war, and that we shouldn't get sidetracked into worrying about the whole range of social issues that could be worried about, because I thought the war was tearing the country apart, and tearing apart the things I cared about."

Nevertheless, Baltimore got caught up in a variety of social issues as a member of the MIT NUC steering committee. Beyond administrative politicking, the committee tried to provide some focus for student anger, as well as simply trying, in Baltimore's words, "to help the students through difficult times, like when they got arrested." In November 1968 Baltimore led a discussion called "What Are We Doing to Them?" regarding "the relevance of radical ideas to teaching the scientist." The radical position on university education in the late sixties was stark:

We have hoped that the university could be a center of work toward [humanist] ends. That hope, however, seems increasingly illusory.

We have all come to realize that through the veil of "official neutrality" and protestations of innocence, the universities—including the "great centers of learning"—are partners with the most pernicious forces in our society.

Our experience at the university has taught us that higher education exists primarily to serve the white middle class. . . . The trend toward the fragmented and impersonal multiversity, existing on the largesse of the large corporations and the permanent war economy, is not merely a product of social complexity. . . .

We [are] forced to observe [that] liberal education has become a sham. College education has taken on the function of accrediting young men and women for personally stifling jobs which maintain the old order. . . . University attendance today is . . . a four-year socialization process which is intended to teach obedience and moderation, and a trained incapacity for creativity.

The NUC declared March 4, 1969, as Strike Day at MIT, protesting what they perceived as MIT's cooperation with the warmongers of the industrial-military complex. NUC managed to empty most of MIT's lecture halls and offices for the entire day, setting a precedent for March 4 protests at the university for years to come.

Baltimore's antiwar activities occupied a substantial amount of his energies without obviously slowing his scientific work. In February 1969, he won the Gustave Stern Award for Excellence in Virology. It was his first major award and cause for celebration in the lab, especially with Alice, who had collaborated on most of the later poliovirus work. Shortly thereafter, Baltimore became an editor of the prominent *Journal of Virology* and launched himself into the larger circles of virology.

Baltimore's first MIT graduate student, Martha Stampfer, arrived in the summer of 1969 and was enlisted to spearhead the VSV work. VSV turned out to be dramatically different from poliovirus. Poliovirus was a "positive strand" RNA virus: the information for protein synthesis could be read directly from the RNA strand contained within the infecting virus. The RNA strand within VSV could not be read directly by a cell it infected. No one knows why a virus would do this, but for some reason viruses like VSV and measles possess "negative strand" RNA, the non-protein-coding strand, encapsulated in their virus shell as their genetic material. The big question was, How does the VSV negative strand RNA start an infection inside a cell if its genetic information is all written ass-backward? Something had to happen to convert the VSV RNA into a readable form, the positive strand, so that VSV's viral proteins could be translated and initiate their predatory assault on the cell. From all of his work on poliovirus, Baltimore knew that there was no RNA-dependent RNA polymerase, an RNA replicase, in an uninfected cell, so he figured that VSV's negative strand RNA couldn't be read by any cellular enzyme. If that was the case, VSV must carry an RNA replicase inside the virus shell along with its negative strand RNA. When VSV infected a cell, the RNA replicase enzyme could then synthesize a positive strand of VSV RNA by reading and copying the negative strand. The infection could then proceed much like a poliovirus infection, with the RNA replicating over and over again as the viral proteins drove the cell to create thousands of viruses in a blitzkrieg of suicidal chemistry.

Baltimore figured out the basics of the VSV system—how to grow it, how long it took the virus to get through different stages of infection—and then peered inside for the polymerase: "No one imagined that this class of viruses had a polymerase in the virion, but I said maybe there is one." He knew how to test for polymerases; he'd done it more often than he'd done his own laundry. With some help from Martha Stampfer and Alice, he found the VSV replicase with little difficulty.

The discovery was unique, and Baltimore wanted to look for RNA replicases inside more viruses. The obvious candidates were other negative strand RNA viruses, including Newcastle disease virus and influenza virus. Newcastle disease virus caused a mumps-like disease in birds; scientists studied it because it was safer than mumps virus. Baltimore found Newcastle disease virus's RNA replicase present inside the virus virion (the virus shell), but he didn't find the influenza polymerase inside the influenza shell.

While working on this variety of RNA viruses, Baltimore's team obtained some sample RNA tumor viruses, cancer-causing viruses, from the National Institutes of Health (NIH) and tested them for RNA-dependent RNA polymerases. The results were negative. This was puzzling. If the tumor viruses didn't make RNA from the RNA, how did they survive? One possible explanation was that Baltimore was simply using the wrong experimental conditions, as he had with influenza virus. (The influenza polymerase was discovered the following year by another virologist, Robert Simpson.) An alternative explanation was that the tumor viruses didn't have RNA replicases but RNA-dependent DNA polymerases. Several published papers suggested the existence of a DNA "intermediate" in certain RNA virus infections. In fact, Howard Temin, Baltimore's friend from Jackson Lab, had become a pariah in virology because since 1964 he had been promoting the idea that RNA tumor viruses actually made DNA. Temin called it his provirus theory. Everyone else called it silly. Michael Bishop, a virologist at the University of California at San Francisco and winner of the 1989 Nobel Prize, described scientists' vehement opposition: "Howard Temin's idea of the provirus wasn't just heretical—it was pornographic!" Biologists ridiculed Temin and generally agreed that his experiments were playing tricks on him. But so far no one had managed to prove him wrong.

Didn't Temin have to be wrong? Couldn't DNA only come from DNA? This problem came up while Baltimore was teaching MIT's virology course that year, and he was forced to grapple with the paradox surrounding RNA tumor virus infections. Years later he reflected on that class: "Teaching is very important. It forces you to learn things in a way that you never learn them otherwise, because you've got to explain them to somebody. And you've got to be prepared to answer all these foolish questions students ask." He smiled and then continued, "It's a much more organized moment of learning than one ordinarily has. Because normally you can skip over things and not notice that there are big holes. When things are just breaking, they tend to be much more complicated than they later turn out to be. So, in order to teach it, I had to go through that—so it was in my mind. The teaching helped, and knowing the people, and knowing the literature, and all those things."

Temin might be wrong, but Baltimore knew he wasn't crazy. Temin had already revolutionized the study of RNA tumor viruses by developing a way to test their tumor-causing ability in cell culture; maybe his provirus theory would revolutionize the field again. Baltimore figured that testing Temin's provirus theory was worth a brief side trip. He switched tracks and tested RNA tumor viruses for a DNA polymerase.

The first virus he tested was Rauscher mouse leukemia virus. "It was a throwaway experiment," Baltimore felt. "If it hadn't worked, it would have cost me a day." After a few days, Baltimore turned up an RNA-dependent DNA polymerase. There it was: the first enzyme to reverse the Central Dogma. This enzyme took information in the opposite direction, from RNA to DNA.

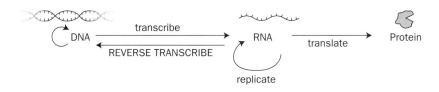

The discovery of reverse transcriptase redefined the Central Dogma. Baltimore and Temin proved that hereditary information could be transmitted in the opposite direction, from RNA to DNA.

The next day, April 30, 1970, the United States invaded Cambodia. Furious, Baltimore and much of the faculty protested; a nationwide university strike was declared. The Vietnam War, already a nightmare, was out of control. On May 4, 1,200 students and faculty members crammed into MIT's

Kresge Auditorium to discuss the strike. Two hundred latecomers sat outside on the lawn and listened to the discussion over loudspeakers. On that same day, National Guardsmen opened fire on one thousand college students protesting at Kent State University in Ohio, killing four of them. After several hours of commentary by MIT students and various professors, including Noam Chomsky, the famous MIT linguist and firebrand political analyst, the students decided to strike for a week. MIT's faculty held a meeting the following day to discuss their options, and they decided to cancel all lectures. Not only did they cancel classes, but Baltimore and numerous other researchers closed their labs for the week following the invasion. Meanwhile, Howard Temin was preparing for an important lecture in Houston.

Baltimore returned to his lab the following weekend, ready to continue his tests. He ran several experiments to characterize the RNA tumor virus's DNA polymerase more accurately. Next he looked for the enzyme in another related RNA tumor virus, Rous sarcoma virus (RSV), an RNA virus that caused monstrous tumors in chickens. He found a DNA polymerase there as well. He quickly wrote a paper and submitted it to *Nature.* Baltimore telephoned Temin at the University of Wisconsin in Madison to tell him the good news: "Howard, there's DNA polymerase in the virion of RNA tumor viruses!"

"I know, but where did you hear that?" Temin asked, puzzled.

"I didn't hear it, I did it," Baltimore replied, also puzzled.

"*You* did it? *We* did it!"

This was the first time their research had overlapped. Since the summer at Jackson Lab they had remained only distant friends. Both men worked on viruses, but Temin was mainly interested in the genetics of cancer viruses, while Baltimore was a biochemist and not interested in cancer. Now, in the first days of June 1970, they were suddenly faced with the fact that they had overturned the Central Dogma simultaneously. The issue was complex. Temin had actually discovered the polymerase before Baltimore, but priority of discovery in scientific research is given to whoever publishes their results first, and Temin had yet to write a paper. Temin had announced his discovery just a few days before, to little fanfare, at a conference in Houston. In fact, Temin thought Baltimore was referring to the talk in Houston when he called. They quickly sorted out the confusion and discussed the details of their independent experiments. Temin had done his work in Rous sarcoma virus; Baltimore had done most of his experiments with the Rauscher mouse cancer virus. By calling the editor of *Nature,* they quickly arranged for Temin to submit a paper two weeks later. *Nature* was so excited about the results that the papers were published back-to-back within a fortnight, in the June 27 issue.

Baltimore was neither downhearted nor upset about Temin's prior discovery. In an interview with *Newsweek* (published in an issue with a front cover portrait of Howard Temin at his lab bench), Baltimore said, "Howard's whole life has been devoted to the understanding of the replication of tumor viruses. I was very much a newcomer to the field." Temin had been attempting to prove the existence of DNA synthesis by RNA tumor viruses for seven years. Why hadn't he discovered the enzyme earlier? First, Temin was not a biochemist, and until a biochemist joined his lab he had made only indirect attempts to reveal the enzyme in action: even in hindsight, most virologists agreed that Temin's early data were fragmentary at best. Second, for years Temin didn't realize that the enzyme might be just sitting inside the virus shell. That realization changed the problem from looking for a needle in a haystack (if the enzyme was only expressed once the virus was inside a cell) to looking for a needle in a matchbox. That was the hint Baltimore got from VSV that allowed him to break open the RNA tumor virus problem in a month.

After the discovery, Baltimore focused the lab's efforts on this new enzyme, which came to be known as reverse transcriptase. He had found a biochemical gold mine. Its significance was grasped immediately by the biological community. This was the first example of an enzyme that reversed the direction of information flow dictated by the Central Dogma. In that respect, the discovery was cataclysmic—a paradigm shift. But the discovery of reverse transcriptase also impacted America's most dreaded disease, cancer.

Cancer was poorly understood in 1970, scientifically, medically, and by the general public. No disease was more feared, and only heart disease took more lives. Simply invoking the word "cancer" ignited memories of friends or relatives slowly devoured by a strange, invisible growth.

The general nature of cancer was known. Cancer was cellular mutiny. Somehow, cells in the body began to grow when they were not supposed to. The cells started multiplying, changing their shape, and changing their metabolism. No longer were they lung cells or colon cells; they were mutant cells, grotesque caricatures of the cells they came from. These mutant cells exploded in number, and as they grew they needed food. So the tumor's tentacles of cells grew toward arteries and pierced the walls of the blood supply. Now the cancer metastasized: the tumor cells entered the bloodstream and spread like hungry termites to colonize other organs.

Medical care saved fewer than one-third of cancer patients in the early

1970s; most cases were discovered too late, or there was simply nothing doctors could do. Medical options were few. A surgeon could cut the growth out with a scalpel and spoon, hoping to remove all of the cancerous cells. If even a few cancer cells were left, they spread like wildfire once the patient was sewn up and sent home. Moreover, surgery only worked while the cancer was a small, solid tumor, before it metastasized. Surgery was useless if the cancer was not localized, as in leukemias, which are diffuse cancers of the blood, or after any metastasis. Surgery could also be impossible because of the tumor's location. Most brain tumors, among others, were impossible to get at without killing the patient. In those cases, doctors resorted to massive assaults with radiation therapy and chemotherapy (cancer drugs) as the only hope.

The goal of these taxing therapies was (and is) to kill off all of the cancer cells without killing so many of the patient's functional cells that the patient died. Both approaches killed normal cells as well as cancerous cells. High-intensity radiation simply destroyed cells outright; its success depended upon the ability to focus the radiation beam precisely at the tumor, avoiding as much general cell damage as possible. Cancer drugs mangled DNA synthesis, causing the cells to die during replication because their genetic blueprints were torn to shreds; these therapies relied on killing the quickly replicating cancer cells in greater proportion than normal cells.

The media, and cancer researchers, were keen on the connection between the Temin-Baltimore discovery of reverse transcriptase and cancer. The big question was, Did RNA tumor viruses cause human cancer? A group of scientists had recently been championing the idea that viruses caused human cancer. They argued that there were known cancer viruses of chickens, mice, ducks, rabbits, and other animals, so surely there were viruses that caused cancer in people. Intoxicated by the idea that they could eliminate cancer, members of the National Cancer Institute convinced Congress in 1965 to start a Special Virus Cancer Program (SVCP). The program was showered with tens of millions of dollars a year. The National Cancer Institute built a massive, high-security laboratory to contain the deadly cancer viruses. They hired the organizers of the Apollo moon landing to orchestrate the program. As soon as someone discovered a virus that caused cancer, this special lab would grow huge quantities of the virus in massive cell culture vats. It could then be killed and injected into the American population as a vaccine to protect against cancer, in exactly the same way that the Salk vaccine for poliovirus was developed to protect people against polio. But first someone needed to find the human cancer viruses.

Baltimore and Temin's discovery of the heart of RNA tumor viruses gave the cancer virus crusaders a powerful new way to hunt for viruses in human cancer patients; they could search for reverse transcriptase activity. Testing for the activity of an enzyme was a much more sensitive way to test for the presence of cancer viruses that any previous diagnostic. Results began coming in even before Baltimore's and Temin's papers were published in *Nature*. Sol Spiegelman of Columbia University, a member of the SVCP, heard about Temin's report in Houston and began running tests of his own. In a few weeks, he had detected reverse transcriptase in eight different tumor viruses, and he failed to find reverse transcriptase in several nontumor viruses. Shortly after the Baltimore and Temin papers came out in *Nature,* another virologist, Bob Gallo, working at the National Cancer Institute of the NIH, found reverse transcriptase activity in three human patients with acute leukemia. He did not find reverse transcriptase activity in patients who were not affected by leukemia. These results led Gallo to theorize that the human leukemia was caused by an RNA tumor virus. Spiegelman then went further and tested for reverse transcriptase in 120 leukemia patients. He found that the enzyme activity was greatest when the disease was the most severe, and it disappeared when patients went into remission. It looked as though a viral infection caused the cancer. This was the breakthrough that cancer researchers had been hunting for, or so they thought.

Members of the NIH and the press hailed the "immense importance" of the discovery of reverse transcriptase, and they envisioned miracle drugs that would destroy reverse transcriptase, or vaccines that would render tumor viruses harmless and wipe out cancer "by the end of the century." Temin and Baltimore didn't believe that reverse transcriptase would lead to a magic bullet against cancer. They tried to explain that it was a great discovery, but it wasn't *that* great. No one had yet discovered any virus that definitely caused cancer in humans. In fact, Baltimore felt that the implications of reverse transcriptase's discovery were purely intellectual: "When I discovered the reverse transcriptase, there wasn't much more to be said. There it was, but that wasn't going to help cancer." He sympathized with medical research, but that wasn't his personal passion. He was a basic research scientist: "My life is dedicated to increasing knowledge. We need no more justification for scientific research than that. My motivating force is not that I will find a 'cure' for cancer. There may never be a cure as such. I work because I want to understand." In addition, the data he saw indicated that viruses weren't a widespread cause of cancer in people; if they were, obvious cancer epidemics would have broken out, and no one had ever seen that happen.

In January 1971, President Richard Nixon announced the start of the "War on Cancer" during his State of the Union address: "The time has come in America, when the same kind of concentrated effort that split the atom and took man to the moon should be turned toward conquering this dread disease." *Newsweek* wrote the following month: "Despite the picture of almost unrelieved gloom projected by the statistics, the war against cancer has entered a new and hopeful phase. There is no cure in sight. That must be said at once. But scientific discoveries in recent years, months, and even weeks have lifted the level of cancer research to a dramatic new plateau."

Baltimore opposed the War on Cancer, and he hated Nixon. He felt that the War on Cancer was politically motivated, and Baltimore didn't believe that a war on cancer could exist in the same way as the Moon mission or the Manhattan Project. Those concentrated efforts had a definite project, a perceivable goal, and tools to attack the problem. Cancer was a big unknown. The fumbling of the Special Virus Cancer Program showed Baltimore that a directed assault on cancer was just a money pit. Cancer was not the singular enemy that the public often considered it. It wasn't a single disease, like the flu or smallpox: it was a group of some two hundred diseases that all exhibited uncontrolled cell growth. It was well known that smoking, UV light from the sun, other radiation, and certain chemicals were all implicated in cancer.

No one knew what caused cancer on a cellular level, much less had any idea how to deal with it. They were making headway, this was true, but their scientific understanding was still in the very early stages. Baltimore commented at the time, "Although much progress has been made, especially during the last few years, we are still so far from the goals that we cannot measure the distance we have left to travel." He lobbied heavily against the War on Cancer. Other prominent biologists rallied behind the project as a unique opportunity and called Baltimore a fool for decrying this massive infusion of federal research funds. Baltimore retorted that the War on Cancer, and Congress's proposed Conquest of Cancer Act, misdirected research funding. He argued in a statement to Congress that it was impossible to attack cancer as a tangible target, because the answers to cancer's secrets would come from basic research. If you wanted to know about cancer, you needed to look everywhere.

> In this circumstance, to maintain progress we need a strong, broadly-based research effort, not a channeled, direct attack. Only when the problem is much better understood will a crash program

be justified. . . . The people who are going to make the breakthroughs, by analogy with history, are going to be young, well-trained scientists working in unpredictable areas. . . . For instance, my own work on a virus of cattle could not have been predicted as the source for a new idea on cancer. Neither was I working on it because of an interest in cancer.

Baltimore's analogy to his own VSV work was a persuasive argument, but it was difficult to turn the tide on such a popular measure. Baltimore wrote letters to the chair of the House committee and other representatives, hoping to convince them to quash the bill. He feared that the sudden popularity of cancer in political circles would lead to bureaucrats tampering with the NIH, allocating all of its funds to diseases of special interest to congressional representatives. And he was concerned about overoptimism. No cure was in sight, and neither was a fundamental understanding of the problem. He insisted that "cancer research is progressing slowly because the problems are difficult and research work is time-consuming, not because of a lack of desire to cure cancer." He feared that false hopes about a cancer vaccine or a cure for cancer would lead to a public backlash against basic research and biological science in general. Physicists had promised in the 1930s that their research would lead to great medical advances, but it didn't happen, and their reputation was tarnished by their overzealousness. Baltimore didn't want to feed the public false promises and unjustified hopes. But his opposition to the Conquest of Cancer Act was to no avail, and it passed into law.

With his opposition to the War on Cancer, Baltimore had consciously shifted his political efforts to his areas of expertise. He and Alice had tired of the ineffectual "intellectual commentary on politics" by radical academic groups and the antiwar movement. There he was just another face in the crowd. If he was going to make a difference, it would have to be in his own field, where he commanded respect and had the power to catalyze change and direct policies. He was determined not only to make basic discoveries that would shape the future of biology but also to define science policies that reflected his belief in the value of scientific knowledge. Involvement in politics was a way to expand his influence.

He believed in the social responsibility of science; and in those radical years of the late 1960s and early 1970s, he freely mixed his leftist political beliefs with his science. In 1971, he won the Eli Lilly Company Award in Microbiology and Immunology, a coveted award to the most promising microbiologist under thirty-five. It was his second major award as a biologist and one considered well-deserved by his peers. At the May national meeting of the American Society for Microbiologists, held that year in Minneapolis, he graciously accepted the honor but then launched into a philippic lambasting Eli Lilly for its "monopoly situations which allow it to set its own prices." He asserted that the drug industry had "taken advantage of its position to make exorbitant profits" from the people "least able to defend themselves—the sick and infirm." He announced that he would give the $1,000 award (then nearly a tenth of his yearly salary) to organizations that would fight the inhuman and unacceptable practices of the pharmaceutical industry, saying that he believed that drug companies sometimes sold "useless or dangerous mixtures of drugs." His homiletic speech made him the talk of the town. His anticapitalism comments were printed in newspapers around the country the following day, making him a topic of conversation for scientists everywhere: Did you hear what Baltimore did? Can you believe it?

It would be many years before he changed his political views. Baltimore took some time to reflect on his radical intellectual past during a 1995 interview:

> I must say that I was *extremely* naïve then. I was a constitutional leftist. I basically did not believe in the capitalist structure—and it was on social grounds. I had grown up in a moderately affluent family, but I saw around me, in America, as everybody does, terrible discrimination, terrible poverty, and I believed—I don't believe anymore [shaking his head with a slight chuckle]—that a more socialist form of government, a government that took an active interest in the needs of people, would help to alleviate the terrible poverty that we saw, and that we can still see around us even today. As modern biology developed and I realized that it was going to be corporations that made it happen, my first reaction was that there ought to be a government corporation that takes over this whole thing and makes it happen for the public, instead of for private gain. And, in an ideal world, I still think that would be wonderful, but no one has figured out how to actually do that. . . .
>
> So I really was anticapitalist, and was quite horrified that there were companies that were earning money from people who were sick—from people who had no choice. [Baltimore winced.] I still agree with that. I still believe that in some ideal world and ideal setting there should be a way to see that people get what they need, without being at the whim

of industrialists. I personally learned, by watching the development of the biotechnology industry and being involved in it, that it simply doesn't work any other way. . . .

Nothing taught me that. I grew up in a family where my father was a manufacturer. He, I suppose, could have taught me those things, but never did. Never once wanted to make it seem that his world was one that I should enter. [Baltimore paused for a long moment.] I'd love to be able to go back and talk to him about these things now. He died many years ago.

CENTER FOR CANCER RESEARCH

Cancer research was receiving amazing amounts of cash from federal and private sources during the 1970s, and molecular biologists were soon well supported. In addition, the 1970s were an extraordinary period for biology at MIT. Salvador Luria and Gobind Khorana had won back-to-back Nobel Prizes in 1968 and 1969. Shortly thereafter, a private benefactor awarded MIT a $1.75 million grant to build and support a new Center for Cancer Research (CCR), to be headed by Salvador Luria. That gift, in combination with major grants from the National Cancer Institute and other sources, provided the future CCR with over $5 million in support. In 1973, Baltimore was awarded an American Cancer Society professorship of microbiology, a major personal windfall worth over $1 million in salary spread over the next thirty years, as long as he stayed in cancer research. The public had enlisted him in the War on Cancer.

Baltimore was rapidly changing his views on the undertaking. Twenty years later, he reflected on the enterprise: "First of all, it worked out much better than I thought it would, because enough of the money went to basic research that, in fact, the War on Cancer fueled the incredible discoveries that we've had about oncogenes and all of the various aspects of cancer we now know about." The excitement of Spiegelman, Gallo, and others about human cancer viruses turned out to be misplaced, as Baltimore and Temin had predicted: their original results were artifacts, the product of imprecise experiments. But Baltimore had been wrong about the Conquest of Cancer Act: "It was not an efficient program, in the sense that there was a whole lot of money that went into things that were not terribly useful, but the positive side of it is very strong. I give credit to the people who were behind the War on Cancer. I, to some extent, underestimated their ability to see that the money went to new initiatives instead of the same old stuff." In the end, the extra funding helped him, and it helped biology. Unfortunately, he had made a number of enemies because of his vociferous opposition.

Baltimore had been wrong, but he was a fighter, in both science and politics. He did not hesitate to get in a fight: "I know what I believe, and I stick by what I believe, and I'll defend what I believe. I understand that I could be wrong about things, but that's what I'm going to stay with." It was not surprising that the words "stubbornness" and "arrogance" always came up when colleagues were asked about Baltimore.

After a few construction delays, the new CCR was completed in December 1973, and David Baltimore moved in. The building, a large, six-story brick block, was situated only a hundred yards from the biology department's Building 56 and Building 16. By the time of Baltimore's move to the CCR, two and a half years after the first reverse transcriptase paper, his name was on forty-seven additional publications. And molecular biology was about to get a lot more interesting, thanks to some experiments in California.

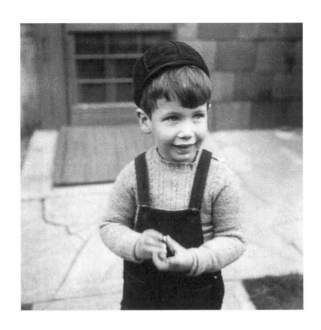

David in New York, circa 1943. (Courtesy Alice Huang)

The Baltimore family at Pompano Beach, Florida, 1948. (Courtesy Katalin R. Baltimore)

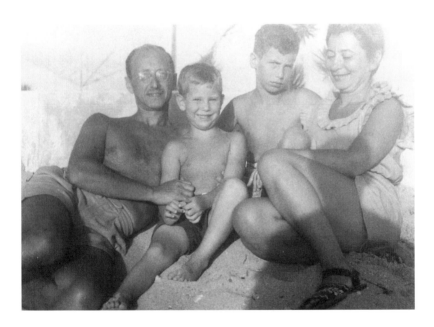

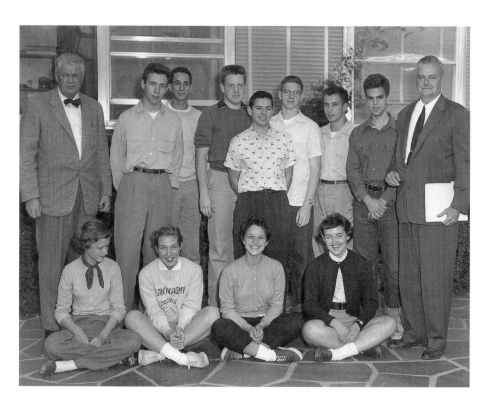

Several of the 1955 Jackson Lab summer program students. David is standing third from the right. C. C. Little, who ran the laboratory, is standing on the far right. (Courtesy Jackson Laboratory)

Howard Temin injecting a mouse at Jackson Lab, July 1955. (Courtesy Alice Huang)

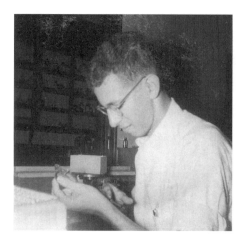

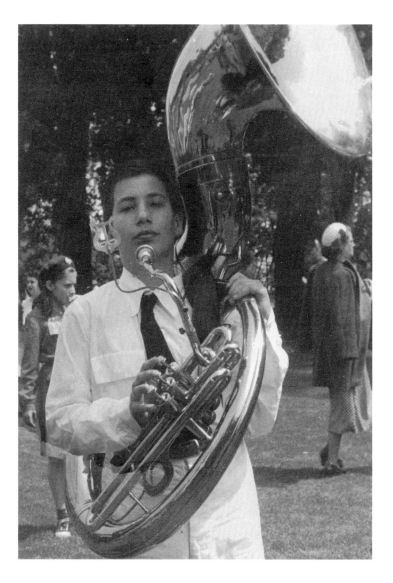

David Baltimore, half of the Great Neck Marching Band tuba section, circa 1954. (Courtesy David Baltimore)

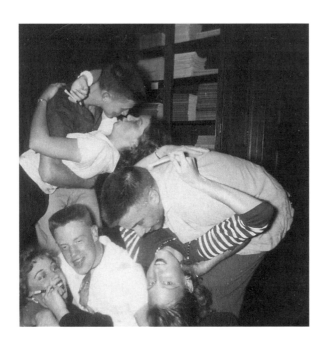

David and friends at Swarthmore, circa 1957. (Courtesy David Baltimore)

David with Swarthmore girlfriend Kay Senegas, behind his parents' house in Great Neck, January 1957. (Courtesy David Baltimore)

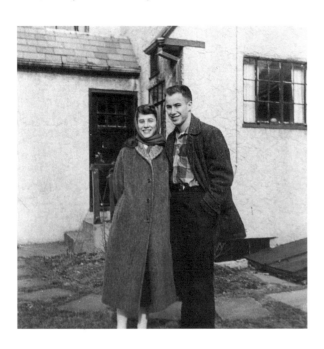

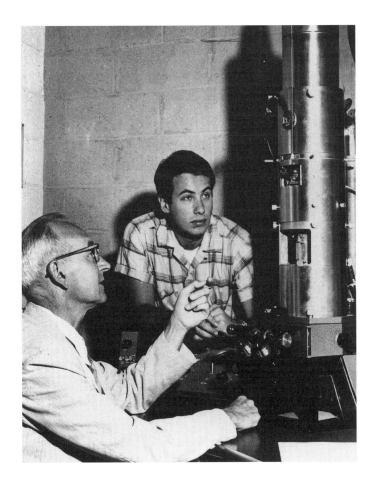

David with Berwind Kaufmann at the Cold Spring Harbor electron microscope, summer 1959. (Courtesy Cold Spring Harbor Laboratory)

Electron micrograph image of poliovirus particles. (Courtesy Raul Andino)

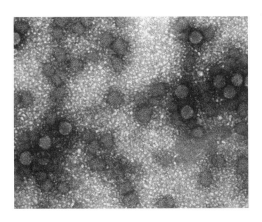

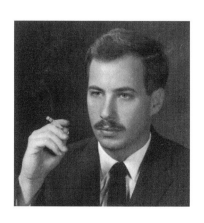

David Baltimore, Rockefeller Institute graduate school portrait, 1962. (Courtesy Alice Huang)

David Baltimore and Alice Huang outside her parents' house in Pennsylvania, circa 1969. (Courtesy Alice Huang)

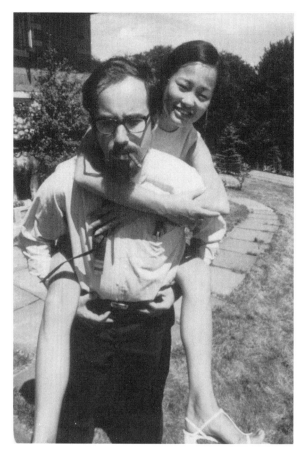

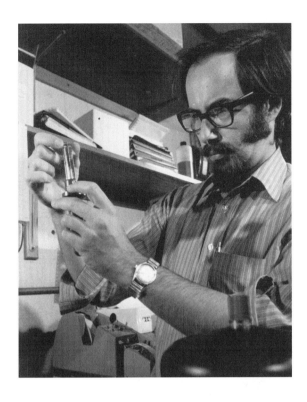

David Baltimore in his laboratory at MIT, 1971. (Courtesy Alice Huang)

Howard Temin at work in lab, 1987. (Photo by Michael Kienitz, courtesy University of Wisconsin—Madison)

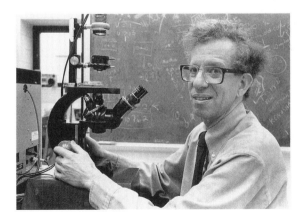

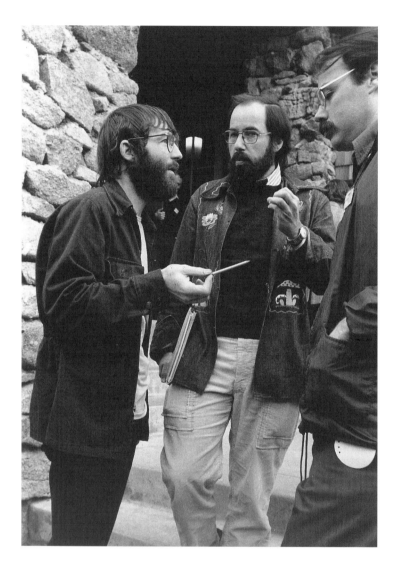

David Baltimore (center) at the 1975 Asilomar meeting, talking with molecular biologist Joe Sambrook (left) and another scientist. (Courtesy National Academy of Sciences)

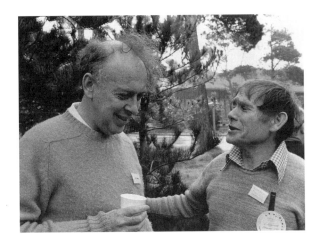

James Watson (left) and Sydney Brenner at the 1975 Asilomar meeting. (Courtesy National Academy of Sciences)

Four of the Asilomar organizing committee members at work in Sand and Surf: Maxine Singer, Norton Zinder, Sydney Brenner, and Paul Berg. (Courtesy National Academy of Sciences)

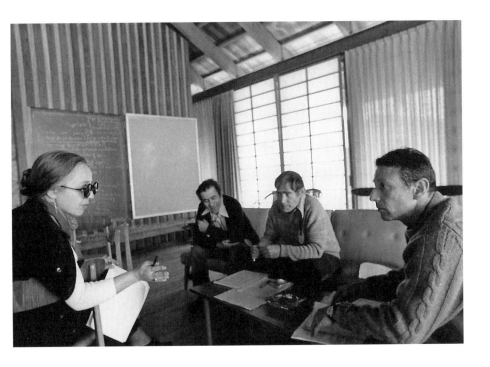

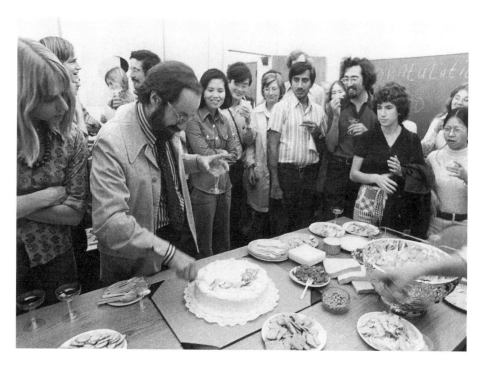

Celebration of the Nobel Prize announcement at MIT, 1975. (Photo by Calvin Campbell/MIT)

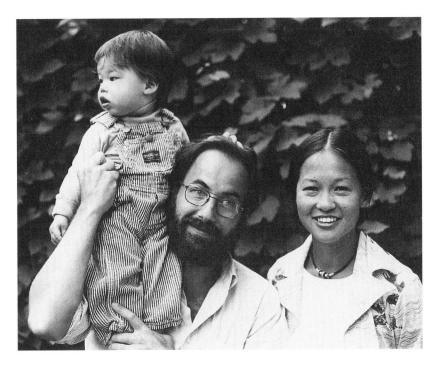

David, Alice, and Teak in Richard Franklin's backyard, Basel, Switzerland, 1975. (Photo © Richard M. Franklin)

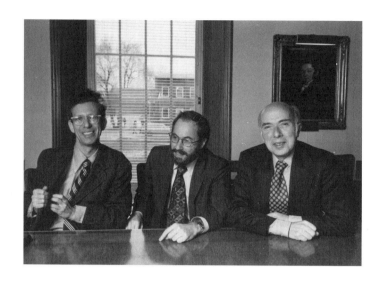

Howard Temin, David Baltimore, and Renato Dulbecco in Sweden for the Nobel Prize ceremony. (Courtesy Svenskt Pressfoto)

David and Alice dancing at the Nobel banquet. (Photo by Ronny Karlsson, Å&Å/Kamerabild)

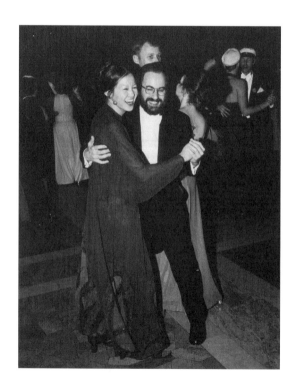

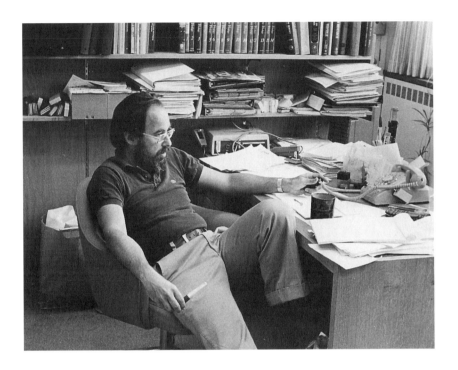

Baltimore in his office, circa 1980. (Photo by Calvin Campbell/MIT)

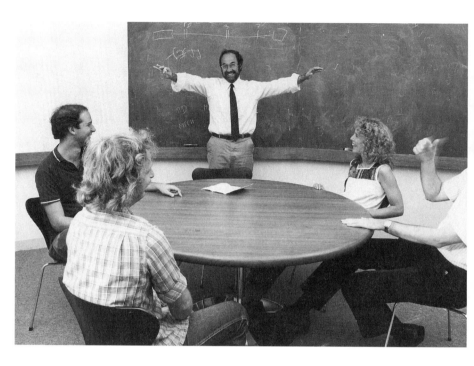

Baltimore with lab members, from left to right: Ronald Prywes, Peter Sarnow, Karla Kirkegaard. (Photo by Calvin Campbell/MIT)

Thereza Imanishi-Kari and David Baltimore. (Photo by BettyAnn Holtzmann Kevles)

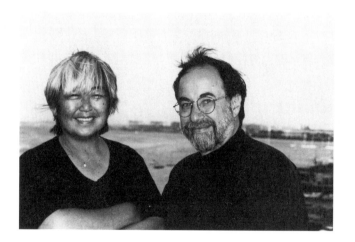

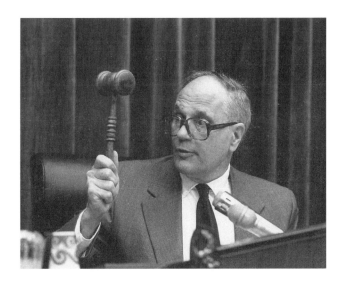

Representative John Dingell of Michigan. (Courtesy AP/Wide World Photos)

Margot O'Toole, Walter Stewart, and Ned Feder at the Dingell subcommittee congressional hearing, April 12, 1988. (Courtesy AP/ Wide World Photos)

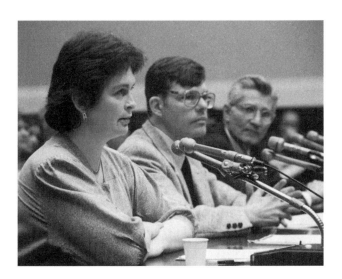

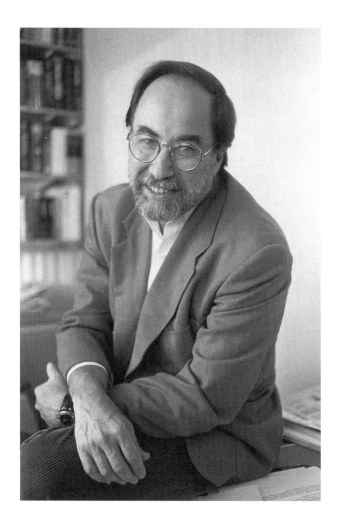

David Baltimore at MIT, 1994.
(Photo by Donna Coveney/MIT)

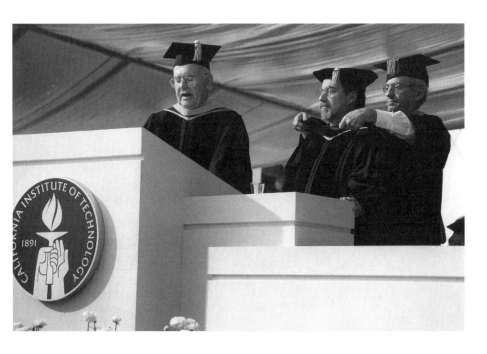

Baltimore's inauguration as president of Caltech, 1997. (Courtesy Caltech)

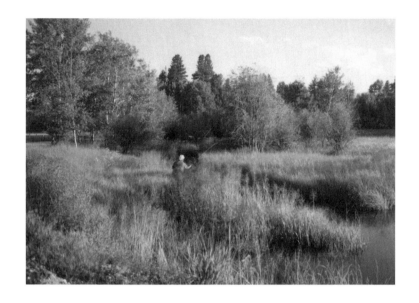

Baltimore fishing. (Courtesy Alice Huang)

Six

RECOMBINANT DNA

I wasn't surprised about much of anything until 1966.
But after that, well, the last ten years have surprised us enormously.
We had no idea. No idea.

FRANCIS CRICK
1983, quoted in Laurie Garrett, The Coming Plague

JANUARY 1971. THE MAIN building of the Stanford University School of Medicine was the ugliest building on campus. The beautiful central quad was a spacious collection of buildings laid out like a vast Spanish villa, all coordinated with terracotta roofs, fine murals, intricate stone carvings, and covered walkways around sun-drenched courtyards. But the medical school, on the western edge of the campus, consisted of a hundred-yard-long, monolithic edifice apparently designed in a bizarre fit of Egyptomania. Constructed of huge concrete tiles with a squared-spiral pattern on them, the outer walls looked more like freeway soundproofing than anything else. Cramped and oversized iron platter chandeliers hung theatrically along the outside perimeter from thirty-foot chains. Luckily, biologists aren't picky about architecture, and the members of the Stanford biochemistry department worked busily inside. Paul Berg was there, and he was planning an experiment that embodied the most revolutionary idea in experimental biology in twenty years.

Berg was forty-five years old and full of vigor. He was a pleasant man with a fatherly manner and sun-worn skin. He still had his naval officer's haircut from World War II. By 1965, he had won the California Scientist of the Year Award, and he still managed to put enough time into his teaching to win Stanford's teaching award twice. Originally, after graduate school and his early successes in the lab of Arthur Kornberg (who won the

1959 Nobel Prize in medicine for the discovery of DNA polymerase and the in vitro synthesis of DNA in a test tube), Berg went on to develop in vitro systems for synthesizing RNA and proteins. In 1967, he decided that he wanted to study animal cell biology by means of tumor viruses, so he took a sabbatical and studied with Renato Dulbecco at the Salk, who was then specializing in tumor viruses.

When Berg returned to Stanford, he began work on SV40, a DNA tumor virus. SV40 was originally isolated from monkeys (SV stands for simian virus), where it lived a peaceful existence; but it caused cancer in mice and in human cells grown in laboratory flasks.* It seemed to have no obvious effects on humans. Berg was initially concerned that if SV40 could cause cancer in laboratory cells, exposure to it would give him cancer; but researchers at the Salk calmed his fears, and Dulbecco swore that SV40 was so harmless he would drink it. Nevertheless, no one could be certain that SV40 would not cause cancer twenty years later. The dishwashers, technicians, and the members of neighboring laboratories at Stanford were all scared of SV40. Contagious cancer was a terrifying prospect, and no one wanted to be part of an inadvertent experiment with a lethal virus. Berg took everyone's fears in stride and built a high-security lab, separate from the main building, complete with sterile laminar-flow hoods and a high-tech air filtration system. The rooms were under negative pressure so that air always flowed into the laboratory rather than out, keeping SV40 from floating out the doors. It was the safest lab Berg could build; and the precautions were virtually worthless. As time went on, Berg had blood tests taken of everyone in the lab. Everyone had been infected with SV40. No one showed any ill effects. They simply hoped SV40 was as harmless as they had claimed.

In search of the SV40 gene that caused cancer in mice, Berg was planning a gene transplantation experiment. He wanted to make a piece of DNA that was part bacterial genes, part bacteriophage genes, and part SV40 genes, and put it into bacteria and animal cells. Animal cells are amazingly complex and difficult to understand; they contain tens of thousands of genes interacting in a complicated fashion. Berg saw that he might be able to take animal virus genes and move them into *E. coli* bacteria, which was an easy system to work in. Berg could study the effects of his single experimental gene. If it worked with an SV40 virus gene, he might be able to use the

---

*When normal cells start growing like cancerous cells in laboratory flasks, as when cells are infected with SV40, biologists call the process "transformation."

technique on actual animal cell genes. It could revolutionize the study of the inner workings of animal cells.

Berg's major leap was to think of the power of moving and studying single genes, combining different pieces of DNA to form recombinant DNA, a process now known as genetic engineering.

First he needed to develop an experimental system that could actually move genes. In 1960, recombinant DNA wasn't thought about and wasn't possible. By 1970, the technology to accomplish it was rapidly accumulating. The development of recombinant DNA would come in four stages: the Hamilton Smith stage, the Berg stage, the Baltimore stage, and the Stanley Cohen and Herbert Boyer stage. Smith, Berg, and Baltimore would win Nobel Prizes; and Boyer would make hundreds of millions of dollars using recombinant DNA technology.

For Berg, making recombinant DNA depended on several technical skills. He needed to cut out a specific gene from a large piece of DNA, isolate the DNA containing the gene, and then paste it into another piece of DNA. In 1969, Hamilton Smith discovered restriction enzymes, molecular "scissors" that cut DNA only at specific points. Previously, the only enzymes known to cut DNA, DNases, did so nonspecifically, chopping up DNA molecules like a child with scissors hacking randomly at a book. Restriction enzymes cut only at specific DNA sequences, as though cutting out specific pages of a book. Smith's discovery was a classic example of chance favoring the prepared mind. During an experiment he noticed that, over time, his experimental DNA prep was chopped into small pieces. Instead of simply throwing out the experiment and trying it again with a fresh preparation, as other scientists had done, he asked, "Why does the DNA only partially degrade?" It was the right question. The answer was that the preparation was cut up not by DNase but by another enzyme, one that cut DNA only at specific sites.

After Smith announced his discovery of a restriction enzyme in *Hemophilus influenzae,* Herbert Boyer, at the University of California at San Francisco (UCSF), realized that other species of bacteria would also have restriction enzymes, and he rapidly proceeded to isolate a restriction enzyme in *E. coli,* which he named EcoRI (shorthand for *E. coli* restriction enzyme number 1). Paul Berg, who knew Herbert Boyer and so had access to the precious enzyme, could use it to cut out a gene from a large piece of DNA, and he could precisely isolate that piece of DNA.

The ability to isolate DNA fragments had existed for several years. Imagine a slab of gray Jell-O (a gel) with electrodes placed at each end. Different-sized pieces of DNA, which carry a small electrical charge, travel at different speeds through an electrified gel. Scientists could separate different sizes of DNA by running them through the gel and then scooping out the DNA of the size they were looking for. The third requirement for making recombinant DNA, the ability to join the gene DNA with another DNA piece, was technically possible for Berg, but only barely. The two molecules had to have special matching overlapped ends, or they would not stick together. And they would hold together only at low temperatures.

Berg had several graduate students working on the project in 1971. The procedure was complicated, but they succeeded in making a recombinant DNA molecule that was composed of several *E. coli* genes, a few bacteriophage genes, and the SV40 genes. One of the students, Janet Mertz, was optimizing the technique for transplanting the recombinant DNA into *E. coli*. She was making good progress and went to the Cold Spring Harbor Tumor Virus Workshop during the summer to learn more about experimenting with SV40. The workshop instructor was Robert (Bob) Pollack, a young tumor virologist who spent a lot of time at Cold Spring Harbor (his wife had nicknamed CSH "Camp Cancer"). In a discussion group at the workshop, Mertz explained the Berg Lab SV40 gene transplantation project. Visions of recombinant DNA research were quickly becoming reality, and the nature of the experiment presented grave safety concerns to Pollack. *E. coli* is a bacterium that lives a prolific but harmless existence in the human colon. SV40 is a virus that is harmless to monkeys, but it causes cancer in mice and hamsters and is also cancerous in human cells grown in culture. Berg wanted to mix the two. The SV40 cancer gene had never evolved in *E. coli,* and it might confer its cancer-causing ability to *E. coli.* What would happen if the new *E. coli* that Berg created was tumorigenic? Laboratory *E. coli* frequently infected researchers, but it never mattered because *E. coli* is harmless. If this new *E. coli* induced cancer, it could escape from the lab through the guts of the researchers and spread through the human population. Because cancers often take years to develop, a carcinogenic *E. coli* strain could cause cancers of epidemic proportion before being detected. Other members of the workshop shared Pollack's fear.

By the end of the discussion, Mertz was convinced of the potential hazard of the SV40 experiment, and she called Berg to discuss it. He dismissed her concerns. Pollack called Berg later in the week and explained the potential dangers he saw. Pollack's intrusion annoyed Berg, who discounted Pollack's objections. When Pollack suggested that Berg cancel the experiment, Berg was infuriated. The notion that his gene transplantation experiment was potentially catastrophic surprised him. He was used to hearing concerns from concerned colleagues in other fields about his experiments on tumor viruses, but Pollack himself was a tumor virologist. Pollack later recalled, "He was absolutely dumbfounded, as far as I could see. I must have sounded like somebody coming and saying, 'God will punish you.'"

Much as Berg wanted to simply dismiss Pollack's concerns, he couldn't. Berg was neither hot-blooded nor a fool, and he knew that his experiment needed to be safe. During the next couple of months, he talked to friends inside and outside the field of tumor virology, asking what they thought of the possible hazards. Summarizing the mood of many scientists, one colleague said, "The Berg experiment scares the pants off a lot of people." Berg discussed the problem with Joshua Lederberg and Bob Pollack, and then he talked with David Baltimore.

Berg and Baltimore met up at Cold Spring Harbor and talked about the recombinant SV40 project over a pepperoni pizza and a couple of beers. They spent the entire evening discussing the turmoil Berg's idea had generated. Berg realized the validity of people's worries, but he still wanted to try the experiment because he was convinced of the usefulness of recombinant DNA. Baltimore advised him to put off the experiment; too little was known about the consequences. Berg still wasn't convinced. Who knew anything about biohazards? Baltimore agreed that biohazard questions needed to be addressed by the scientific community.

Berg was not the only researcher to have people complain about the safety of his work. Baltimore had similar problems: "This specific issue of biohazards became a concern to me because I was a newcomer to a field which presented the greatest potential hazards at that time, which was tumor viruses." Berg, Baltimore, and other animal virologists were forced to reply to the concerns with arguments they could not substantiate. There simply wasn't enough information about biohazards.

Berg was changing his mind about the experiment: "The more and more I talked to people, and the more and more I thought about it myself, I realized that while I could argue that the probability was low, I could never say that the probability was zero. And it was certainly finite. And then . . . I must have realized that I'd been wrong many, many times before in predicting the outcome of an experiment, and that if I was wrong about my assessment of the [SV40] risk, then the consequences were not something that I would want to live with."

Berg and Baltimore decided they would hold a conference on biohazards in which they would attempt to determine the true dangers of Berg's experiment and other recombinant DNA experiments. Though Berg's SV40 recombinant DNA molecule was ready to be put into *E. coli,* with perhaps extraordinarily valuable results, he decided to postpone the experiment until after the biohazards conference, which was almost two years away.

CDNA

A photo taken of Baltimore in the early 1970s by an MIT undergraduate photographer for the student newspaper, the *Tech,* shows him in his office chair, wearing a suit, and relaxing in a comfortable slouch. He is smoking a pipe and staring at a point somewhere far beyond the sunlit window. He received tenure in 1972 as a full MIT professor of biology at the young age of thirty-four. Life was good; every Saturday he and his lab would play volleyball and then go out for Chinese pastries. He threw parties at his house and went hiking with lab friends in the New Hampshire mountains.

All of Baltimore's pretenure research had worked to destroy the idea that animal viruses were the boring cousins of bacteriophage, an idea he helped replace with the much more elaborate truth. Animal viruses were extraordinarily diverse, from poliovirus, an RNA virus that synthesizes a polyprotein, to VSV, a negative strand RNA virus that held an RNA polymerase inside the virion, to Rauscher mouse leukemia virus, a retrovirus (as RNA tumor viruses became known after Baltimore and Temin discovered reverse transcriptase) that turned the Central Dogma on its head. RNA tumor viruses were a new challenge for Baltimore, and therefore all the more intriguing. When was the RNA reverse-transcribed into DNA? When and how did viral protein synthesis take place? Could reverse transcriptase convert only virus RNA into DNA, or did it work on normal animal RNAs as well? This last question was answered in 1972 by Baltimore's postdoctoral fellow Inder Verma. He reverse-transcribed rabbit hemoglobin RNA (the messenger RNA that codes for the oxygen-carrying blood protein hemoglobin) into DNA. DNA that had RNA as its origin became known as cDNA.

When Phillip Sharp and Richard Roberts discovered introns and the complexity of animal genes in 1977 (work that won them a Nobel Prize), Verma and Baltimore's cDNA work would provide a way to deal with that complexity, a crucial step for the broad application of genetic engineering. cDNA copies of genes have been the source of virtually all the mouse and human genes that have been discovered and studied by biologists.* This is because most human genes (and animal, plant, and fungal genes, but not bacterial genes) have a series of large gaps in them, called introns. Biologists tend to call introns "junk DNA" because they have no known function.** This junk DNA makes it difficult to figure out where genes begin and end and to identify the "coding sequence" (the sequence that actually codes for the protein) that scientists care about. Using cDNA solves this problem, because when a gene is transcribed from DNA into RNA, the junk sequence is cut away by the cell, leaving "messenger RNA" that is easy to analyze because it mainly contains the RNA coding sequence of the protein of interest. This messenger RNA is normally what molecular biologists convert into cDNA and then use in recombinant DNA studies.

BIOHAZARDS

In the summer of 1972, Paul Berg flew to Sicily for a NATO conference, teaching young European scientists current molecular biology philosophy and techniques in a resort hotel near the Mediterranean. There he introduced his SV40 gene transplantation project as a model of future molecular biology research. The students were amazed, shocked, and concerned. Berg was opening up a new era of biology, and they immediately saw the dangerous possibilities of genetic engineering: human modifications, behavioral control, eugenics, biological warfare. Berg was unprepared for the social, political, and ethical problems the students threw at him. They pressed him to hold a session later to discuss the ramifications of recombinant DNA. Surprised but willing, Berg agreed.

The session was organized as an informal evening meeting on the ramparts of a castle above the city of Erice, overlooking the dark Straits of Sicily. Pearls of lights were strung along the streets below. Lit by the cool glow of a full moon, Berg and the group of eighty Europeans sat around in the warm night drinking beers and pondering genetic engineering: Should we do it or not? Berg wasn't so interested in the ethical issues; he was fixated on health hazards. Everything else could be sorted out by society when the time came; the immediate question was that of safety. But he was unable to pull the students away from their uneasy ethics questions. The possibilities were fas-

*cDNAs have also been used to discover new viruses, such as hepatitis C.
**That doesn't mean introns are useless. As Sydney Brenner has observed, "Introns are junk DNA, not garbage DNA; garbage you throw out, junk you keep."

cinating and disturbing. What if we could cure genetic diseases? What about creating entirely new species of microorganisms, ones that could kill ten thousand people a day and others that could make better beer? What if we could program people's eye color? Intelligence? Height? Giant corn plants? Fruit that didn't freeze? Blue roses? Prettier women?

Francis Crick was there, sitting to one side, silently drinking his beer. When the debate broke up around midnight and the excited but tired mob walked back into the city, Berg asked Crick his opinion of recombinant DNA. Crick said very little. Berg later recalled, "It just seemed like an issue that he didn't want to have to worry or think about." Or perhaps he was reticent to talk about an issue with which he felt such a tight kinship but which disturbed him profoundly.

In the autumn of 1972, a year after Berg and Baltimore had discussed biohazards over pizza at Cold Spring Harbor, Berg called Baltimore and several other colleagues and asked them to help organize the biohazards conference. To be held in January 1973 at Asilomar, California, it would be the first conference on biohazards. It would look at the available information on biohazards and try to assess the risks. Berg and Baltimore obtained funding for the conference through the National Science Foundation (NSF) by asking their friend Hermann Lewis, an NSF administrator who was a former professor at MIT (and on whom they would call again for help later). They planned to use the conference to list known and potential biohazards and summarize the scientific understanding of those dangers, and then they would hold a larger conference with the broader biological community. It didn't work out that way. "We considered there would be a second meeting," Baltimore recalled, "and the second meeting would be, 'Given this baseline of data, what do you do?' But we never got to that meeting, because we just couldn't figure out what could happen at it. The baseline of data was so slim that we knew it would be a meeting in a vacuum."

Even in the absence of data, the conference generated epic arguments about biohazards. Some people who worked with highly infectious and pathogenic organisms had to defend their safety practices. There were arguments about a recently discovered hybrid virus found in several labs, part adenovirus (a cause of the common cold) and part SV40. Could this hybrid virus give you cancer when you caught a cold? There were heated discussions about the safety of SV40, often focusing on the people who had inadvertently been infected with SV40 by contaminated batches of polio vaccine made before 1962. None of those people had developed cancer yet, but might they in ten years? Should laboratory workers be more wary of the long-term effects of SV40? There was only one documented case of a laboratory accident leading to a cancer fatality, and that was a French medical student in 1926 who pricked his hand with a needle that contained fluid from a cancer patient. A tumor grew on his palm, and he died months later when the tumor spread.

Dulbecco was willing to drink SV40, but others weren't so cavalier. George Todaro at the National Cancer Institute declared, "I have no doubt that if you gave enough of some of these agents to a susceptible person, he would get a tumor." At the same time, Todaro said, "It's entirely a guess as to risk, but my guess is that it is considerably less dangerous than smoking two packs of cigarettes a day." Another researcher said, "We're in a pre-Hiroshima situation." Berg considered the SV40 question to be virtually moot, because even in his highly sterile laboratory everyone had been infected with SV40 despite his precautions. But another researcher argued that 90 percent of safety comes from good technique, not safety equipment.*

They also argued about the significance of the recent Marburg incident. In 1967, twenty-three German employees at a vaccine company, and six more who worked in the government's Paul Ehrlich Institute, became sick with an unknown illness. They developed fevers and fiery rashes and began vomiting blood. After three weeks in quarantine, their skin peeled off with agonizing pain and, as the doctors in charge wrote, "Blood is pouring from all apertures." Seven of them died. All had caught a virus from a shipment of monkeys. Years later, the virus would be named Ebola. Could similar viruses be hiding in the monkey cells that researchers used? It was doubtful, but no one could measure the risk.

Someone from Harvard announced that they were planning on growing lymphocytes (white blood cells) that produced Epstein-Barr virus, which causes mononucleosis (mono). Jim Watson stood up, raised a lanky arm, and said that he would sue the researcher if he even tried to do that experiment.

The conference did generate the book *Biohazards in Biological Research,* but Paul Berg later summed up the feeling of everyone who attended: "What came out of it, frankly, was a recognition of how little we know." They did not know how dangerous many of their experiments might be in the long term; they knew only that nothing disastrous had happened yet. Perversely, perhaps the most comforting announcement at the meeting was from scientists from Fort Detrick, the secret Army germ warfare base, who announced

*Twenty-five years later, the safety of SV40 is still debated. Epidemiological studies indicate that SV40-infected people are not at higher risk for cancer.

that they had tried to create new monster microbes (manipulating strains of anthrax, encephalitis virus, and other microscopic predators) and failed.* Nature might be more difficult to subvert than they had thought. But this was all before recombinant DNA technology.

Berg had been in communication with Herbert Boyer since beginning his recombinant DNA work, and Stanley Cohen found out about the SV40 recombinant DNA project through both Berg and Boyer. Cohen worked near Berg at Stanford. Cohen's specialty was plasmids, small circular pieces of DNA in bacteria that carried a fascinating assortment of "extra" genes, genes that weren't often used but were essential every once in a while. For example, many bacterial genes on plasmids convey resistance to antibiotics.

In 1973, the enzyme DNA ligase was purified, a useful tool that hadn't been available to Berg two years earlier. It provided an excellent means of joining DNA fragments. With Boyer's EcoRI restriction enzyme expertise and Cohen's expertise with plasmids, in spring 1973 they designed the world's first full recombinant DNA experiment. They had isolated two different plasmids, each of which contained an antibiotic resistance gene. The first plasmid contained the gene for resistance to ampicillin. When grown on petri plates coated with ampicillin, E. coli containing this plasmid will flourish, and all other E. coli will die. The second plasmid contained the gene for resistance to tetracycline, which has the effect of allowing bacteria to grow on tetracycline-coated plates. Cohen and Boyer cut both plasmids once with the restriction enzyme, mixed the two plasmids together, used the DNA ligase enzyme to connect them into one plasmid, and inserted the composite plasmid into E. coli. The results: the E. coli grew on petri plates coated with both ampicillin and tetracycline, showing that the bacteria contained Cohen and Boyer's genetically engineered plasmid. Recombinant DNA technology was now a reality. The technique was so straightforward that in ten years undergraduates and even high school students would be repeating Cohen and Boyer's experiment.

When Boyer announced their results at the 1973 Gordon Conference on nucleic acids, the news hit like a tidal wave. The future was here. The power

*Fort Detrick's biological warfare program was closed in 1969 after the signing of the Biological and Toxin Weapons Convention treaty between the United States and the Soviet Union. The Russians ignored the treaty and developed biological warfare agents through the 1990s.

of recombinant DNA was both exhilarating and disturbing. Some of the Gordon Conference participants had heard of Berg's early recombinant DNA plans, but most thought that recombinant DNA was a pipe dream. Now some were scared. Couldn't this new technology be dangerous? Couldn't those *E. coli,* which might be thriving right then in the gut of Herbert Boyer, transfer their newfound antibiotic resistance to less pleasant bacteria, perhaps pneumonia bacteria, that could then become resistant to medical treatment? Ethical problems were raised, as they had been in Sicily the year before. Maxine Singer and Dieter Söll, the conference cochairs, decided that the safety of genetic engineering demanded attention, even though such concerns were clearly not the purpose of the Gordon Conference. On the last day of the meeting, in a short improvised session, the researchers voted to send a letter to the National Academy of Sciences asking for an investigation of the implications of recombinant DNA. In an unusual move, they decided to publish the letter in *Science,* making their concerns public. The letter, which was published three months later, came to be known as the Singer-Söll letter. It began: "We are writing to you, on behalf of a number of scientists, to communicate a matter of deep concern." Though the Singer-Söll letter did not attract much media attention when it was published in September, it announced the worries of the scientific community, and the American public, journalists, and even Congress gradually began to watch the recombinant DNA debates much more closely.

Immediately after the publication of the Singer-Söll letter, the NAS called Paul Berg and asked him for his opinion on the safety of recombinant DNA research. He refused to make a statement off the top of his head; but, with reluctance, he agreed to organize a committee to review the issue. He recruited seven prominent molecular biologists, including David Baltimore, to meet at MIT in six months' time.

In the meantime, Boyer and Cohen expanded their initial genetic engineering results. By late fall, Cohen and his student Annie Chang had taken genes from *Staphylococcus aureus* (a mildly infectious bacterium causing boils or blood poisoning) that gave resistance to penicillin, erythromycin, cadmium, and mercury and put them on a plasmid in *E. coli.* The Staph genes were expressed in *E. coli,* they conferred their drug and heavy metal resistances, and the antibiotic genes were inherited by the *E. coli* progeny. Cohen and Chang had transferred functional genes across species. They wrote that their results "now suggest that interspecies genetic recombination may be generally attainable. Thus, it may be practical to introduce into *E. coli* genes specifying metabolic or synthetic functions (e.g., photosynthesis, antibiotic production) indigenous to other biological classes [such as plants and animals]."

Cohen and Boyer had managed to change the genetic makeup of a bacterium by adding new genes from another species. They had an even bigger experiment planned. With postdoc John Morrow doing the brunt of the work, Cohen and Boyer tried to express a frog gene in *E. coli*. By New Year's Day 1974, they had succeeded. The frog gene was stably inherited by subsequent generations of *E. coli*, and its gene product was expressed. Cohen and Boyer had changed nature.

MORATORIUM

I think every age is interesting if you get yourself involved in it.

DAVID BALTIMORE

January 20, 1995

Morrow corresponded with a variety of people about the frog gene transplantation during the winter of 1974, before the Berg Committee met, and Cohen, Boyer, and Berg began receiving phone calls from researchers around the world requesting the *E. coli* genetic engineering plasmids used in their different experiments; they wanted to try genetic engineering for themselves. Berg was boggled by the requests: "When they called me and I would ask what experiments they were doing, I was really shocked because . . . [many] were exactly the kind of experiment that we had been forewarned [about] a couple of years earlier. [There were] people wanting to cut up herpes virus DNA and put that into *E. coli!*" Berg refused to send the plasmid out. Upset to the point of distraction, Cohen called Berg and related similar experiences. They agreed that they wouldn't disseminate the plasmids until after the Berg Committee meeting.

Berg flew to Boston on April 17 for the meeting. All seven of the other invited professors were there; it was a high-powered biohazards team. The group was heavily weighted with tumor virologists, because those were the colleagues Berg knew best, and he felt that tumor virology was the area where recombinant DNA would be of most serious concern. Dan Nathans was a respected SV40 researcher who would win the Nobel Prize in 1978. Sherman Weissman, both an M.D. and a Ph.D., was a renowned infectious disease specialist who worked with SV40 as well. Norton Zinder had been invited on the basis of his sheer brilliance. Richard Roblin was a passionate and vocal speaker about genetic engineering ethics, as well as an old friend; he had been at the Salk Institute around the time that Baltimore and Berg were there. Hermann Lewis was a respected *Drosophila* geneticist, and he had pushed through the original biohazards conference funding at the NSF. David Baltimore was the most prominent virologist in America, and James Watson was perhaps the most famous biologist in the world.

Baltimore was deeply interested in a forum where scientists might come to a consensus about the real dangers of genetic engineering, and with any luck they could decide on appropriate actions. The essential questions were, What was the probability of creating a dangerous organism, and what could they do to protect against that? Baltimore suggested that one way to handle the safety problem was to develop "safe" viruses, plasmids, and bacteria, which would be crippled so that there was no way they could infect lab members or the public, even if someone's recombinant DNA experiment resulted in a potentially dangerous genetic combination. The idea was a crucial one. Hermann Lewis later said, "I thought it was most ingenious, and most imaginative, and so befitting that Dave Baltimore made the suggestion."

Within an hour the group agreed that an international conference discussing the safety of recombinant DNA should be held in February 1975, ten months away, in Asilomar. Berg knew the conference wouldn't come soon enough. He looked around the table and asked, "Has anybody heard about Morrow's results?" "No" was the unanimous response. He described Cohen and Boyer's frog gene transplantation experiment to the group, along with the requests he had received for plasmid. A startled hush fell over the room. What should they do? If they waited until the conference before they acted, action would be moot because people would certainly expand on Cohen and Boyer's results before then. Norton Zinder said gruffly, "Well, if we had any guts at all, we'd just tell people not to do these experiments. Maybe what we ought to do is make some public announcement." The group was disturbed by the idea. It seemed rather reactionary. Eventually they decided that, given the unknown dangers posed by indiscriminate genetic engineering, a letter asking people to refrain from certain risky experiments was in order. Experiments they blacklisted included manipulating genes involved in producing bacterial toxins (like botulin, the cause of botulism), viral cancer-inducing genes, and antibiotic resistance genes. The letter would be a personal appeal from them to their thousands of colleagues, and its effectiveness would rest on the respect the individual committee members commanded.

Berg, Baltimore, and most of the rest of the committee were politically naïve, and they harbored only dim notions of the significance of their action. As May and June slid away, the importance of the informal Berg Committee grew. Berg showed an early draft of the letter to Arthur Kornberg, his former mentor. Kornberg, old, wise, and politically savvy, looked Berg straight in the eye and told him that he shouldn't mislead himself: this letter would create quite a stir. Kornberg suggested Berg take a global scope in the letter, appealing to scientists all over the world, otherwise the moratorium would be flawed. Berg then showed the letter to the president of the NAS, Philip Handler. Handler realized that this was a major event and, after some thought, told Berg that the NAS would adopt the recommendations of the moratorium letter as its own. The Berg Committee was now the official Recombinant DNA Molecules Committee of the National Academy of Sciences. This move was a big leap for the group, because now they had the full weight of the academy behind them.

The moratorium letter went through four major revisions as it circulated among scientists in the United States and Europe. Baltimore made the first U.S. announcement of the committee's recommendations in mid-June at the 1974 Cold Spring Harbor symposium on tumor viruses. It was an obvious choice, since tumor virologists were likely to try some of the more dangerous applications, and Baltimore wanted to gauge their response. By all accounts, the audience was surprisingly receptive. The tumor virologists did not aggressively defend their stomping ground. There were no fights, no totalitarian accusations.

The committee finished the statement in June and published it in *Nature, Science,* and the *Proceedings of the National Academy of Sciences* in July and August. It announced a moratorium on recombinant DNA experiments posing "fairly obvious risks" and publicized the Asilomar conference next February. The NAS held a press conference on July 18, the day before the committee letter was published in *Nature,* attempting to prevent any hysterical news coverage. Baltimore was there to answer questions, along with Paul Berg and Richard Roblin. Baltimore was worried about the public response to their announcement. Would public fear grow out of hand? Safety needed to be insured, but Baltimore did not want recombinant DNA research hobbled any more than absolutely necessary: "What I hope is that the dangers in the work will be made small enough so that we can go forward with it, without having to be careful not to step over certain boundaries. But I'm not sure that's going to be possible." Baltimore was torn between two desires: the need for safety and the scientific need for recombinant DNA. These two desires would become cornerstones of the scientists' self-regulatory efforts, and the specter of unknown dangers would plague those efforts for years.

Though Baltimore had participated in group political activities, like the antiwar efforts, he had never assumed a leadership role. Somewhat unwittingly, Baltimore was placing himself at center stage, alongside a few of his colleagues, in what would become a four-year public controversy. By the time the dust settled, Baltimore and a number of other participants had gone through a considerable evolution of their beliefs and their understanding of biological research.

But for now the moratorium was on, and the Berg group would have to see if the respect they and the NAS commanded was enough to restrain independently motivated scientists. Both the publication of a moratorium letter and the press conference were unprecedented in science. No scientific group had ever asked their colleagues to stop basic research. It seemed an extreme step, and one that conflicted with the philosophy that no subject should be off limits to scientific research. During a talk Baltimore gave several months later, a member of the audience challenged that the Berg Committee moratorium conflicted with the fundamental belief that scientific curiosity should be the driving force of research. Baltimore replied sadly: "Yes, it does. And that bothered a lot of people. . . . Should there be certain experiments about which we say no, which would violate the traditions of academic freedom in principle? Certain kinds of experiments are just too dangerous to do, and you should just say no—principles be damned. That seemed like the appropriate way to go."

Baltimore was plagued by nagging questions about the safety of recombinant DNA. They distracted him from his work and complicated his planning for Asilomar. He would often sit in his office, stroking his beard slowly, and just think. "We can always argue that any specific experiment would not be dangerous, and yet when you consider them in aggregate, probably somewhere in there there's a serious danger, and you don't know where it is." He thought about plasmids, he thought about politics, he thought about viruses, and he thought about how biologists had always been limited by what evolution had created naturally, until now. "By allowing DNA to be moved from any organism to any other organism, we are effectively allowing genetic combinations that have never existed before on the planet to come into existence. That's where we're talking about a qualitative difference from any other biohazard that's been around," he later said. "In a sense, we had gone beyond the barrier we had all believed in, which was the barrier of evolution."

It was time for a sabbatical. Baltimore had been researching long hours for ten years. He and Alice decided that they would take their sabbaticals together during the following academic year. They considered a number of exotic locations, including Australia and Switzerland. Baltimore was particularly tempted to travel to the Basel Institute of Immunology in Switzerland and study with Niels Jerne, the world's preeminent theoretical immunologist. But, in the end, he was unable to tear himself away from the excitement of the East Coast academic community—the Power Corridor—as he wrote in a letter to Niels Jerne in December: "My wife and I have thought long and hard about what we wanted to do on our sabbaticals, and have made the conservative, but, I believe, wise decision to stay reasonably close to home by going to the Rockefeller University for the next academic year."

"SCIENCE AGAINST ITSELF"

After the NAS press conference, the recombinant DNA debate was in the public forum, and the controversy was suddenly expanded to include *all* recombinant DNA research. Genetic engineering seized the public imagination, and people pontificated on the scary possibilities of human genetic engineering and other fantastical things, much as the European students had done after Berg's lecture in Sicily. Berg and Baltimore thought the ethical issues could wait for many years, because the technology was still nowhere near that stage. The only issue that needed discussion, for Berg and Baltimore, was the immediate safety of a small subset of recombinant DNA experiments, which was a problem that should be handled by the scientific community. But some observers felt that the Berg Committee was a facade to protect recombinant DNA from federal scrutiny. To this, Hermann Lewis said, "I would never accuse Berg or Dave Baltimore of being devious, because I don't think they're that kind of people. I think they're as authentic as anybody I've ever met. . . . Their motivations are of the highest order." They felt that it was imperative to show the public and the government that science could regulate itself, so that the public didn't get scared and the government didn't create counterproductive restrictions. As Baltimore saw it:

The big question involved behind all this is, how science should be regulated—if we accept the principle that it should be regulated at all, and I think most people will accept that. In this situation, the group of us who met were acting formally as policemen. We were saying, "We see a problem. We want to flag that problem, but we don't want to act as judges. We simply want to stop it for a moment, and then allow a larger group of people—the meeting in California—to act as judges."

In October, two months after the initial press conference and six months before the Asilomar conference, CBS News ran a program called "The DNA Debate: Science against Itself," in which they interviewed Baltimore. They pushed him to explain the value of recombinant DNA and justify its risks. Baltimore responded with an earnest enthusiasm:

Although we've had enormous successes in dealing with diseases that come from microorganisms: viral diseases, bacterial diseases—we have vaccines, we have antibiotics—we have made very little fundamental progress in understanding diseases that have, as their origin, cellular misfunction. And cancer, heart disease, and immune defects are diseases of that sort. To understand those diseases, we have to understand the nature of normal cell function and the nature of malfunction. And to get at that requires the whole armamentarium of modern molecular biology, including recombinant DNA work.

I think before the recombinant DNA methodology became evident, people were predicting *very* long times before we could make any fundamental advances on cellular diseases. I think because of recombinant DNA research, we can see a pathway toward success. That doesn't mean success is around the corner, but it means that success is a predictable event, rather than being a hope.

That interview was the first time Baltimore publicly argued that recombinant DNA research should go forward because of its medical value. That argument, in a variety of forms, would become a cornerstone of the scientists' debate with Congress and the public over recombinant DNA.

BEACON ON THE BEACH

Berg and Baltimore's "motivations of the highest order," as their friend Hermann Lewis put it, were generating a lot of work for each of them. The Asilomar organizing committee had Berg and Baltimore as coordinators.

The NAS had provided them with $75,000 for the meeting, enough to allow about 150 scientists to attend. But many more wanted to come. It took the organizing committee months to decide whom they would invite as representatives of the world's biological research community. They needed to invite scientists from all major countries. Would the Soviet Union let anyone come? They also needed scientists from a variety of specialties: epidemiologists, microbiologists, ecologists, biochemists, and molecular biologists were all invited. How to deal with the press was another issue. Should they even invite reporters? The public was becoming more and more aware of the recombinant DNA controversy. The media was slowly scaling up its coverage, intrigued by a story in which scientists were so scared of their own research that they stopped it themselves. Yes, they would have to invite reporters. One reporter told them bluntly: "A secret international meeting of molecular biologists to discuss biohazards? If the press isn't allowed, I'll guarantee you nightmare stories." But how could they avoid negative press? They would have to select the reporters carefully and give them strict instructions not to publish anything until after the conference.

The temporary moratorium on recombinant DNA was holding; labs voluntarily refrained from experiments posing "fairly obvious risks." Baltimore was impressed with scientists' restraint:

> The response of the biological community to it has been, as far as I can tell, extremely positive. No one has come up to me, or anybody I know for that matter, and said, "You're nuts. We're going to go out and do these things. You guys are just raising red flags." And I think that's very interesting. It indicates that maybe the climate which was created by the continual raising of these questions in a more general way over the last five years—often as not, at any given university, by the students or the younger faculty—has created a climate where people were willing to accept the idea of limitation very easily. But it happened that way.

On February 22, 1975, the three panels in charge of the International Conference on Recombinant DNA rolled into Asilomar. Baltimore and the other four members of the organizing committee arrived early. The Asilomar Conference Grounds sprawled along Asilomar State Beach on the Monterey Peninsula. The monarch butterfly migration was passing through, heading for Canada. Millions of tiger-striped butterflies hung from the trees. As described in the Asilomar brochure, "the rooms all have individual lanais and lovely marine views," just a few hundred feet from the sea. (*Lanai* is Hawaiian for porch.) Baltimore and Berg stayed in a unit called "Sand & Surf." Their room faced north; James Watson was in the room on their right, and Sydney Brenner was on their left. On that first day, Brenner and Watson sat on the lanai, watching monarchs flutter by. Watson was an ungainly-looking man, long and lanky. His hair, initially combed across his scalp to cover his baldness, flopped around comically in the wind. Brenner's hair was brushed forward and down his forehead. Brenner was a great talker, and he probably had the best sense of humor of anyone at the conference. An older man with a lively face, he spoke with a mild South African accent, his bushy eyebrows constantly accentuating his speech. The Sand & Surf enclave shared a large separate living room with floor-to-ceiling panoramic windows, a Steinway grand piano, a stone fireplace, and a wooden deck. The organizing committee would spend much of the week in that living room, arguing out the future of recombinant DNA.

Two days later, 140 biologists crammed into Asilomar's stone chapel to listen to Baltimore give the opening remarks. As one scientist put it, "Here we are, sitting in a chapel, next to the ocean, huddled around a forbidden tree, trying to create some new Commandments—and there's no goddamn Moses in sight."

The conference included sessions on technical issues, followed by debates on potential biohazards and safety precautions. Discussions were loosely grouped into plasmid/bacterial, viral, and plant and animal issues. Suppressed tensions filled the rooms. Many at Asilomar oscillated between feeling overwhelmed—as though they were looking into a great unknown and making a guess—and regressing into selfish protection of their own research. Baltimore, Berg, Brenner, Lederberg, and Watson dominated the discussions. Lederberg and Watson had already won Nobel Prizes. Watson strongly and repeatedly pronounced that he wanted no regulations—a surprise announcement from the man who swore at the first Asilomar Conference that he would sue a Harvard colleague if he pursued the development of a cell line that produced Epstein-Barr virus.

Lederberg argued vigorously against a wide variety of regulations as well, but it was sometimes tough to tell what he wanted. A large, older man with a healthy professorial look, he would stand up in the meetings and speak off the cuff for several minutes in brilliantly obfuscated language and then sit down, leaving scientists around the room whispering to their neighbors,

"What did he say?" Then Lederberg would change his mind, stand up again, and say something else equally confusing. "It's hard to know what Josh Lederberg's comments mean sometimes," shrugged Berg. Some of the younger scientists confided that they were intimidated by Lederberg and Watson: "If you're a Nobel laureate in this country, then there's nobody who can touch you."

Berg and Baltimore were tensely focused on success and control. Baltimore frequently went head-to-head with Lederberg or Watson in the discussions, arguing the importance of caution. Baltimore put his case articulately, exposing fine points and implications in precise and lucid language, but he was not a passionate speaker; no one was particularly impressed with his opening speech. As one reporter summarized, "He's a bit too downbeat." His arguments were poignant, but he was not moving. Brenner, on the other hand, came full of charisma and humanity. One participant recalled, "He always used to bring the meeting back to center," getting the group to focus on their obligations

One session focused on whether or not laboratory *E. coli* was still capable of infecting people. To test this, a group of British researchers mixed laboratory *E. coli* into half-pints of milk, drank it, and then analyzed their own feces. They charted the results and showed them to the Asilomar participants with comments like "A nice, quiet, boring person, as far as his colon is concerned." In the end, their entertainment value was clearer than their scientific results.*

The meeting schedule was demanding, and discussions continued between meetings as the scientists mingled outside. Various people argued that DNA recombination happened all the time in nature, so why should it be a problem in laboratories? One scientist countered, "Nature does not need to be legislated, but playing God does." One conference photo shows Baltimore wearing a coarse, embroidered windbreaker with large wooden buttons, standing in the sunlight on the deck of the stone church with a group of colleagues. He holds a folder full of notes and a legal pad in his right hand, and he gestures emphatically with his left hand.

Redwoods ringed the area, and surreal numbers of monarchs floated on the steady wind. Scientists strolled on the wooden walkways that meandered through the conference grounds while they debated plasmid structures. Some walked along the beach discussing the differences between an-

---

E. coli strains that can cause food poisoning, such as strain 0157:H7, are a relatively new concern and weren't an issue in the 1970s.

imal and bacterial gene expression, or held animated arguments about virus genes while sitting on worn, grey benches carved from whole tree trunks. Ragged scrub pines stretched up from the sand.

Tensions regularly exploded into bitter arguments. After one session Stanley Falkow, an excitable and passionate scientist from Brooklyn, stormed up to Baltimore in the main hallway and shouted, "I think you *fucked* the plasmid group!" Heads turned. "You twisted around the plasmid group recommendations!"

"I don't understand you," Baltimore replied calmly but icily.

"You twisted our recs into your recs!" Falkow retorted, and they launched into a long and terrible argument.

In one session, Berg asked, "Can we measure the risks numerically?" and Watson exploded, "We can't even *measure* the fucking risks!" Berg, fed up with Watson's contrarian behavior, eventually pegged him: "Jim, you could be sued on the following grounds: you are a signatory to a public statement which said that you agree that there *is* a potential risk to this line of work, and for you to get up here and now say that you are not willing to institute any procedures which would protect the staff of Cold Spring Harbor—and you're the director. If anybody has the responsibility for the people at Cold Spring Harbor, you do." He shook an accusing finger. "And if you say publicly now that you are not prepared to undertake any of the kinds of arrangements because people won't observe them, you don't have the money, you don't have the space, and all of that; then as far as I'm concerned, and according to what the law says, I could bring suit against you for being irresponsible, and I will!"

The organizing committee spent many hours on Wednesday sitting in the Sand & Surf living room with piles of notes spread out across the coffee tables, trying to forge a biohazard safety statement. A large stone chimney was flanked on both sides by chalkboards covered with scribbles:

> Is the "war" over?
> What do we do now?
> What about industrial applic?
> What about construction of m.o. (viable) for intentional release?

The five members of the organizing committee, Paul Berg, David Baltimore, Sydney Brenner, Norton Zinder, and Maxine Singer, took turns wandering around the room, scratching their heads, silently fumbling with their hands, or pausing to lean on the grand piano. Baltimore wore faded jeans and a dark navy blue sweater. The sweater had a big, ragged hole in the left side, through which you could see his striped button-up. He stayed slumped in an armchair, a pile of notes on his lap, and his leg resting on the nearby table. His coffee-colored hair was matted, and he wore thin-rimmed metal glasses. His dark beard was short but brambly; he wore no rings, no jewelry. He thought and talked with all the intensity he could summon. Sydney Brenner sat on one of the couches with Norton Zinder and smoked voluminously while scrawling on a thick legal pad. There were about half a dozen crumpled cigarette butts in the glass ashtray. Zinder wrung his hands. His lips were slightly pushed out as he stared distantly, brow furrowed, thick dark hair slicked back. Every once in a while one of them would leave to go find an expert on a specific question or pick up a six-pack of beer from the social hour. Berg sat in a wicker chair, clean-cut and fatherly. Singer sat in a tall wooden chair across from them all, next to a cluttered table. Her thick black, greying hair was tied up; it was coarse in the crisp light. She wore dark sunglasses over her tight face and periodically nibbled on the end of a pen. Sometimes she would stroll outside and sit on the wooden railing of the deck and look out across the ocean.

While the organizing committee spent their evenings worrying in their glass living room, the rest of the scientists hung out drinking beers inside one of the conference halls, and it was here that individuals engaged in the most intense debates. At beer hour battles were won and lost. People adamantly disagreed about the potential hazards of experiments they desperately wanted to do. It became painfully apparent through such free-for-alls, as the days went on, that the participants were selfishly motivated, each defending their potential experiments as safe but readily agreeing to regulate any other area of research. Arguments went on and on. Some people got sick of it all and went out on the beach to smoke marijuana.

Despite their disagreements, they all felt a strong impetus to insure that they regulated themselves adequately. One obvious reason was safety. The other was to "keep the Feds out," as one participant put it. Senator Edward Kennedy had announced that he planned to reevaluate biomedical research policy, and the scientists didn't want anything to do with government regulation. Baltimore understood the problem crisply:

> In the United States the government could take action, if it felt it necessary, but I want to avoid that. And in fact, a large amount of what we have done has been ways of avoiding governmental response, because governmental response is going to be too rigid, it's going to be

too hard to reverse, it's going to be too hard to work within, and I think that's likely to impede research seriously—probably without really stopping the hazards.

A third strong reason for self-regulation was raised by a session on legal responsibilities in the final evening. It was organized by Maxine Singer's husband Daniel Singer, a lawyer. He broke the ice with a joke: A scientist and a lawyer were arguing about whose profession was older, and they argued for a while and worked their way all the way back to God. The scientist said that God was clearly a scientist, because he had created order out of chaos. "Yes," replied the lawyer, "but where do you think the chaos came from?"

Singer then brought in four attorneys who established that scientists could be held personally liable for any infectious biohazards from their labs. They could be sued by lab technicians, postdocs, or grad students exposed to danger, and if anything managed to get out of the lab there could be catastrophic legal consequences. The ramifications were deeply troubling. The scientists present could not help but reflect on the recent disaster in England.

In March 1973, within the Tropical Disease Research Unit of University College London, a plain concrete building in the middle of the city, scientists were handling smallpox rather casually. One researcher unknowingly became infected with the virus and continued about her normal routines. During the next week, several smallpox infections were discovered in London. Two women died. The outbreak was contained, but the scare left Britain edgy.

The possibility of creating new infectious diseases, no matter how remote, was terrifying. And the notion that you could be sued for it did not improve the situation. Yet again, Sydney Brenner brought the discussion back to center. He stood up, looked around at his colleagues, raised his eyebrows, and pronounced that if people were going to act only out of fear of lawsuits, then the conference had failed. He swept his arms out and said, "It is your responsibility, as a matter of conscience, to not endanger yourself, your colleagues, or anyone else." After this declaration there was a different tone at the social hour that final evening. A participant later said respectfully, "He reminded the scientists that they were dealing with cosmic matters, and to forget their parochial interests."

That last evening, the organizing committee stayed up all night in their Sand & Surf living room, a beacon on the beach, drafting a statement. As it grew later, they ate Chinese takeout and drank gallons of coffee while sitting around tables inundated with paper. Brenner smoked. No definite consensus had arisen during the conference, and the organizing committee was concerned about obtaining general approval for measures they felt were necessary. Around midnight, several people from each of the three biohazard groups came round and made suggestions. Each group sat in a different part of the room—plasmid by the fireplace, virus by the piano, and plant and animal over by the north windows—and they passed drafts around, talking and revising. Paul Berg's personal secretary typed drafts all night. Clickclickclickclickclick . . . in a room full of chattering geniuses.

As the night wore on, the statement accumulated a slurry of technical explanations, criteria for ranking hazards, and recommendations for safety equipment. The group decided that physical containment strategies were important, but, as Paul Berg summarized, "Frankly, most of us who work with these kinds of facilities have known for a long time that they're not foolproof. They're really only as good as the people who work with them. And the history of people working with nasty organisms is filled with accidents," like the London smallpox outbreak. Therefore they emphasized the importance of Baltimore's idea from the original Berg Committee meeting: develop "safe" viruses, plasmids, and bacteria, crippling them so that they could not infect humans. As Sydney Brenner whimsically explained, there were two options: "One, we should make the bug so safe that nothing could happen; or, two, we should make it so dangerous that everybody would be petrified to work with it." So he proposed, with a wink and a smile, that either the experimental bug be *Pasteurella pestis*—the plague bacterium—or they design a bug so safe that nothing could go wrong. The Asilomar statement also set up a four-level scheme of physical containment, which required security precautions commensurate with the severity of the biohazard.

The committee wanted to present the statement to the conference without a vote, fearing that it might be rejected as too restrictive by the conference members. Maxine Singer recalled, "We thought we would be voted down. And yet we felt very strongly that we had to have *something,* that we couldn't just leave with nothing."

They finished the statement at 5:30 A.M. Paul Berg presented the draft to the crowd of scientists. Baltimore and the other organizers passed out copies and gave everyone an hour to sit in the chapel and read it. The organizing committee sat up on the dais and waited quietly. Baltimore slumped in his chair. His clothes were disheveled, and his hair was tussled. Dark bags drooped beneath his eyes. As people finished reading, they kept filtering up to the stage and congratulating Baltimore and the others with comments like, "God, I don't understand how you guys could have put this thing together. It was just fantastic." Some people pointed out quibbles or, humorously, corrected the grammar. At the end of the hour the statement was forced to a vote. It passed with a show of hands; there were only half a dozen dissenters.

The organizing committee was startled. They had expected much more resistance. Surprised and happy, many of the scientists who left that day, including David Baltimore, felt that the worst was past, and it was simply a matter of time before the measures were revised and adopted by the National Institutes of Health and genetic engineering experiments could proceed. Then scientists could wield the powerful recombinant DNA techniques. A large number of experiments would be restricted by the safety guidelines, so researchers geared up their facilities to meet those guidelines.

Baltimore understood that this was the turning point for modern biology, both technologically and sociologically:

> It was the beginning of the industrial application of modern biology, medical application of modern biology, and the real revolution in the *concept* of what you could learn from it, and medicine for that matter, which we are still in the process of seeing [in 1995]. Now that meant that we, as molecular biologists, went from being woolly-headed intellectuals to being at the center of a major societal movement. And so our science suddenly became important in issues of ethics and industry and all sorts of things.

That "major societal movement" was intrinsically tied to the publicity and debate started by the Berg Committee. The public was made aware of the new power of biology through the massive press that Asilomar and the recombinant DNA controversy generated from 1975 to 1978. The concept of recombinant DNA was easy to understand: you can take a gene out of one living thing and put it in another. Even the most pedestrian mind could imagine grotesquely evil and fantastically beneficial applications. As Baltimore realized, "The whole Asilomar process opened up to the world that modern biology had new powers that you had never conceived of before."

The public was scared of this power. Public faith in just about everything hit rock bottom in 1975. Richard Nixon had resigned the presidency in August 1974, after the nation had suffered through two years of the Watergate scandal. The Vietnam War finally ended in April 1975 after a decade of public turmoil and government duplicity. More important, science's reputation had been tainted by a number of technological horrors in the previous two decades. Rachel Carson's *Silent Spring*, published in 1962, exposed the dangers created by the chemical industries, most prominently represented by DDT and PCBs, and later Agent Orange and asbestos. Her stories about the deadly effects of chemicals helped start a massive environmental movement in the United States, one that focused on the devastating results of the ignorance and complicity of scientists and the self-serving short-sightedness of the chemical industry. Millions of Americans participated in Earth Day in 1970, celebrating the earth and condemning pollution. By the time of the Asilomar conference, environmental groups such as the Natural Resources Defense Council and the World Wildlife Fund were mobilizing to lobby against recombinant DNA.

Exacerbating public fears, Michael Crichton's novel *The Andromeda Strain* had been published in 1969 and spent thirty weeks on the *New York Times* bestseller list. His horror story tracked a deadly virus that kills the residents of an Arizona town by turning them into heaps of powdered bone. It included a slew of authentic touches, including long scientific explanations, computer printouts, historical facts, and references to actual scientific papers. It was made into a motion picture within eighteen months of publication. *The Andromeda Strain* did for biology what *Jaws* did for beaches. Americans are afraid of diseases and fascinated with their invisible power. On the day after the Asilomar conference, the *Boston Globe* ran a front-page headline, "Scientists to Resume Risky Work on Genes: Danger of Andromeda Strain Posed."

Meanwhile, another scientific monster, thermonuclear war, hung over the world like a giant, unpredictable guillotine. The public was well aware that nuclear energy was the most awesome destructive force on the planet, and they also knew that it had been created by scientists. They lived with the threat of complete annihilation in an extremely short World War III. No one wanted to hear that biologists were building another destructive monster.

The parallels between recombinant DNA and nuclear energy were drawn early by both scientists and the public. Before the Asilomar conference, in correspondence on the hazards of recombinant DNA, Daniel Singer sent Baltimore a copy of the 1939 letter from Albert Einstein and Leo Szilard to Franklin Roosevelt on the danger of the atomic bomb. In 1972, Baltimore had given a lecture at a faculty lunch meeting about the dangers of biology "commonly analogous to the atom bomb." When the recombinant DNA controversy began to heat up, Baltimore was also involved in a public discussion at MIT with Philip Morrison, the physicist who armed the *Enola Gay's* atomic bombs on Tinian Island and had since been vocal in efforts to eradicate nuclear arms. The discussion, titled "When Does Molecular Biology Become More of a Hazard Than a Promise?" explored the parallels between the development of atomic weapons and recombinant DNA. Morrison found only a few historical parallels, but he strongly believed that the power created by the new technology needed careful assessment. A number of the physicists involved in the Manhattan Project were at MIT. "Those people were around here—Vicki Weisskopf and Philip Morrison and Jerry Weisner—and were friends," Baltimore noted. "So we were very conscious of that as a precedent. I think it's fair to say that they had set a very good example of scientific responsibility—of looking coldly at what they had done and saying, 'There are implications for this in society, and we have to carry those implications in society—on our own terms, and not simply the politicians'.'" Baltimore chuckled as he continued, "They had been notably unsuccessful in doing that, but they were the conscience of a country. It takes a long time for things to come around, but I think that they, in the end, had a very salutary influence in the country. And yes, we were certainly aware of that parallel. Even though it was a very different situation than nuclear war. No weapons of mass destruction. We hoped, anyway," and Baltimore smiled faintly.

Even though the Berg Committee had publicized the moratorium letter in an attempt to instill public trust, the public, the media, and the government remained worried. If scientists were concerned enough to put a moratorium on some of their own work, and restrictions on most of it, perhaps it was dangerous enough to ban altogether. Complicating things further, scientists did not agree among themselves regarding the safety of experiments. The majority of biologists supported recombinant DNA research as carried out under the NIH guidelines. However, a number of other scientists advocated prohibitive recombinant DNA regulations, and they quickly became central public figures. Several biologists felt that recombinant DNA experiments should not be done under any circumstances. Harvard's George Wald and MIT's Jonathan King explained the potentially disastrous consequences of recombinant DNA research to the press and to Congress. King said that letting biologists decide on the safety guidelines of recombinant DNA research was like "having the chairman of General Motors write the specifications for safety belts." The battle over recombinant DNA was just warming up.

Seven

It's about time the scientists began to throw all their goddamned shit
right out on the table so that we can discuss it.

ALFRED VELLUCCI
Mayor of Cambridge, Massachusetts, 1977

IN THE FALL OF 1975, BALTIMORE was starting his year-long sabbatical at
Rockefeller University, working with Jim Darnell. He needed a break from
MIT, and he wanted to be near his parents in New York. His father had
had his first heart attack that summer and was in and out of Mt. Sinai Hospital for months. Concerned, David, Alice, and their newborn daughter
Lauren, whom they nicknamed "Teak," moved to New York. Alice was taking a sabbatical from Harvard to work at Rockefeller. They lived in the on-
campus Rockefeller faculty housing, at 1500 East 63rd Street, and they hired
a nanny for Lauren.

With administrative and teaching commitments aside, Baltimore's goal
was to return to the laboratory bench, but those plans were soon curtailed.
First, Baltimore and Darnell went on a two-week trip to the Soviet Union,
sponsored by the National Academy of Sciences and the Russian Academy
of Sciences. They met with a number of Russian scientists, and Baltimore
recalls, "We talked an awful lot of nonscience, I can tell you—a lot about
their lives." He was amazed to see the despotic conditions under which the
scientists worked, and he also saw how a theoretically ideal social structure
could go bad:

> It was very, very interesting. It was an eye-opening experience for me. I
> never saw the Soviet Union the same way since. I grew up in a family

that was quite left-wing, and quite sympathetic to socialist movements—although never to the Communists, per se. And I had, still have, many of those instincts myself. I understood then how wrong it could go, how bad it could be. I never thought politically the same way again. None of us did. . . .

Countries like the Soviet Union that have tried to do just what I was talking about [at the Eli Lilly Award Convocation in 1971], have failed because of a lack of public accountability. Accountability is what it all comes down to. . . . The notion that people will simply work for the public interest and not their own private interests is wrong. They're going to take advantage of a situation in which they're not accountable, and work for their own private interests—as we've seen so grossly in the Soviet Union and generally in Eastern Europe.

On his way back from Russia, Baltimore passed Alice in New York's Kennedy Airport, on her way to a Leukemia Society conference in Copenhagen. Two days later, Baltimore flew to Boston to visit his brother Bob, then at Harvard Medical School. He had just become Uncle David to Bob's newborn son. But their father suffered another heart attack and was hospitalized at Mt. Sinai. David and Bob, along with Bob's wife and the baby, rushed back to New York to visit their father in the hospital. When David finally made it back to his apartment at Rockefeller for some much-needed sleep, he wasn't prepared for the phone call from Alice the following morning.

On October 16, Alice was in a conference session chaired by a member of the Nobel committee. The session ended at noon, Denmark time, and the chair began to give his discussion summary, a speech that normally lasts five to ten minutes. But he kept talking on and on, glancing frequently at his watch, clearly stalling. Finally, after apologizing profusely, he confessed that he wanted to make a very important announcement. Although it was too early in the day to be official, he told the group that David Baltimore, Renato Dulbecco, and Howard Temin had won the 1975 Nobel Prize in medicine and physiology.

Alice rushed to the nearest phone in Copenhagen and called David. It was about 7:30 A.M. in New York, and he woke groggily to the ringing of the telephone. Alice gave him a minute to wake up while she made small talk. Then she blurted out the news. Baltimore was stunned. He wasn't expecting the prize at all; at thirty-seven he was young to be winning the

Nobel.* He was ecstatic, but it came as a very strange surprise, and tough to grasp a minute after waking. In fact, the early morning Nobel phone calls have generated a number of funny stories. When the 1995 medicine winner, Eric Wieschaus, was woken up at Princeton, he said, "I think you have the wrong number."

The day would prove a whirlwind of elations and uncertainties. His wife was in Europe, and he was far away from his close friends at MIT. When he tried to call his father at Mt. Sinai Hospital, he couldn't get through: they didn't turn the patients' phones on until eight o'clock in the morning. As a result, his father saw the Nobel announcement on the *Today Show* before David could talk to him, and he was back in intensive care the same day.

The Nobel committee awarded the 1975 Nobel Prize to Dulbecco, Temin, and Baltimore specifically for their "discoveries concerning the interaction between tumor viruses and the genetic material of the cell." The award would become a testament to the overwhelming importance of cancer research worldwide.

By nine that morning, a *New York Times* photographer had come and gone, taking a photograph of Baltimore holding fourteen-month-old Teak that would be on the front page of the next day's paper. Before flying to MIT, shortly after ten, David stopped by Mt. Sinai to talk with his father. His brother and mother were there. Bob wanted to fly up to Boston with David, but their father's condition was deteriorating. Bob decided to stay behind, but his wife and son went with David. Teak stayed behind in New York with the nanny.

At MIT, a news conference was held in the Center for Cancer Research with about a dozen reporters, half a dozen video camera crews, and at least three photographers, along with numerous professors and students from the biology department. Baltimore's graduate students were ready to celebrate. The press conference swelled with optimism. Baltimore sat at a plain collapsible table, confronted by a bank of microphones. He laughed during nearly all of the questions and answers. The air was buzzing with euphoria, coupled with an awkwardness about the press. No one there was used to this sort of celebrity, and most of them just wanted to get to the champagne party afterwards. Still, everyone recognized the importance of the media attention. People fidgeted, with smiles filling their faces, barely suppressing giggles. The questioning began.

*In medicine and physiology the average age of recipients is mid to late forties. In physics it is five to ten years younger. The youngest recipient was William Bragg, who won the physics prize in 1915 at age twenty-five.

"When your wife called, you . . . were asleep?"

"Yes," Baltimore replied, smiling.

"What was your first reaction?"

"Try to wake up." He smiled again, and everyone laughed.

"What is your first reaction to all this attention that, apparently, you are getting for the first time and possibly may never ever get again?"

Baltimore laughed heartily, rocking back in his chair. He smiled at the reporter and playfully said, "Amusement?" raising his eyebrows with a nod to the reporter.

"Have you thought about what you're going to do with the money?"

"No."

"Hello, I'm a Swedish reporter."

"Welcome!"

"Will you be going to Sweden to accept the prize?"

"I presume so," with a smile.

"Do you know when they are?"

"I'd expect you to know. You're the Swedish reporter!"

"Dr. Baltimore, would you outline the nature of your studies?"

"Ummm," Baltimore said, scratching his head. He paused and raised his eyebrows. "Hopefully that's in here," flipping through the MIT press release, "but I can try." He quickly slipped into a comfortable lecturing mode, more sure of himself. He spoke clearly, spending several minutes explaining his work.

"Do you know what you're going to do with the money?

"No." Then, on second thought, "Ask the other guy who asked."

"Are you still concerned about genetic engineering?"

Overnight, Baltimore had become the figurehead of the recombinant DNA controversy. "My interest was, and still is, to see that that technique is used in a way which is responsible. That is, that it's used to further the development of molecular biology, but at the same time doesn't portend a risk to the public outside." He played with the hair on the back of his hand. "We don't want to be in the position, two years, ten years from now, whenever it happens, when the public says, 'You never told us what you guys were doing!'"

"When do you think cancer as we know it will no longer be a threat?"

"I have absolutely no idea." Even though *Time* magazine had chosen him as one of two hundred rising leaders of America the previous year, based on his advances in cancer research, he was not fond of prognosticating. Howard Temin's standard answer set the mood of most cancer biologists: "I'll tell you the same thing I tell everybody else. I'm not a psychic, and I don't like trying to predict the future."

"Could you sum up for the layman the significance of your discoveries?" another reporter asked Baltimore.

"Ummm . . . I tried before . . . "

"We're talking about people who don't really know what the DNA, RNA are."

All of the scientists in the room audibly winced. The question seemed insurmountable. A reporter from *Time* once told the physicist Richard Feynman, in an aside, that he should answer such questions with, "Listen, buddy, if I could tell you in a minute what I did, it wouldn't be worth the Nobel Prize." But Baltimore honestly tried to explain his work, knowing that the hopes for cancer cures lay submerged beneath these questions. "All I can really say is that . . . what we found was that a class of viruses that cause cancer has very unique properties, and these unique properties . . . allow one to get a wide appreciation for the role of the virus in animals. Since cancer is a disease that's on everybody's mind much of the time, an advance in the understanding of cancer . . . is one that catches the fancy of people very easily. Had this been a discovery that was made about a virus that causes warts or moles or something else, it would not [have] been the same hoopla surrounding it." He explained that cancer-causing viruses have a small role in human cancers, and he stressed the importance of cutting down on the environmental causes of cancer, such as chemicals and smoking. His mother and his dying father, heavy smokers all their lives, were surely on his mind.

One of Baltimore's students, Ellen, had created a humorous, loosely symbolic poster, which hung behind the table. A reporter asked, "At the risk of displaying further scientific ignorance, could you explain the significance

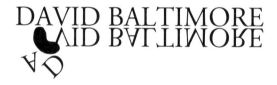

From the Nobel Prize press conference: Ellen's poster of reverse transcriptase (the black, bean-shaped box) writing Baltimore's name.

of the sign that Ellen made for you?" Baltimore turned toward the poster, and slowly grabbed his bottom lip. Now he was stuck. "Maybe she should explain it," he said hopefully. Ellen moaned, "David," realizing he hadn't figured it out.

"It looks like Russian," he guessed. His graduate students groaned. He was stumped. "My problem really is, what happened at the end there?" pointing at the drifting A and D. People started shouting out encouragements.

"You're reading in the wrong direction!"

"Go to the 5' end!"

Another colleague demanded playfully, "Is this the man who won the Nobel Prize?"

"Look at that black box."

He looked. "Oh, it's the enzyme!" It was reverse transcriptase writing his name. The room filled with laughter, the press conference ended, and Baltimore and his friends went on to the party. That night, Baltimore had a quiet dinner with Professor Maurice Fox and his wife and then spent the night at their home, since his own Cambridge house was rented out.

Baltimore enjoyed the publicity and acclamations, but felt somewhat guilty about it. His tax-free quarter of the $143,000 award was certainly a windfall,* but Baltimore believed that the public unjustly differentiated Nobel-winning scientists from a faceless sea of other deserving researchers. The media, as was usual with fundamental science, overemphasized the medical importance of the Nobelists' research. *Time* magazine applauded the laureates for their implication of viruses as "prime suspects in human cancer," when in fact they were less and less convinced that viruses were anything more than a footnote to human cancer. For years after the announcement, Baltimore received a stream of letters from cancer victims or their spouses, begging him for help.

On his death in 1896, Alfred Nobel endowed the Nobel Prizes with a gift equivalent to $23 million in today's dollars. Almost all of that money was acquired through his invention of dynamite. It was, in fact, nearly all the money he ever earned; he had no heirs. The prizes were to go to those who "conferred the greatest benefit on mankind" in literature, peace, physics, chemistry, and physiology or medicine (economics was added later), most of whom are selected by Swedish academicians. Today, each of the six Nobel prizes is selected by a small panel, which accepts nominations in different ways depending on the field. In literature, anyone can be nominated, as long as they don't nominate themselves or offer bribes (like one suitor

*Dulbecco received half the prize money, and Baltimore and Temin shared the remainder. Of some note, the United States recently became the only country in the world to tax the Nobel Prize.

who sent the academy eighteen crates of pistachio nuts). In the sciences, the selection committees maintain a group of fifty or so "nominators" in the United States and other countries, of whom a fraction are asked to submit nominations each year. The nominations are given to a subcommittee that quickly trims the number of candidates down to a dozen or so, and this short list of nominees is presented to the full academy in April or May. The process is conducted in absolute secrecy. After the summer, the subcommittee members present their individual choices for the award, and then every week thereafter they argue about who the winner should be, until a clear majority is reached. The winner is usually announced in mid-autumn. All the proceedings and winners are kept secret until the actual announcements are made, and even then no one can look at the records of the selection meetings for another fifty years.

The Nobel celebrations climaxed for Baltimore in December, at the ceremony in Stockholm, where King Carl XVI Gustaf awarded the three scientists their prize. Afterwards, there was a royal banquet and ball. David and Alice loved it. Peter Temin, who was in Stockholm to celebrate with both Howard and David, said, "I spent much more time there with David than with my brother. David was a friend. Howard was, really, quite tense, and his wife was even more tense. Whereas David enjoyed himself very much—he had a *very* good time." David and Alice hired a chauffeur to take them out to parties, and Peter went along to relive the days when he and David cruised jazz bars in Philadelphia: "We went out in the evening to Old Stockholm, to hear jazz. And we tried to get in [to a club], but it was very crowded. And so the question was, he won a Nobel Prize, could that get you into a nightclub?" It took some talking, but they did manage to get in.

The next day, the Nobelists gave their respective lectures, which were delivered at the Karolinska Institute in Stockholm. Baltimore talked about "bringing molecular biology to bear on the awful and awesome problem of cancer," but he also took the opportunity to speak about the beauty of basic research. He explained molecular biology as an exercise in natural aesthetics, saying that virologists are perhaps the most fortunate of these aestheticians because they can fully explore the intricacies of their subject. Temin's lecture was titled "The DNA Provirus Hypothesis: The Establishment and Implications of RNA-Directed DNA Synthesis," and his lecture did not stray far from its stated title. Dulbecco, a writer as well as a scientist, spent most of his time on the history of animal virology. But the last portion of his lecture was devoted to the possibilities of curing cancer, and he focused on the nonscientific factors. He asserted that most cancers were the result of environmental causes, chemicals and radiation, and that it was the responsibility of governments to reduce the incidence of cancer by eliminating those carcinogens. He urged scientists to maintain a social conscience, and he urged governments to strongly discourage the use of tobacco, which caused the highest proportion of cancers. He expressed the frustration of scientists attempting to cure cancer while "society merrily produces oncogenic substances and permeates the environment with them." Dulbecco later committed himself to studying breast cancer as a model human cancer, in hopes of finding a cure.

All three Nobelists stressed the importance of research into the environmental causes of cancer. They were convinced that environmental factors were more significant than viruses or other pathogens. In this regard, Baltimore had a clear view of himself as a public spokesman. "It's interesting, both Howard Temin and I, really independently, felt that, as people involved in cancer research, that we had to try and make it understood to the world that there were some very simple things you could do to decrease cancer. And that although we were trying to do some fairly complicated things, and ultimately trying to get at the basis of cancer, there was no reason to sit around waiting for that. There was a more obvious road to success. And I guess both of us felt that we had a certain responsibility to make that clear, and to spend some time on it."

Baltimore later took part in a high-profile antismoking campaign by the American Cancer Society. Temin, too, strongly opposed smoking—so strongly that, according to one account, on receiving the Nobel award from King Carl, he turned to the crowd and virulently chastised the members of the audience who were smoking, including the queen of Denmark. In truth, there is no opportunity to say anything when the king hands you the Nobel Prize; everything is ceremonially silent. The story was jumbled in the press. It even appeared in Temin's *New York Times* obituary. Temin did in fact speak against smoking at the Nobel dinner later that evening, where each Nobel Prize is entitled to a two-minute speech. There he spoke against the environmental causes of cancer and admonished the smokers present. The queen of Denmark, the consort of King Carl, was smoking at her table.

CAMBRIDGE FEARS

The recombinant DNA controversy was growing in public and government arenas. Baltimore's unique qualifications as one of the organizers of Asilomar and a Nobel laureate placed him in a critical position in the biological community. His plan for a sabbatical year doing solitary research was shelved.

In early spring 1976, the Cambridge City Council, led by Mayor Alfred Vellucci, proposed a moratorium on genetic engineering research within the Cambridge city limits, which would effectively shut down labs at both MIT and Harvard. Relations between the universities and the city had always been strained; from time to time Vellucci threatened to turn Harvard Yard into a parking lot. With Harvard planning on building a high-hazard-level recombinant DNA facility, the Cambridge City Council was extremely concerned. Vellucci declared, "It's about time the scientists began to throw all their goddamned shit right out on the table so that we can discuss it." Until Vellucci could be convinced otherwise, recombinant DNA work in Cambridge was postponed.

Scientists from the two universities were summoned before the city council to discuss the safety of genetic engineering. Baltimore was heavily involved, as were a number of biologists in the area on both sides of the issue. *Science* described the Cambridge City Council hearings as an "interesting phenomenon of a 'public' debate on recombinant DNA that really amount[ed] to a debate between two scientific camps slugging it out in public." Baltimore went before the city council on June 23, defending genetic engineering research and attempting to prevent the Mayor's proposed ban. Mark Ptashne of Harvard also testified, stressing that "no known dangerous organism has ever been produced" by recombinant DNA. To this a city councilor shot back, "Just what the hell do you think you're gonna do if you *do* produce one?" No one would give an inch. Mayor Vellucci declared, "I have learned enough about recombinant DNA molecules in the past few weeks to take on all the Nobel Prize winners in the city of Cambridge!" Vellucci even wrote a letter to the president of the National Academy of Sciences:

> In today's edition of the *Boston Herald American* . . . there are two reports which concern me greatly. In Dover, MA, a "strange, orange-eyed creature" was sighted and in Hollis, New Hampshire, a man and his two sons were confronted by a "hairy, nine foot creature."
>
> I would respectfully ask that your prestigious institution investigate these findings. I would hope as well that you might check to see whether or not these "strange creatures" (should they in fact exist) are in any way connected to recombinant DNA experiments taking place in the New England area.
>
> Thank you in advance for your cooperation in this matter.

Things were getting out of hand, and Baltimore was getting a taste of real politics: "The recombinant DNA debates really were a watershed, because we learned—I at least learned—for the first time what it meant to be in real politics, not just in intellectual commentary on politics, which is much of what we were doing in the period of the Vietnam War. And so, when we had to come up against Mayor Vellucci in Cambridge it was a wholly different view of politics, and I began to understand what the word politics meant. And it's messy, and it's really not a world for intellectuals," he smiled, "who are used to thinking of things in much clearer terms, and much less emotional terms."

National public concern about genetic engineering continued to increase, and in 1976 President Ford and Congress established a Federal Interagency Committee on Recombinant DNA Research. Functioning much like a presidential commission, it was charged with analyzing the problems posed by recombinant DNA. The committee was led by Donald Fredrickson, head of the National Institutes of Health (NIH). Senator Edward Kennedy held the first congressional hearings on the subject in mid-1976. This was a critical turn; many scientists felt seriously threatened by such inquiries. They were afraid that if outside regulation began, the government might shut down recombinant DNA research and also react to other issues that were potentially hazardous, such as the handling of tumor viruses. In 1884, Louis Pasteur's neighbors tried to shut down his new laboratory, claiming that it could create "a horrible plague impossible to imagine." If they had succeeded, Pasteur might not have developed the rabies vaccine. Baltimore and others saw amazing promise in recombinant DNA techniques, and they had no intention of allowing their hands to be tied by outside regulators.

Baltimore was concerned about the political reaction to the situation: "I think that we had a responsibility to do it [bring up the concerns and make them public], and I don't see how we could have avoided that responsibility. But we haven't provided what we wanted to provide, which was a smooth transition from a kind of laissez-faire policy in science to a rational evaluation of hazards. . . . I think the situation has escalated to the point where it's an inappropriate response." Protesters disrupted a National Academy of Sciences meeting with a giant poster stating: "We will create the perfect race—Adolf Hitler, 1933." In the face of this overwrought response, prominent molecular biologists organized a highly effective informal congressional lobbying group. Given his prominence as a Nobelist, Baltimore's opinions carried substantial weight among congressional representatives at private lunches and public hearings. On September 22, 1976, on one of several trips to Washington to try and keep the government out of scientific regulation, Baltimore testified before the Kennedy Committee. At that hearing, the members of the Asilomar organizing committee convinced the Kennedy Committee to let the NIH guidelines regulate recombinant DNA research. However, Kennedy announced later that he would continue to pursue regulatory legislation, in large part because of widespread public concern and the lobbying efforts of public interest groups. The opponents of the NIH guidelines were mainly organizations like Science for the People, consumer groups led by Jeremy Rifkin, and environmental groups such as the Environmental Defense Fund and Friends of the Earth.

In April 1977, Kennedy introduced three bills to regulate recombinant DNA research and held a new hearing on recombinant DNA hazards. A lawyer for the National Resources Defense Council testified, "It needs emphasis that wise exploration of the effects of novel substances prior to their distribution to individuals, or release into the environment, might have averted serious and sometimes tragic effects. One thinks, for example, of DES, thalidomide, DDT, asbestos, etcetera." Later the same lawyer brought up the specters of nuclear fission and the Andromeda Strain. Jeremy Rifkin and Massachusetts governor Michael Dukakis also testified, making similar references to the atomic bomb and the dangers of technology.

Scientists at the hearing responded that those fears were based on hysteria, not on a scientific understanding of the issues. Scientists had a comfortable monopoly on understanding recombinant DNA. That knowledge commanded respect.

The opponents of recombinant DNA argued that outside regulation was essential, reviving Jonathan King's analogy that having biologists regulate recombinant DNA research was like letting GM regulate automobile safety. It was an issue of accountability. Scientists defused this argument in the Kennedy hearing, and in private conversations with representatives, by pointing out that they had implemented a moratorium on recombinant DNA research and developed regulations by themselves.

The Interagency Commission on Recombinant DNA presented its views at Kennedy's hearing as well. Donald Fredrickson, as head of the NIH, gave a lengthy statement supporting Kennedy's legislative proposals to set up a new recombinant DNA regulatory board that would have a majority of nonscientists on it. Fredrickson was a doctor, not a scientist. Norton Zinder protested: "I can't believe that I was here just six months ago, when we agreed to use the NIH guidelines, and now you want to do something different. Give the guidelines a chance!" Zinder hammered home the point that biologists had recognized a threat and responded by developing the NIH guidelines. He assured Senator Kennedy that scientists could govern themselves. Behind the scenes, Baltimore and other scientists did the same.

Several other recombinant DNA regulatory bills were introduced in Congress in 1977, one in the House Committee on Interstate and Foreign Commerce, one in the House Committee on Science and Technology, and one in the Senate Committee on Commerce, Science, and Transportation. The Senate committee held hearings similar to the Kennedy Committee hearings. There, Philip Handler, president of the National Academy of Sciences, testified that the NIH guidelines had been established in a timely, informed, and respectable manner, and that the government had no reason to interfere with them. He lectured the senators on the promise of recombinant DNA. He showed them a chart listing every known genetic disease and pronounced that recombinant DNA had the potential to cure all of them by gene therapy—replacing the bad genes with good genes. He then warned the senators that if recombinant DNA guidelines were written into law, it would be very difficult to change the law to allow promising new DNA technologies to be used as they emerged. The NIH Committee was already having difficulties keeping pace with the changes.

Back in Cambridge, after months of haggling, Baltimore and numerous other professors managed to convince Mayor Vellucci to let a panel of Cambridge citizens decide the fate of recombinant DNA research at Harvard and MIT. In this experiment in democracy, the professors spent hours with the members of the panel explaining DNA, viruses, restriction enzymes, and cancer-causing genes in an effort to convince them that the scientists were making an honest assessment of the dangers. The citizen panel recommended a moratorium only on the most dangerous recombinant DNA experiments (those involving the kinds of agents used in biological warfare), a restriction to which MIT and Harvard completely agreed. The day the ban was lifted, Baltimore's lab raced to clone the genes of several viruses.

The national public relations campaign lasted longer. Scientists used every resource available to settle public fears about recombinant DNA. Baltimore even wrote an article for *TV Guide* in 1976 defending recombinant DNA. The article was crammed onto a back page, amid a series of glamour photos of the supermodel Lauren Hutton. In the end, no recombinant DNA federal legislation was even brought to a vote. All of it was stalemated by the scientists. The only regulations in place were the NIH regulations drafted by the Asilomar committee.

As the years passed, Baltimore saw recombinant DNA as less and less dangerous. "There were times there when we realized what we had let loose, when we said, 'Jesus, maybe we were wrong in letting it loose.' And it's only now that everything had calmed down and that we can look with perspective and say, 'No, I think we were right . . . ' It took up just an incredible amount of our time and energy, and . . . it was emotionally draining." Baltimore and the rest of the scientists who originally brought up the issue were convinced that recombinant DNA work was safe. They had learned a lot about bacteria and viruses. The strains of *E. coli* used in modern biology had adapted to life on petri plates and lost their ability to survive in the human colon, rendering them completely innocuous. The scientists also decided that viruses were too specialized to pose a problem. In addition, they encountered massive biological barriers to inserting genes into mammalian cells, let alone getting genes to do anything harmful once they were inserted. The use of recombinant DNA was growing exponentially, with new applications appearing as rapidly as scientists could think of them; it was becoming an almost mandatory technique in biological research. To encourage the growth of biology, Baltimore felt that it was essential for scientists to have maximum access to recombinant DNA techniques, which meant to him that the NIH safety requirements, virtually unchanged since the Asilomar committee's initial document, needed to be relaxed. With this in mind, Baltimore joined the Recombinant DNA Advisory Committee at the NIH in 1979. By the time he left the NIH committee in 1982, the guidelines no longer regulated 95 percent of the recombinant DNA research in the United States. When it was clear that none of the nightmare scenarios would be realized, Baltimore could look back on Asilomar and the years that followed and note what happened: "It was a learning process. . . . It was partly a matter of experiment and partly of thinking things through. It took time. And I think it has served the public and the scientific community extremely well, that we were the ones to call for a moratorium, not some politicians. Therefore we took the tempo of the situation. We couldn't control it completely, God knows! But at least we were there in the beginning. And that really, I think, gave us a lot of credibility. Still does."

Baltimore's views on genetic engineering and recombinant DNA evolved a great deal as new information became available and as scientists found themselves publicly defending their intellectual territory. By the early 1980s, the debate had shifted entirely away from safety issues to the question of whether various genetic engineering experiments should be restricted for ethical reasons, and these questions began to come before the NIH Recombinant DNA Advisory Committee. Baltimore didn't want much to do with those messy problems. A 1983 interview with Baltimore on the ethical implications of recombinant DNA research illustrated his now consistent stance for minimal control of scientific research:

> What this all boils down to is that we don't live in a perfect world. If scientists want to be active participants in that world, then we have to have a fundamental belief that the interplay of forces within the society will, at a minimum, not be disastrous.
>
> Personally, I feel that scientists really have only two choices: Either stop doing science entirely or take the risk that your work will be misused. Science finds what it finds and hands that over to society. It's up to the society to use it intelligently. Scientists can play a major role in interpreting and explaining their results, but in the end, we have consequences that are very unpleasant to us. That's the chance we take.

The results of recombinant DNA research have been extraordinary by any scientific or public measure, but those gains have only just begun to be realized. Twenty-five years from now they will have far surpassed atomic energy in cultural significance and medical and economic value. In Baltimore's opinion, atomic energy on one hand brought "a certain fear of atomic explosion, and on the other hand, an alternative form of energy. [That] is . . . just really an increase in style, but not really an increase in a qualitative sense in our lives." Recombinant DNA biotechnology is different. Human insulin is now mass-produced inexpensively by giant vats of bacteria in biotechnology companies. Valuable growth hormones, blood clotting factors, and blood proteins are similarly cultivated. The major hepatitis B vaccine was developed using recombinant DNA, and if there is ever an HIV vaccine, it will be based on recombinant DNA technology. New plant strains have been developed, generating fruits that don't freeze, firm tomatoes, higher-yielding grains, more nutritious rice, and better cotton. In strictly biomedical terms, new medical tests have been developed and genetic factors identified for diseases such as cystic fibrosis, breast cancer, Alzheimer's disease, some infertility conditions, Huntington's disease, and spinal muscular atrophy. The first successful gene therapy to treat a human genetic disease has recently become a reality. In fundamental research the return has been phenomenal, impossible to quantify. The ability to isolate single genes has revolutionized biology research: cancer genes, viral genes, immune system genes, transcription genes, cell-to-cell signaling genes, hormone receptor genes, structural protein genes, brain genes.

The fanfare of the Nobel Prize and the battles of the recombinant DNA controversy didn't stop Baltimore's research. In fact, things moved faster than ever. His lab grew from five students and postdocs in 1970 to fifteen in 1978. The growth of a laboratory is a curious process. Researchers contact a professor and request to join his or her lab. However, there are only a few positions available, and as the reputation of a professor grows, the pressure to accept more researchers increases, as does the talent of the applicants. If a professor increases the size of her lab, she has to increase the lab's funding, decrease the amount of lab space allocated to each researcher, and reassess the time she has available to mentor all of the students.

Running a laboratory is not easy. Many scientists with great hands or brilliant ideas fail at leading a research group. When Paul Berg was asked in 1997 what he considered Baltimore's greatest scientific accomplishment, he replied:

> In the long run, his influence has been through the people he's trained. In the course of doing that, of course, they all did some terrific science. But, you know, science has a tendency to fade after a while. What you think was so critically important in one time becomes old hat five years from now. . . . Is reverse transcriptase Dave's monument? I don't think so. . . . He's influenced a lot of people, and he's inculcated them with a style, a rigor, a way to do science, which I think has got to be seen as a very significant accomplishment.

Berg then added with a laugh, "And the science is sort of a freebie." Baltimore has trained what must be viewed as a school of biologists. Great virologists, immunologists, cancer biologists, and molecular biologists have all come out of his lab. Dozens of his students are now professors at major universities, and four are already members of the exclusive National Academy of Sciences.

Baltimore taught these people very clear lessons in how to do science and run their own labs. Inder Verma, a Baltimore postdoc who is now a professor of gene therapy at the Salk Institute, recalled, "The model was clear: You do the best science you can do, and good people [in the lab] will work hard. Bad people won't work anyway, so why waste your time? Give people their freedom. You are not a taskmaster, you are not a nanny, you are not a policeman. You just create an atmosphere where people can work." Verma found that out when he succeeded at the first cDNA synthesis experiments while Baltimore was out of town: "He wasn't originally involved in it, but, you know, David has an influence." Part of that influence was Baltimore's ability to analyze data: "I mean, he can look at your data [and see] more things than you can, which was, of course, as a student, very annoying; because you worked so hard to do the experiment, and then he comes and tells you things you should have known, and [you] missed. . . . David certainly was arrogant. He was more clever than you, and he made it clear to you." This was how David pushed his students toward excellence. And his students attested that Baltimore's arrogance was not oppressive; he encouraged people to challenge him, which gave the lab an open atmosphere.

As his lab grew, Baltimore sought out new questions. How did viral proteins allow a retrovirus to wreak havoc with the growth of cells, sending them into the vicious cycle of cancer? Cancer weighed more and more on his mind. How did it happen? What did it do to cells at the molecular level? He redirected part of his lab to study the molecular nature of cancer. Viruses were exciting, but he had been working on them for over a decade, and ultimately his interest in viruses had come from his belief that they were the best way to understand human cells. Now, with the tools of recombinant DNA, Baltimore could begin to study animal cells directly.

The in vitro and cell culture experiments he had concentrated on for years were not the right framework for dealing with cancer. Cancer needed to be studied in a living system. The most obvious choice was chickens. Howard Temin had worked with chickens for most of his career, as had many cancer researchers, and they were the best-understood model for cancer studies. Cancer-causing retroviruses of chickens, including Rous sarcoma virus, were well-known. People had virus stocks that caused consistent, obvious, and rapid cancers in chickens. It takes a long time to develop an organism as an experimental model, and that groundwork had been done on chickens.

But Baltimore didn't want to work with chickens; he just didn't like them. He imagined smelly, flapping birds, with feathers all over the lab. So he looked at other possibilities and decided on mice: "It's interesting, I never really thought about it at the time. I just said, 'mouse,' and there it was. It seemed right and I followed it." A huge amount of genetics work had been done in mice in labs around the world, and at Jackson Lab in particular. Since the 1950s, a series of scientists had studied cancer-causing viruses in mice. However, there were no mouse retroviruses that were known to cause cancer rapidly. Baltimore wanted a virus that would make it possible to carry out quick experiments in mice and perhaps even in cell culture, one that would cut down on the time spent waiting for the cancer to develop. After a lot of work, Baltimore's lab finally developed a mouse leukemia virus, the Moloney strain, but it caused a slow leukemia, and he decided against working with it much.

Around 1973, Herbert Abelson came to MIT. A young physician who had stayed out of the Vietnam War by signing up with the Public Health Service, he had been working at the NIH for several years. Given the military draft, entry into that program was amazingly competitive, and only the best physicians were admitted. Those doctors were then trained as scientists at the NIH. Abelson had been working on leukemia viruses in mice. As a pediatrician, he was interested in leukemias because they are a common childhood cancer. For one experiment, Abelson took a Moloney virus, which was known to cause a cancer of the thymus, and asked the straightforward question, "What happens if you take out the thymus? What will the virus do then?" He ran the experiment in mice and discovered that one animal out of over one hundred he tested developed a bone cancer. The cancer infected the bone marrow of the skull so profoundly that it caused the skull to bulge. This was odd, because Moloney wasn't supposed to cause bone cancer. Curious, he took those leukemia cells out of the animal, purified the virus, and injected it into another animal. The animal developed the same bone marrow cancer. Abelson realized that he had developed a new virus; the original Moloney virus had mutated somehow so that it now infected bone marrow cells. He had created Abelson virus. Though uncommon, creating a new virus was not unheard-of; Rous sarcoma virus was another famous example of the extraordinary ability of viruses to evolve.

What was Abelson to do with this new creature? He was not a virologist, so when he left the NIH after his service time was completed and came to MIT, he contacted David Baltimore. Abelson knew about the reverse transcriptase work, and he thought perhaps Baltimore would be interested in Abelson virus. Baltimore was very interested.

Baltimore took on a new postdoc, Naomi Rosenberg, in 1974, and recommended that she work on developing the Abelson virus. He knew that one of Abelson's colleagues, Charles Scher, who was working at the Children's Hospital Medical Center associated with Harvard Medical School, was attempting to develop the potential of Abelson virus to infect cultured mouse skin cells. Baltimore was interested in Scher's work, but he really needed Abelson virus to transform lymphoid cells—bone marrow and blood cells. So Rosenberg and Scher set about developing a strain of Abelson virus that could transform cultured lymphoid cells. In autumn 1974, Scher succeeded in transforming skin cells, and several months later Rosenberg succeeded in transforming lymphoid cells. Baltimore had what he wanted now: a rapidly transforming cancer virus in mice. It even transformed cultured cells, making the cancer accessible to detailed laboratory study. The mouse was now a viable system for intensive cancer studies using a retrovirus. Since the virus infected blood cells that are a major component of the immune system, Abelson virus was also a viable system for studying the immune system—yet another major accomplishment for Baltimore. A new model was created. In the coming years, hundreds of papers on cancer-causing mouse retroviruses would be published that would help propel the fields of cancer biology, immunology, and retrovirology.

"He has an almost uncanny ability to pick the right problem," said Owen Witte, a former postdoc of Baltimore's. Again and again, Baltimore pushed the problem-solving limits of molecular biology. There are two kinds of great experimenters: those who identify a critical path and run swiftly along that path, posting signs pointing to major landmarks; and those who innovate to leap across chasms where other scientists have fallen. In his early polio work, and in his reverse transcriptase work, Baltimore had run quickly. Now, with the creation of a rapid retroviral lymphoid cancer model in mice, he proved his ability to innovate.

The mouse work grew vigorously, both inside and outside his lab. With Abelson virus, Baltimore's cancer interests gradually merged with a newfound interest in the immune system, as immunology was quickly becoming the hottest field in biology.

POLIOVIRUS

An Interlude

ONCE THE CAMBRIDGE BAN on recombinant DNA was lifted, one of the first pieces of DNA that the Baltimore laboratory cloned was the poliovirus genome. This work was done by Vincent Racaniello, a postdoctoral fellow in the lab. Since poliovirus is an RNA virus, Racaniello first made a DNA copy (cDNA) of the poliovirus RNA using reverse transcriptase. He then pasted the poliovirus DNA copy into a plasmid using the recently developed recombinant DNA cloning techniques. He used a new DNA sequencing technique developed by Frederick Sanger (who won his second Nobel Prize in chemistry in 1980 for this powerful technology) to determine the entire genetic sequence of poliovirus.* The poliovirus genome was published in early 1981. This is all of the information necessary to create poliovirus:

TTAAAACAGCTCTGGGGTTGTACCCACCCCAGAGGCCCACGTGGCGGCTAGTACTCCGGTAT
TGCGGTACCCTTGTACGCCTGTTTTATACTCCCTTCCCGTAACTTAGACGCACAAAACCAAGTT
CAATAGAAGGGGGTACAAACCAGTACCACCACGAACAAGCACTTCTGTTTCCCCGGTGATGTCG
TATAGACTGCTTGCGTGGTTGAAAGCGACGGATCCGTTATCCGCTTATGTACTTCGAGAAGCC

---

*Sanger won his first Nobel Prize in chemistry in 1958. The 1980 Nobel Prize in chemistry was shared by Sanger, Walter Gilbert, and Paul Berg. Gilbert developed a different DNA sequencing technique. Berg's award was for his contributions to recombinant DNA technology.

CAGTACCACCTCGGAATCTTCGATGCGTTGCGCTCAGCACTCAACCCCAGAGTGTAGCTTAG
GCTGATGAGTCTGGACATCCCTCACCGGTGACGGTGGTCCAGGCTGCGTTGGCGGCCTAC
CTATGGCTAACGCCATGGGACGCTAGTTGTGAACAAGGTGTGAAGAGCCTATTGAGCTACATAA
GAATCCTCCGGCCCCTGAATGCGGCTAATCCCAACCTCGGAGCAGGTGGTCACAAACCAGT
GATTGGCCTGTCGTAACGCGCAAGTCCGTGGCGGAACCGACTACTTTGGGTGTCCGTGTTTCC
TTTTATTTTATTGTGGCTGCTTATGGTGACAATCACAGATTGTTATCATAAAGCGAATTGGATTG
GCCATCCGGTGAAAGTGAGACTCATTATCTATCTGTTTGCTGGATCCGCTCCATTGAGTGTGTT
TACTCTAAGTACAATTTCAACAGTTATTTCAATCAGACAATTGTATCATAATGGGTGCTCAGGTT
TCATCACAGAAAGTGGGCGCACATGAAAACTCAAATAGAGCGTATGGTGGTTCTACCATTAAT
TACACCACCATTAATTATTATAGAGATTCAGCTAGTAACGCGGCTTCGAAACAGGACTTCTCTCAA
GACCCTTCCAAGTTCACCGAGCCCATCAAGGATGTCCTGATAAAAACAGCCCCAATGCTAAACT
CGCCAAACATAGAGGCTTGCGGGTATAGCGATAGAGTACTGCAATTAACACTGGGAAACTCCAC
TATAACCACACAGGAGGCGGCTAATTCAGTAGTCGCTTATGGGCGTTGGCCTGAATATCTGAGG
GACAGCGAAGCCAATCCAGTGGACCAGCCGACAGAACCAGACGTCGCTGCATGCAGGTTT
TATACGCTAGACACCGTGTCTTGGACGAAAGAGTCGCGAGGGTGGTGGTGGAAGTTGCCTG
ATGCACTGAGGGACATGGGACTCTTTGGGCAAAATATGTACTACCACTACCTAGGTAGGTCCGGG
TACACCGTGCATGTACAGTGTAACGCCTCCAAATTCCACCAGGGGGCACTAGGGGTATTCGC
CGTACCAGAGATGTGTCTGGCCGGGGATAGCAACACCACTACCATGCACACCAGCTATCAAAA
TGCCAATCCTGGCGAGAAAGGAGGCACTTTCACGGGTACGTTCACTCCTGACAACAACCAGA
CATCACCTGCCCGCAGGTTCTGCCCGGTGGATTACCTCCTTGGAAATGGCACGTTGTTGGGG
AATGCCTTTGTGTTCCCGCACCAGATAATAAACCTACGGACCAACAACTGTGCTACACTGGTACT
CCCTTACGTGAACTCCCTCTCGATAGATAGTATGGTAAAGCACAATAATTGGGGAATTGCAATAT
TACCATTGGCCCCATTAAATTTTGCTAGTGAGTCCTCCCCAGAGATTCCAATCACCTTGACCATAG
CCCCTATGTGCTGTGAGTTCAATGGATTAAGAAACATCACCCTGCCACGCTTACAGGGCCTG
CCGGTCATGAACACCCCTGGTAGCAATCAATATCTTACTGCAGACAACTTCCAGTCACCGTGTG
CGCTGCCTGAATTTGATGTGACCCCACCTATTGACATACCCGGTGAAGTAAAGAACATGATGG
AATTGGCAGAAATCGACACCATGATTCCCTTTGACTTAAGTGCCACAAAAAAGAACACCATGG
AAATGTATAGGGTTCGGTTAAGTGACAAACCACATACAGACGATCCCATACTCTGCCTGTCACT
CTCTCCAGCTTCAGATCCTAGGTTGTCACATACTATGCTTGGAGAAATCCTAAATTACTACACAC
ACTGGGCAGGATCCCTGAAGTTCACGTTTCTGTTCTGTGGATTCATGATGGCAACTGGCAAA
CTGTTGGTGTCATACGCGCCTCCTGGAGCCGACCCACCAAAGAAGCGTAAGGAGGCGATGTTG
GGAACACATGTGATCTGGGACATAGGACTGCAGTCCTCATGTACTATGGTAGTGCCATGGATTAG
CAACACCACGTATCGGCAAACCATAGATGATAGTTTCACCGAAGGCGGATACATCAGCGTCT
TCTACCAAACTAGAATAGTCGTCCCTCTTTCGACACCCAGAGAGATGGACATCCTTGGTTTTGTG
TCAGCGTGTAATGACTTCAGCGTGCGCTTGTTGCGAGATACCACACATATAGAGCAAAAAGCGC

TAGCACAGGGGTTAGGTCAGATGCTTGAAAGCATGATTGACAACACAGTCCGTGAAACGGTGG

GGGCGGCAACATCTAGAGACGCTCTCCCAAACACTGAAGCCAGTGGACCAACACACTCCAAG

GAAATTCCGGCACTCACCGCAGTGGAAACTGGGGCCACAAATCCACTAGTCCCTTCTGATACAG

TGCAAACCAGACATGTTGTACAACATAGGTCAAGGTCAGAGTCTAGCATAGAGTCTTTCTTCG

CGCGGGGTGCATGCGTGACCATTATGACCGTGGATAACCCAGCTTCCACCACGAATAAGGATAA

GCTATTTGCAGTGTGGAAGATCACTTATAAAGATACTGTCCAGTTACGGAGGAAATTGGAGTTC

TTCACCTATTCTAGATTTGATATGGAACTTACCTTTGTGGTTACTGCAAATTTCACTGAGACTAA

CAATGGGCATGCCTTAAATCAAGTGTACCAAATTATGTACGTACCACCAGGCGCTCCAGTGCC

CGAGAAATGGGACGACTACACATGGCAAACCTCATCAAATCCATCAATCTTTTACACCTACGG

AACAGCTCCAGCCCGGATCTCGGTACCGTATGTTGGTATTTCGAACGCCTATTCACACTTTTAC

GACGGTTTTTCCAAAGTACCACTGAAGGACCAGTCGGCAGCACTAGGTGACTCCCTTTATG

GTGCAGCATCTCTAAATGACTTCGGTATTTTGGCTGTTAGAGTAGTCAATGATCACAACCCGAC

CAAGGTCACCTCCAAAATCAGAGTGTATCTAAAACCCAAACACATCAGAGTCTGGTGCCCGCGT

CCACCGAGGGCAGTGGCGTACTACGGCCCTGGAGTGGATTACAAGGATGGTACGCTTACAC

CCCTCTCCACCAAGGATCTGACCACATATGGATTCGGACACCAAAACAAAGCGGTGTACACT

GCAGGTTACAAAATTTGCAACTACCACTTGGCCACTCAGGATGATTTGCAAAACGCAGTGAACG

TCATGTGGAGTAGAGACCTCTTAGTCACAGAATCAAGAGCCCAGGGCACCGATTCAATCGCAAG

GTGCAATTGCAACGCAGGGGTGTACTACTGCGAGTCTAGAAGGAAATACTACCCAGTATCCTTCG

TTGGCCCAACGTTCCAGTACATGGAGGCTAATAACTATTACCCAGCTAGGTACCAGTCCCATAT

GCTCATTGGCCATGGATTCGCATCTCCAGGGGATTGTGGTGGCATACTCAGATGTCACCACGG

GGTGATAGGGATCATTACTGCTGGTGGCGAAGGGTTGGTTGCATTTTCAGACATTAGAGACTT

GTATGCCTACGAAGAAGAAGCCATGGAACAAGGCATCACCAATTACATAGAGTCACTTGGGGC

CGCATTTGGAAGTGGATTTACTCAGCAGATTAGCGACAAAATAACAGAGTTGACCAATATGGT

GACCAGTACCATCACTGAAAAGCTACTTAAGAACTTGATCAAGATCATATCCTCACTAGTTATTA

TAACTAGGAACTATGAAGACACCACAACAGTGCTCGCTACCCTGGCCCTTCTTGGGTGTGAT

GCTTCACCATGGCAGTGGCTTAGAAAGAAAGCATGCGATGTTCTGGAGATACCTTATGTCAT

CAAGCAAGGTGACAGTTGGTTGAAGAAGTTTACTGAAGCATGCAACGCAGCTAAGGGACTG

GAGTGGGTGTCAAACAAATCTCAAAATTCATTGATTGGCTCAAGGAGAAAATTATCCCACAAGCT

AGAGATAAGTTGGAATTTGTAACAAAACTTAGACAACTAGAAATGCTGGAAAACCAAATCTCAAC

TATACACCAATCATGCCCTAGTCAGGAACACCAGGAAATTCTATTCAATAATGTCAGATGGTTATCC

ATCCAGTCTAAGAGGTTTGCCCCTCTTTACGCAGTGGAAGCCAAAAGAATACAGAAACTAGAG

CATACTATTAACAACTACATCAGTTCAAGAGCAAACACCGTATTGAACCAGTATGTTTGCTAG

TACATGGCAGCCCCGGAACAGGTAAATCTGTAGCAACCAACCTGATTGCTAGAGCCATAGCTGA

AAGAGAAAACACGTCCACGTACTCGCTACCCCCGGATCCATCACACTTCGACGGATACAAA

CAACAGGGAGTGGTGATTATGGACGACCTGAATCAAAACCCAGATGGTGCGGACATGAAGCT

GTTCTGTCAGATGGTATCAACAGTGGAGTTTATACCACCCATGGCATCCCTGGAGGAGAAAG
GAATCCTGTTTACTTCAAATTACGTTCTAGCATCCACAAACTCAAGCAGAATTTCCCCCCCCAC
TGTGGCACACAGTGATGCATTAGCCAGGCGCTTTGCGTTCGACATGGACATTCAGGTCATGAAT
GAGTATTCTAGAGATGGGAAATTGAACATGGCCATGGCTACTGAAATGTGTAAGAACTGTCACC
AACCAGCAAACTTTAAGAGATGCTGTCCTTTAGTGTGTGGTAAGGCAATTCAATTAATGGACA
AATCTTCCAGAGTTAGATACAGTATTGACCAGATCACTACAATGATTATCAATGAGAGAAACAGA
AGATCCAACATTGGCAATTGTATGGAGGCTTTGTTTCAAGGACCACTCCAGTATAAAGACTTGA
AAATTGACATCAAGACGAGTCCCCCTCCTGAATGTATCAATGACTTGCTCCAAGCAGTTGACTCC
CAGGAGGTGAGAGATTACTGTGAGAAGAAGGGGTTGGATAGTCAACATCACCAGCCAGGTTCA
AACAGAAAGGAACATCAACAGGGCAATGACAATTCTACAAGCGGTGACAACCTTCGCCGCA
GTGGCTGGAGTTGTCTATGTCATGTATAAACTGTTTGCTGGACACCAGGGAGCATACACTGGTT
TACCAAACAAAAAACCCAACGTGCCCACCATTCGGACAGCAAAGGTACAAGGACCAGGGTTC
GATTACGCAGTGGCTATGGCTAAAAGAAACATTGTTACAGCAACTACTAGCAAGGGAGAGTTCA
CTATGTTAGGAGTCCACGACAACGTGGCTATTTTACCAACCCACGCTTCACCTGGTGAAAGCA
TTGTGATCGATGGCAAAGAAGTGGAGATCTTGGATGCCAAAGCGCTCGAAGATCAAGCAGGA
ACCAATCTTGAAATCACTATAATCACTCTAAAGAGAAATGAAAAGTTCAGAGACATTAGACCACA
TATACCTACTCAAATCACTGAGACAAATGATGGAGTCTTGATCGTGAACACTAGCAAGTACCCC
AATATGTATGTTCCTGTCGGTGCTGTGACTGAACAGGGATATCTAAATCTCGGTGGGCGCCAAAC
TGCTCGTACTCTAATGTACAACTTTCCAACCAGAGCAGGACAGTGTGGTGGAGTCATCACATGT
ACTGGGAAAGTCATCGGGATGCATGTTGGTGGGAACGGTTCACACGGGTTTGCAGCGGCCC
TGAAGCGATCATACTTCACTCAGAGTCAAGGTGAAATCCAGTGGATGAGACCTTCGAAGGAAGT
GGGATATCCAATCATAAATGCCCCGTCCAAAACCAAGCTTGAACCCAGTGCTTTCCACTATGTG
TTTGAAGGGGTGAAGGAACCAGCAGTCCTCACTAAAAACGATCCCAGGCTTAAGACAGACTTT
GAGGAGGCAATTTTCTCCAAGTACGTGGGTAACAAAATTACTGAAGTGGATGAGTACATGAAAG
AGGCAGTAGACCACTATGCTGGCCAGCTCATGTCACTAGACATCAACACAGAACAAATGTGCTTG
GAGGATGCCATGTATGGCACTGATGGTCTAGAAGCACTTGATTTGTCCACCAGTGCTGGCTACC
CTTATGTAGCAATGGGAAAGAAGAAGAGAGACATCTTGAACAAACAAACCAGAGACACTAAGG
AAATGCAAAAACTGCTCGACACACATGGAATCAACCTCCCACTGGTGACTTATGTAAAGGATG
AACTTAGATCCAAAACAAAGGTTGAGCAGGGGAAATCCAGATTAATTGAAGCTTCTAGTTTGAAT
GACTCAGTGGCAATGAGAATGGCTTTTGGGAACCTATATGCTGCTTTTCACAAAAACCCAGGAG
TGATAACAGGTTCAGCAGTGGGGTGCGATCCAGATTTGTTTTGGAGCAAAATTCCGGTATTGAT
GGAAGAGAAGCTGTTTGCTTTTGACTACACAGGGTATGATGCATCTCTCAGCCCTGCTTGGTTC
GAGGCACTAAAGATGGTGCTTGAGAAAATCGGATTCGGAGACAGAGTTGACTACATCGACTAC
CTAAACCACTCACACCACCTGTACAAGAATAAAACATACTGTGTCAAGGGCGGTATGCCATCTG
GCTGCTCAGGCACTTCAATTTTTAACTCAATGATTAACAACTTGATTATCAGGACACTCTTACTGA

AAACCTACAAGGGCATAGATTTAGACCACCTAAAAATGATTGCCTATGGTGATGATGTAATTGCT
TCCTACCCCCATGAAGTTGACGCTAGTCTCCTAGCCCAATCAGGAAAAGACTATGGACTAAC
TATGACTCCAGCTGACAAATCAGCTACATTTGAAACAGTCACATGGGAGAATGTAACATTCTTGAA
GAGATTCTTCAGGGCAGACGAGAAATACCCATTTCTTATTCATCCAGTAATGCCAATGAAGGAAAT
TCATGAATCAATTAGATGGACTAAAGATCCTAGGAACACTCAGGATCACGTTCGCTCTCTGTGC
CTTTTAGCTTGGCACAATGGCGAAGAAGAATATAACAAATTCCTAGCTAAAATCAGGAGTGTGC
CAATTGGAAGAGCTTTATTGCTCCCAGAGTACTCAACATTGTACCGCCGTTGGCTTGACTCATTTT
AGTAACCCTACCTCAGTCGAATTGGATTGGGTCATACTGTTGTAGGGGTAAATTTTTCTTTAATTCG
GAGAAAAAAAAAAAAAAAAA

Eight

The test you will face is the toughest one imaginable:
can the published experiments be replicated by others and,
even more importantly, do your experiments provide a basis for
further scientific development? This is how we ascertain truth.

DAVID BALTIMORE
Testimony to congressional committee, May 1989

EDWIN "JACK" WHITEHEAD started a biomedical company called Technicon in 1939. Over the next forty years he led the company to success, and he sold Technicon to Revlon for $400 million in 1980. Whitehead, an energetic and persistent man, wanted to use some of his wealth to found a biomedical institute, and in 1974, with the help of his advisers, he began searching for a suitable location. The search was complicated. He commented many years later, "It's easier to make $100 million than to give it away." Several medical schools rejected his offer because Whitehead burdened the gift with too many special conditions: Duke University initially accepted, but then found the restrictions too cumbersome. Whitehead insisted that the research facility be set up as a company, for various tax and business reasons, and that the Whitehead Institute, not the university, would own the company. Jack Whitehead himself would thereby be able to maintain close control of the company and the institute. No university wanted to build a new institute that they couldn't control, and so no one would touch the money. After five years of frustration, Whitehead gave up and began exploring broader possibilities.

In August 1980, Whitehead's advisers suggested that he approach David Baltimore as a possible consultant for the philanthropic project. Baltimore had a history of rejecting such administrative proposals. He had been approached innumerable times to become a dean or department chair at various universities. He turned down all these offers because he knew that they would burden him with petty politics and the drudgery of fundraising. However, the Whitehead project had a very different flavor to it. Baltimore saw in it the possibility of starting an important institution for biological research. Baltimore agreed to meet Whitehead and his advisers at Rockefeller University, an obvious model for a new institute.

At Rockefeller, Whitehead asked Baltimore outright what he would do with a research institute if he had one. Baltimore said that he would focus it on the molecular aspects of development, because he felt that this was going to be the era of developmental biology, the study of the procession from fertilization to adult organism. Whitehead liked Baltimore's style. His energy and confidence were traits well suited to the director of an institute. In Whitehead's mind, the research challenges Baltimore outlined were the kind that could energize a research facility.

He invited Baltimore back a few days later and made an offer: if Baltimore agreed to design and establish the institute, Whitehead would provide $35 million for the building and an additional endowment of $100 million. No inherited administrative baggage, no fundraising, just pure opportunity. Baltimore was confident that he could maintain the momentum of his own laboratory while directing the Whitehead Institute, but he still hesitated, reluctant to commit himself. He knew the history of Whitehead's attempts in philanthropy, and he wasn't going to be stuck in a project with unreasonable special conditions. He also didn't want to leave MIT. Baltimore refused to commit to being the director of the institute until he knew where it was going to be located, what its specific focus would be, and which university it would be connected with. Whitehead agreed to the conditions, Baltimore signed on as a consultant, and they became good friends.

Baltimore began formulating plans, drawing on his past experience with various universities and institutes. He immediately decided to try to establish the institute at MIT. The Whitehead Institute wouldn't have the intellectual critical mass necessary to survive on its own. Baltimore viewed MIT as a down-to-earth, honest institution, and he was comfortable there. He also felt that the university focused on research and did it well. He wanted to establish a viable research community, much as Cyrus Levinthal had done with the MIT biology department and Salvador Luria had done with the Center for Cancer Research. Baltimore set his goal:

It was a consciously very simple, conservative goal. I wasn't out to do something brand new; although, it turned out to be brand new, but that wasn't what I was out to do. I just wanted to do very good science along the lines that I saw science developing in the next ten years. I wanted to get people who were going to be important to the next ten years of science. And the developmental biology rubric was in the air. It was just what was going to happen. Everybody knew it.

Developmental biology involved the hunt for the genes and the mechanisms that determined left or right, up or down, arm or leg, heart or lungs, eye or antennae in a maturing organism. There is a famous *Drosophila* fruit fly mutation named aristopedia, in which a pair of legs grow out of the fly's head. Therein lie the fascinating and often grotesque complications of developmental biology.

Baltimore wanted the Whitehead Institute to be a self-governing research institute with independent professors and researchers, but one that also had access to the resources of MIT. His proposal met strong resistance among the MIT faculty. They worried about where the loyalties of the Whitehead faculty would lie, and they were worried that the Whitehead might have commercial objectives. They knew that MIT worked well, and they didn't want to endanger it with a massive and complicated new component of the biology department. What would happen if Whitehead dropped his support five years down the road? What if the Whitehead faculty were not MIT caliber? For almost a year Baltimore worked, with the help of provost Jerome Weisner and biology chair Gene Brown, to convince MIT professors that the Whitehead Institute would be an asset. The faculty demanded compromises. For example, researchers would be jointly appointed by the Whitehead and MIT, thereby allowing MIT to control the quality of the faculty. Baltimore brought these issues to Jack Whitehead and, in the words of Weisner, "charmed him into making many concessions." With these compromises agreed to, the MIT faculty voted on November 18, 1981, to create the Whitehead Institute for Biomedical Research. The label "Biomedical Research" was a nod to Whitehead's earlier dream.

With that battle behind him, Baltimore began personally recruiting the Whitehead faculty. His reputation was impressive, his demeanor persuasive, his voice confident and convincing. The Whitehead Institute quickly developed from an extension of MIT in 1982 to a fully functional institute in 1984, complete with its $35 million building and two hundred people. It succeeded because it was well-organized. Baltimore took a strong interest in the work and well-being of the younger professors. Peter Kim, a biochemist, said that no grant application left the building until Baltimore had reviewed it: "I remember getting my first grant application back with red ink all over it." Richard Young, another recruit, said that Baltimore was "utterly unforgiving," but he "had a way of offering the most brutal criticism to young faculty and then going out of his way to have you out for a beer or over to his house, so you would know that it was not personal."

Under Baltimore's stewardship, the Whitehead Institute became "established as a centre of intellectual power in molecular biology," as *Nature* described it. When Jack Whitehead died in 1992, at the age of seventy-two, while playing squash, he had donated over $140 million to the institute, at that time one of the largest gifts to a single institution from a private donor. In 1992, ten years after its founding, the Whitehead Institute produced the most cited papers of any biological research institute. The MIT biology department ranked second, and together they far surpassed any other institution in the world.

A NEW INFECTIOUS DISEASE

A new and lethal retrovirus appeared in 1981, known by different people as lymphadenopathy-associated virus (LAV), human T-cell lymphotrophic virus type III (HTLV-III), AIDS-associated retrovirus (ARV), or the "gay plague." Baltimore learned about acquired immune deficiency syndrome a few months after the first cases were discovered in 1981. Diagnosis: The disease "induces slow and irreversible destruction of the patient's immune system, resulting in the inability of the patient to prevent devastation from rare infections, normally easy to ward off, now fatal." The existence of this new and feared disease caught Baltimore's attention. "As a virologist, the idea that there was a new infectious disease, and that it could be so devastating, was—intriguing. I followed it from a distance."

The initial identification of the acquired immune deficiency was complicated. AIDS apparently could lie dormant for years before symptoms developed, and they weren't consistent. Some patients contracted chronic, incurable pneumonia, whereas others contracted rare infections and infections never before witnessed: strange growths that, when analyzed by pathologists, revealed normally harmless bacteria or viruses. Why wasn't the body's immune system destroying them? Some patients died from bizarre forms of cancer, like the blotchy red Kaposi's sarcoma, rarely observed in non-AIDS patients. Once these symptoms were linked to the disease named AIDS, a flood of new cases was reported. The AIDS epidemic had begun.

At a scientific meeting early in 1982, researchers discussed the state of clinical knowledge, public health knowledge, and scientific knowledge about AIDS. Doctors were quickly improving at diagnosing the disease, but they could do nothing to stop it or even slow it down. They didn't even know how it was transmitted. On the public health side, the Centers for Disease Control knew the virus was spreading quickly, but they couldn't track it, and they couldn't explain why a large number of the cases were emerging from gay communities. On the scientific side, nothing was known. There was a hunch that the disease was caused by a virus. No one was yet calling it HIV, the human immunodeficiency virus. At the meeting, Baltimore encouraged Bob Gallo to try to find the virus for AIDS. Gallo was reluctant. After a ten-year search, he had finally discovered a virus that caused a human cancer, HTLV-I retrovirus, and his lab was deeply involved in studying it.* He didn't particularly want to turn his lab over to what he knew would be a very difficult search for the AIDS virus—if it was a virus at all. The future of AIDS research was uncertain.

ONCOGENES

Baltimore's lab was on the third floor of the Whitehead Institute. More students worked for him now than any other time in his career, swelling his lab to thirty researchers. Although he was Whitehead's director, he did not allow himself more lab space than anyone else. Benches were cramped, to say the least, but people were willing to live with the tight quarters in exchange for being exposed to some of the best science in the world. Keeping in touch with the experiments of all thirty students required all the efficiency he could muster. But, as he noted, "The nice thing about being in charge is that you can define your time. Everyone else responds to you. I could decide when meetings were held, and I could decide how I proportioned my time." He spent his days between the office and the lab.

Baltimore's group was large and diverse enough to require two separate group meetings: one for the immunology group, and another for the virus and cancer people (which was held jointly with Robert Weinberg's cancer lab). The lab would publish two hundred papers during Baltimore's eight years at the Whitehead, many of them focused on the molecular nature of cancer. The breakthroughs for understanding the genetic paradigm of cancer came in the 1970s, particularly with the 1976 isolation

*HTLV-I, human T-cell leukemia virus 1, causes a rare, contagious leukemia.

of *src* (pronounced "sarc"), the first cancer gene. It was called an "onco-gene" because of its ability to cause cancer. *Src* was discovered in Rous sarcoma virus by Harold Varmus and J. Michael Bishop. Surprisingly, Varmus and Bishop soon found cellular relatives of the *src* oncogene in humans, chickens, and even fruit flies; and they would win the Nobel Prize in 1989 for these discoveries. But if *src* caused cancer, what was it doing in normal human cells and bodies?

In 1978, the *src* protein was shown to be a protein kinase, an enzyme that modifies other proteins by adding an extra phosphate group, a scant five extra atoms, to certain amino acids on specific proteins in the cell. This was generally understood to be a mechanism for regulating signaling in the cell. For example, a protein with no attached phosphate group was "off," not signaling. Once a phosphate group was added to the protein, the protein was turned on, sending certain signals through the cell. What those signals were for, where they went, and their possible role in cancer were not clear. There was only one way to find out. The race was on to find more oncogenes. In 1980, Owen Witte in Baltimore's lab isolated the Abelson virus oncogene, *abl*, and showed that its protein product was a protein kinase, like *src*. Also in 1980, Owen Witte discovered that the *abl* protein added phosphate groups to the amino acid tyrosine, making the *abl* protein a new type of kinase, a tyrosine kinase. Simultaneously and independently, Tony Hunter at the Salk Institute showed that *src* was a tyrosine kinase.

The field of cancer research was electric with the discoveries. What was the difference between a cancer cell and a normal cell? A third oncogene, *ras*, which activates a kinase, became the protein that revealed the secret. In 1982, the DNA sequence of the *ras* gene in normal cells was contrasted with the DNA sequence of the *ras* gene in cancer cells by three different labs in a frantic race, and they showed that the dramatic difference was caused by a single change, a single mutation, in the DNA sequence of the *ras* gene. Part of the four-thousand-letter sequence of the *ras* gene in normal human cells is GGTGGTGGTGGGCGCCGGCGGT. The same part of the cancer-causing mutant *ras* oncogene is GGTGGTGGTGGGCGCCGTCGGT. (Did you miss it?) A one-letter change in the human molecular blueprint made the *ras* gene code for a protein with a valine amino acid instead of a glycine amino acid in one particular spot. A change of nine atoms somehow converted this normal protein into the cause of cancer. Those nine extra atoms short-circuited the protein into always being turned on.

A genetic theory of cancer fell into place. Oncogenes were normal human genes (often referred to as proto-oncogenes in their normal state), like *ras* and *src,* that were responsible for control of cell growth. Oncogenic growth hormones were found, along with oncogenic hormone receptors, oncogenic tyrosine kinases, and oncogenic transcription factors (proteins that bind to DNA and turn on the RNA transcription of certain genes by bringing RNA polymerase to the gene). Under normal circumstances, a growth hormone binds to a hormone receptor on a cell, turning on the receptor. That receptor then turns on other proteins inside the cell by adding a phosphate group to them. Those proteins, some of which are tyrosine kinases, activate other kinases, which activate still other kinases, propagating signals through the cell in complex patterns. The effect is like one of those large, improbable cascading contraptions in which a marble rolls down a ramp and hits the next marble, knocking it off a ledge and down a spiral slide and into the bucket of a balance, lifting a gate that releases the next marble, and so on; when a marble reaches the bottom, it hits a button that turns on a flashing neon sign. Except, in the cell, it turns on a gene that is part of the cell's program for growth. The whole pathway is crammed inside a cell and interconnected with a byzantine collection of other contraptions regulating the cell, which together orchestrate hundreds, if not thousands, of genes and proteins. *Abl,* the protein Baltimore's lab discovered, is one of the marbles. *Src* is another marble, *ras* a third. And people were finding more all the time as they discovered the complexities of the pathways controlling cell growth and replication.

With a crucial mutation, an oncogene becomes active all the time; it can no longer be turned off. The mutant marble is no longer dependent on the marbles above it; it is always pressing the button that turns on the neon sign. Before the mutation, the *ras* or *src* or *abl* protein was regulated by other proteins, which turned it on and off depending on whether the cell should replicate, but once it mutated it was turned on all the time, sending the constant signal: REPLICATE. Cancer is caused by good genes gone bad.

All kinds of cancer now began to make sense. Hereditary cancers were understandable: a person could inherit a mutant oncogene from a parent. However, it generally takes more than one mutant oncogene to cause cancer (cells have built-in redundancy to double-check errant proteins). Hereditary cancers are therefore said to "predispose" people to cancer: the mutant gene bypasses one of these checks and gets them one step closer to full-blown cancer. Cancer-causing viruses like Abelson virus appear to have kidnapped a cellular oncogene, *abl,* some time in the evolutionary past and changed it into a mutant cancer-causing form. The virus apparently carried this mutant oncogene so that it could wreak havoc in the cells it infected, screwing up their internal signaling pathways.

Consider skin cancer: ultraviolet light from the sun penetrates the skin, damaging the DNA in cells. Cells are exceptionally good at fixing the damage, but every once in a while they make a mistake in an oncogene, like the tyrosine kinase *abl*. The cell can sense when a tyrosine kinase like *abl* has mutated and is continuously active. So the cell uses a sophisticated self-destruct system to commit suicide so that the cancer cannot spread. But sometimes these safety mechanisms fail, and the *abl*-mutant cell begins to multiply uncontrollably. Cancer then crawls its way through the skin.

David's mother was dying of cancer. He still professed to be interested in biology research for the sake of pure knowledge: "I think all of us [cancer researchers] would say honestly that it's the normal processes of the cell that are our real concern." But he nevertheless found himself pondering the connections tying his work to his life. His dispassionate interest in HIV as a new, "intriguing" retrovirus became more personal as he contemplated the world in which his teenage daughter would live. His academic interest in cancer became strained as well. His father had possibly had cancer, and now his mother was succumbing to the disease. Her condition tore him apart. Over a two-year period her mind deteriorated. Cancer became a very personal enemy. But he refused to fool himself with hopes of magic bullets emerging from his oncogene research. In his 1986 speech at Massachusetts General Hospital, he said, "We must, I believe, answer that the problem is difficult and the solutions will come slowly and in a piecemeal fashion. . . . In my view, cancer is a problem that will be part of human life for a long time, if not forever."

The crux of the problem was clear: because oncogenic proteins were only slightly altered versions of their normal counterparts, it was extremely tough to develop therapies to identify and attack them while leaving the normal cells unharmed. Additionally, Baltimore noted, "The genetic properties of cancer cells are notoriously plastic, and it seems likely that while we are killing the cells that express a given oncogene, new oncogenes will appear." As Baltimore's lab worked furiously throughout the 1980s characterizing *abl* and analyzing its oncogenic potential, he harbored no hopes of saving his mother.

IMANISHI-KARI

Baltimore's curiosity about cell biology and immunology had grown rapidly after the discovery of Abelson virus. In the 1980s, nearly three-quarters of Baltimore's laboratory was dedicated to studies of genes expressed in the cells of the immune system. One of the more interesting immunology questions Baltimore pursued was antibody diversity. The genius of the immune system lies in its ability to store a huge library of different antibodies capable of detecting foreign molecules—so many antibodies that if each were a book, the library would fill a thousand Empire State Buildings. In 1981, as part of his ongoing efforts to characterize the antibody genes, Baltimore collaborated with Klaus Rajewsky's lab at the Institute of Genetics in Cologne, Germany. By then, Baltimore routinely collaborated with laboratories throughout the world. In 1981 alone he collaborated with the Gefter, Sharp, Eisen, and Weinberg labs at MIT, Marian Koshland's lab at UC Berkeley, the Rajewsky lab in Germany, and the Ruddle lab at Yale. Some of his most exciting discoveries were published in the joint papers resulting from these efforts. The collaboration with Rajewsky's lab was driven by one of Rajewsky's postdoctoral fellows, Thereza Imanishi-Kari, who had developed an important immunological system.

The immune system is made up of two general groups of cells, B-cells and T-cells. B-cells make antibodies. When human B-cells detect the presence of a natural antigen—a foreign substance or organism, such as a virus or bacterium—they multiply vigorously to mount a huge antibody response and destroy the invader. Imanishi-Kari and Baltimore were studying B-cells. Imanishi-Kari had developed a synthetic antigen that was potent enough to stimulate a vigorous and highly specific B-cell response in mice. If Imanishi-Kari gave her artificial antigen to ten different mice, they would all develop virtually the same antibodies. This allowed her to do reproducible experiments and characterize a variety of aspects of the antibody immune response.

As the result of collaborative work using Imanishi-Kari's antigen (called NP^b), Baltimore, Imanishi-Kari, and Rajewsky published a valuable paper on antibody diversity in the journal *Cell,* entitled "Heavy Chain Variable Region Contribution to the NP^b Family of Antibodies: Somatic Mutation Evident in a γ_{2a} Variable Region." At the time, perhaps a hundred scientists in the world could understand that baroque title. The question for molecular biology was how a small number of human genes (fewer than a dozen) could generate a trillion unique antibodies when normally one gene codes for only one protein. To be more specific, the genes generate antibodies with a trillion unique "idiotypes." An antibody is a protein shaped like a Y, and an antibody's idiotype is the unique shape of the arms of the Y, the ends of which bind to the antigen. If an antibody were a key, the idiotype would be the notches and grooves, and the antigen would be the keyhole.

Susumu Tonegawa, a senior member of MIT's Center for Cancer Research, would win the Nobel Prize in 1987 for his pioneering work in the mid-1970s determining the primary mechanism that generated antibody diversity: the few antibody genes are actually broken into dozens of interchangeable pieces that can shuffle around in any given B-cell to make vast combinations of novel genes (about a million) that form novel antibody idiotypes. Baltimore's 1981 *Cell* paper with Imanishi-Kari and Rajewsky helped show that an additional important factor generating antibody diversity was "somatic mutations"; that is, DNA mutations (for example, changing a G to an A in the DNA sequence) generated in different B-cells (which are a type of somatic cell) led to unique antibody genes. The mutations created antibodies with different idiotypes. By making lots of mutations in its antibody genes, each B-cell customized its antibody idiotype, so that it could attack the tuberculosis bacterium, poliovirus, the malaria parasite, or NP^b, Imanishi-Kari's antigen.

Besides the fact that this was the first time he collaborated with Imanishi-Kari, there was nothing about the research procedure that separated it from any of the hundreds of other papers Baltimore coauthored. The results of the research were exciting, and Baltimore and Rajewsky continued collaborative work on the project for a year, publishing another impressive paper on somatic mutations in *Nature.* Baltimore's lab did significant work in the early 1980s studying the creation of antibody diversity by the mechanisms of shuffling (the mechanism Tonegawa discovered), imprecise joining (in which the ends of the shuffled antibody gene fragments join imprecisely and create more diverse antibody possibilities), and somatic mutation (including the work with Imanishi-Kari and Rajewsky). These studies frequently used the tools of recombinant DNA technology and the Abelson virus, which infected B-cells and could change B-cell antibody production in ways that made it possible to study questions about antibody development that other laboratories couldn't approach.

By the summer of 1981, Thereza Imanishi-Kari had joined MIT as an assistant professor in the Center for Cancer Research. The professorship was offered independently of her association with Baltimore; he had never met her. When she was initially considering MIT's offer, she asked Rajewsky for advice, and he told her, "Well, MIT is a very competitive place. It's like a sea full of sharks, and they eat the little ones very fast." She came anyway. Imanishi-Kari was not afraid of sharks. She grew up in Brazil as the daughter of Japanese immigrants. After her sister ran away because her parents would not let her go to school, Thereza was allowed to attend high school and college. Her sister later died of the autoimmune disease lupus; and Thereza Imanishi-Kari became an immunologist in part to avenge her sister's death. Thereza went to Kyoto University, Japan, for graduate studies. Part way through, to escape the political riots on campus, she moved to Finland, where she developed her potent antigen. She continued to work with the antigen in Germany with Rajewsky. On her arrival at MIT, she set out to do mainly independent work, worried that collaborating with the senior faculty would dim her reputation as an independent scientist.

Susumu Tonegawa wanted to collaborate with Imanishi-Kari—badly. He knew that his lab could accomplish some powerful immunological research with a reagent Imanishi-Kari was developing to study T-cells, and so he suggested that they collaborate to use her reagent. His conditions were unacceptable to her, and she refused. This infuriated him, and, according to some colleagues, a huge argument ensued. They smashed glassware and screamed at each other in Japanese so loudly that nearby labs overheard.

Imanishi-Kari said Tonegawa was indeed furious, but the argument took place quietly in his office. Imanishi-Kari was not surprised by the emergence of the apocryphal story:

> Susumu can be *very* charming, but he can be very obnoxious too. There are lots of stories about Susumu. Poor Susumu. There are a lot of things that may be true, but a lot of it is this, "One person talks to another person talks to another person talks to another person." It gets bigger and bigger. It's so blown out of proportion. We never threw glass. I never yelled. I heard a story that he threw a chair at a technician! I mean, I heard *that* story from somebody in *California* who called me at MIT and asked me, "Did you see that!?" I mean, give me a break. . . . So, no, we didn't throw each other.

She added with a laugh, "But I bet I would beat him, because I was bigger than him!" Nevertheless, when Imanishi-Kari refused to collaborate with Tonegawa, he immediately set out to do competing T-cell experiments. And he refused to speak to her for two years. Despondent, Imanishi-Kari destroyed her T-cell reagents. She recalled, "I got very upset. I said, 'This is too much.' So I dumped everything [I was doing with T-cells]. It's hard enough to be at MIT without being in a fight with this guy. . . . I don't like fights; it's very uncomfortable. It's not worth it. But that's science. There are lots of people like that." After this incident, her reluctance to collaborate with senior faculty members became well known.

During the next two years, Baltimore's lab, largely through the work of the postdocs Rudolf Grosschedl and David Weaver, made great progress with their transgenic mice and their hybridomas used to study antibody idiotypes. Transgenic mice have altered DNA: researchers use recombinant DNA techniques to add or delete a gene from the mouse. Transgenic mice are used for a variety of experiments. One researcher at Osaka University made a transgenic mouse that fluoresces green all over: eyes, ears, skin, liver, brain.* Grosschedl and Weaver made transgenic mice with changes in their immune system: for example, in certain mice they added an extra antibody gene. They also used hybridomas, combinations of a normal B-cell with an immortal cell that result in a cell that continuously pumps out antibodies. Given their success in creating transgenic mice and hybridomas, Baltimore approached Imanishi-Kari in 1983. He explained their work and suggested that there were some real opportunities for her to study his transgenic mice and hybridomas, looking at issues of interest to them both. After some thought, she agreed.

David Weaver organized the collaborative work. Imanishi-Kari would handle the cell biology and antibody approaches to the problem, using hybridomas, and Weaver would take care of the molecular biology, analyzing the DNA and RNA. In 1985 they published one well-received paper in *Cell*, and in April 1986 Weaver, Imanishi-Kari, Moema Reis (Imanishi-Kari's postdoc), and Baltimore coauthored another *Cell* paper presenting evidence supporting a nontraditional model for the immune system response, known as the "network theory." This was a provocative immunological hypothesis developed by Niels Jerne that helped win him the 1984 Nobel Prize in medicine. The network theory proposed that antibodies could stimulate the creation of more, identical (or nearly identical) antibodies by first causing the formation of "anti-idiotypic" antibodies, which could then cause the creation of anti-anti-idiotypic antibodies that looked like the original antibodies. It follows the same principle as casting a mold. If you want to create a cast of your hand, first you make an imprint mold of your hand (in this analogy, an anti-hand). Then you cast a new hand (an anti-anti-hand) from the anti-hand mold. If the immune system could do the same trick, it could rapidly amplify its responses to pathogens.

*The green fluorescent mouse was just a test case, not an end in itself. The gene encoding the green fluorescent protein could be applied in other experiments: for example, it could be attached to an unknown mouse gene to help determine its function. If the mouse's brain subsequently glowed green, the researcher would know that the unknown gene (and the protein that the gene codes for) was some sort of brain gene.

The Weaver paper presented evidence that when a transgenic antibody gene (a nonnative antibody gene) was introduced into a mouse, the mouse started generating antibodies that looked like the transgenic antibody (had the idiotype of the transgenic antibody) but were apparently made by the mouse's native antibody genes. This was an extraordinary discovery, because it indicated that you could set off a sort of chain reaction inside an organism generating antibodies that mimicked each other. Over the next ten years, the paper, titled "Altered Repertoire of Endogenous Immunoglobin Gene Expression in Transgenic Mice Containing a Rearranged μ Heavy Chain Gene," escalated into the most famous scientific fraud controversy in the history of biology, a controversy pitting Nobel laureates against each other, throwing the U.S. Congress and the scientific community into a dogfight, generating seven different investigations, and creating hundreds of newspaper and magazine articles.

Shortly before the paper was published, Baltimore went on a wilderness fishing trip with Irving Weissman, an immunologist at Stanford. The two had been good friends since the early 1970s, when Baltimore's growing interest in immunology took him to many of the same conferences as Weissman. Weissman, who grew up in Montana, loved fishing, and he convinced Baltimore to come to Montana and give it a try. Weissman recalled, "He'd never fished before, but he picked it up fast." Montana immediately became Baltimore's favorite summertime retreat; he took his family fishing there nearly every year. Eventually Baltimore and Weissman jointly bought a Montana ranch outside Hamilton. They named it Cutthroat Ranch. They went fishing together several times every year, sometimes in Montana, sometimes in Alaska. They talked a lot of science on these trips, and Baltimore told Weissman about the lab's new antibody results on this particular trip in 1986. Weissman recalled saying, "God, David. Are you really going to get in to this immunology that's networks and idiotypes and anti-idiotypes and all this sort of stuff?" In Weissman's opinion, the data supporting the network theory was beginning to crumble, and immunologists were becoming critical of studies supporting the network theory. As Weissman recalled, "David was aware of [the negative atmosphere about network theory], and he was nervous about it, but they went ahead and published it," because, as Weissman remembered Baltimore replying, "There's the data. How can you get around the data?"

Margot O'Toole, a postdoc working in Imanishi-Kari's lab, was having difficulties with the results of the Weaver paper. She could not repeat one of the experiments that postdoc Moema Reis had completed with Imanishi-Kari. She had difficulty using the BET-1 reagent that Reis had used, and she didn't feel that it was trustworthy. The BET-1 reagent was a tag of sorts that identified transgenic antibodies but not the mouse's normal, endogenous, antibodies. Distinguishing between the two types of antibodies was important in the Weaver paper, because it tried to show that endogenous mouse antibodies (those that were not detected by BET-1) had the idiotype of the transgenic antibodies. O'Toole argued with Imanishi-Kari about BET-1's specificity and the experiments she was running. Imanishi-Kari, who kept careful track of the daily efforts of her students, didn't feel that O'-Toole was spending enough time in the lab to do good science. O'Toole agreed that she was definitely not committed to the "all day, every day" schedule Imanishi-Kari demanded.

When O'Toole continued to complain that Reis's results must be wrong because she could not replicate them, Imanishi-Kari yelled at her. O'Toole asked to see the original data for Reis's experiments. Imanishi-Kari never produced them for her. Later, Imanishi-Kari said she felt that O'Toole was just whining. When O'Toole's complaints didn't abate, Imanishi-Kari pulled her off the project and instructed her to write up the results she had. O'Toole refused.

The history of their personality conflict is difficult to sort out, as the two women present very different accounts. Imanishi-Kari's recollections reflect a disappointment with O'Toole, who had been a postdoc for eight years, in four different labs, and had yet to produce a single paper. Extending the work of Weaver was O'Toole's big chance, but, frustrated with her results, she kept complaining about BET-1, when Imanishi-Kari believed her complaint was foolish. Other researchers in the lab, O'Toole included, had succeeded with BET-1 before. Admittedly O'Toole's project required the greatest finesse in BET-1 handling, but Imanishi-Kari had seen O'Toole's data and found it reasonable.

O'Toole told a different story. Looking over the data, she claimed, Imanishi-Kari scanned some pages and crossed out all the results she didn't like. Imanishi-Kari happily concluded that the remaining data showed a real trend. O'Toole recalled:

> Until that moment I was frantic trying to make myself get the data.
> I was frantic trying to understand why I am not able to be a scientist.
> Watching her, I just had this utter feeling of tranquility that I was
> not partaking because I would not partake. She [Imanishi-Kari] said,
> "Bring me your data." And then she went through my data and made
> them conform. She turned around to me and she said, "So, what do
> you think?" Then she turned back. And this word came out of my

mouth, spontaneous and genuine. It just escaped in a whisper out of my lips: "Fascinating." And she turned around to me and she looked in my eyes, and her eyes were smiling at me. And she liked me. And she pitied me. And she welcomed me back into the fold.

O'Toole said in interviews that she "was instructed several times to simply omit some of the facts in order to bolster the conclusion," and therefore she refused to write anything.

Imanishi-Kari drove herself hard. She had been separated from her husband for four years and was getting a divorce. Meanwhile, she took care of her ten-year old daughter and worked seven days a week. Adding to the stress, she suffered from an unknown ailment. Her joints ached, she felt weak all the time, and she had developed puffy lumps on her face and skin. A doctor at the MIT Medical Center diagnosed her with a skin rash; later, a specialist informed her she had lupus, the autoimmune disease that killed her sister. Her own condition was not lethal, but it was physically draining. Also, she was in the process of moving from MIT to Tufts University Medical Center in Boston, starting as an associate professor in June 1986. After the move, O'Toole would no longer be her concern.

On May 7, 1986, two weeks before the end of her one-year position in Imanishi-Kari's laboratory, desperately looking for a reason besides ineptitude to explain her experimental failures, O'Toole pulled out Moema Reis's old lab notebooks and examined the records of the original mice used in the *Cell* paper. The data in seventeen pages of the notebook indicated that one of the mice used in the published experiments was of the wrong type. The notebook said the mouse was a normal mouse, but the data indicated that it was a transgenic mouse. O'Toole knew that such a mistake would skew the *Cell* paper's results. She recalled that the discovery elated her. In a conversation with a journalist, she remembered declaring, "It's not me!" to no one in particular. O'Toole did not mention her discovery to Imanishi-Kari.

Believing that fraud might be involved, two days later O'Toole called Professor Brigitte Huber of Tufts, who had been on O'Toole's thesis committee there. Huber was concerned. Fraud is the most serious allegation possible in science, and she knew that O'Toole, as a postdoc, would not be able to handle an allegation of scientific fraud on her own.

Concern about fraud in science had been growing since the early 1980s, when the bizarre case of Elias Alsabti came to light, along with the less bizarre and more disturbing cases of John Darsee, Mark Spector, and John Long.

Alsabti survived in science for a while by copying scientific papers from obscure journals and resubmitting them to other obscure journals with new titles. His ruse didn't last long, and the papers were not significant. Darsee's fraud was much bigger. As a researcher at Harvard Medical School, he published almost a hundred papers and abstracts in a single year. His secret was that he fabricated 90 percent of the results. When a supervising scientist taught him a new laboratory technique, Darsee quickly picked it up. Once he had showed his colleagues that he could generate real data, he started faking nearly identical data. He was a highly intelligent, highly motivated charlatan, and he kept up the ruse for seven years before being exposed. The NIH barred Darsee from federally funded studies for ten years, essentially ending his scientific career, and the NIH demanded that Harvard repay $750,000 spent in a fraudulent study. That was the harshest sentence the NIH has ever given.

The case of Mark Spector was similar. This seemingly brilliant graduate student purified and characterized five proteins of a signaling pathway in six months, whereas most people took a year to purify one such enzyme. Four of the proteins were kinases, and he claimed that the kinases were the cellular relatives of the viral oncogene *src,* the first oncogene discovered by Varmus and Bishop. His announcement was huge news in the field of cancer research. Baltimore himself quickly arranged for a collaboration with the upstart genius. Nine months later, the tumor virologist Volker Vogt proved that Spector was a fraud. Spector's reagents didn't work for Vogt, who had a laboratory upstairs from Spector at Cornell University, and so Vogt, skeptical, asked to see Spector's data. Spector showed Vogt beautiful results on an X-ray film that, in theory, showed where a protein had been labeled by a protein kinase enzyme labeled with radioactive ^{32}P. But Spector wouldn't show Vogt the original gel that held the radioactively labeled protein. Later in the day, a labmate of Spector's showed Vogt the drawer where Spector kept his original data. While Spector wasn't watching, Vogt analyzed the original gel with a Geiger counter and discovered the secret. The radioactive signal came not from a ^{32}P-labeled antibody but from a decoy radioactive chemical, iodine-125, that Spector had slipped into the preparation. It was a sophisticated biochemistry card trick. Vogt said, "It was obvious to me as soon as I found it that this was not a casual mix-up, because [radioactive] iodine labeling is not involved in any place in this experiment." Soon, Ed Scolnick at the National Cancer Institute found that Spector had slipped a radioactive iodine decoy into an experiment at the National Cancer Institute as well. Spector's well-respected adviser, Efraim Racker, was devastated. Racker said, "What this shows is that there is no defense against fraud. If we tried to run science as to protect ourselves from fabrication, I think we would ruin the whole enterprise." Later, a background check showed that Spector was a convicted felon.

John Long's career was the most mainstream of the three. He participated in a variety of respectable cancer research projects, working his way up to a position at Massachusetts General Hospital in Boston, but then he turned to chicanery. He produced fraudulent papers and grants based on an immortal cell line he claimed to have developed from a Hodgkin's disease patient: a remarkable feat, since no one else had managed to grow Hodgkin's cells. Prominent cancer researchers, including Baltimore, arranged for collaborations with Long. The only catch was that Long was culturing an immortal cell line from an owl monkey; it had nothing to do with Hodgkin's disease. Quickly enough he was caught and banished, leaving scientists to ponder what had gone wrong. Baltimore was equivocal: "There is no question that the pressure on research workers grows because of the limitation of funds and the increasing formalism of the academic world, with its demands to produce and appear successful, and I am sure that everyone has a cracking point. But whether any of this has to do with John Long or not, I have no idea."

Fraud seems so antithetical, even stupid, to most scientists that they have difficulty figuring out how to deal with it. Was Imanishi-Kari acting fraudulently with BET-1? It would be a foolish idea, but then scientific fraud always appeared foolish to others. At Tufts, Huber arranged for herself and two other scientists to review O'Toole's concerns. The others were Robert Woodland, an experienced friend from the University of Massachusetts Medical School, and Henry Wortis, head of the Tufts immunology division and O'Toole's Ph.D. mentor. All three were friends with both Imanishi-Kari and O'Toole. They met with Imanishi-Kari and O'Toole to review the problems. O'Toole immediately brought up the issue of the mistyped mouse. Annoyed, Imanishi-Kari agreed that the mouse was mistyped; she had known that since they had started the study. Concerned that the mouse was transgenic, Imanishi-Kari and Reis had confirmed that fact and then used a different mouse, a true normal, in the subsequent experiments. Imanishi-Kari showed plenty of evidence that this was true. The data made sense when compared with similar experiments, and the panel decided that the seventeen pages were accounted for and accurate.

The panel understood all along that there was a severe personality conflict between Imanishi-Kari and O'Toole that clouded their relationship. Many months earlier, O'Toole had talked privately with Wortis about her concerns regarding the "tenor of life" in Imanishi-Kari's lab. Her comments worried Wortis because this was the third time O'Toole had made such a complaint about a postdoctoral position soon after starting in a lab.

O'Toole further complained to the panel that the BET-1 reagent was unspecific: it sometimes reacted with antibodies that it shouldn't have. Imanishi-Kari claimed BET-1 was fine, and she presented data to support her position. Wortis was well aware of the data; BET-1 was used by various labs he knew. Moreover, if the BET-1 reagent had been unspecific in the experiments, the outcome would have been opposite to what O'Toole claimed—it would have worked against the paper's results, not in favor of them. The panel decided that O'Toole's complaints were insubstantial; she and Imanishi-Kari disagreed about scientific interpretations, and they suffered from a personality conflict.

By the end of the meeting, Imanishi-Kari was convinced that O'Toole was simply being vindictive. She refused to shake O'Toole's hand and said choppily, "You caused so much trouble. If you have scientific issues, come to me." O'Toole claimed that Imanishi-Kari angrily called her on the phone threatening her career and shouting about legal action. Imanishi-Kari denied the allegation and responded that she had no reason to threaten O'Toole. In her mind, the matter was settled; they no longer worked together. O'Toole's postdoc position with Imanishi-Kari had ended, and Imanishi-Kari had left MIT and moved on to Tufts.

O'Toole however, was not satisfied, and she brought the problem to David Baltimore's attention. She did not receive much sympathy. He dismissed her concerns, believing simply that O'Toole differed with Imanishi-Kari in the scientific interpretation of the results; she was free to disagree, but he didn't share her view. As John Maddox, the editor of *Nature,* later wrote diplomatically, "Baltimore has said that he heard her out courteously, explaining why she was mistaken. O'Toole's account is that he dismissed her version peremptorily. Those who know Baltimore's emphatic way of making a case he believes to be correct will readily acknowledge that the two accounts can be reconciled."

Unwilling to accept the original review panel decision, O'Toole then asked for an MIT panel to review Imanishi-Kari's work. O'Toole did not bring up the charge of fraud; this omission was important, because it would have changed the nature of the hearings. In a case of fraud, MIT opens a formal investigation of the investigator. Otherwise, a single reviewer is appointed to handle the problem. In this case, the reviewer was Herman Eisen, an experienced and highly respected MIT immunologist. In his first conversation with O'Toole, she spoke incomprehensibly about μ^a and μ^b and BET-1 and a jumble of her experiments. Confused, he asked her to write everything down and come back.

O'Toole then produced a detailed memo that raised four issues. Interestingly, she did not bring up the seventeen pages of data or the mistyped mouse in the memo. In Eisen's view, three of the four issues seemed to be "matters of judgment and could not be described as evidence of misconduct," but he considered the fourth issue serious: "One of O'Toole's allegations was disturbing because it raised a serious question about deliberate misrepresentation of data. This allegation concerns a [reagent] termed 'BET-1.'" O'Toole stated, "In all my experiments and in data from others in our laboratory, the BET-1 reagent easily detects both μ^a and μ^b." That is, the reagent did not specifically distinguish the transgenic and endogenous antibodies. Eisen took this issue to Imanishi-Kari, who told him what she had told the Tufts review board: BET-1 was able to detect μ^a twenty-five times better than μ^b. She showed Eisen data that matched that assertion. To determine who was right, Eisen contacted Bill Paul at the NIH, who originally developed the BET-1 reagent. Paul agreed with Imanishi-Kari. Other members of Imanishi-Kari's laboratory reported the same, reliable specificity of BET-1, contradicting O'Toole's claim.

Nevertheless, Eisen was unhappy that the paper had stated that μ^b antibodies "bound only to the anti-μ^b allotype reagent." This was not true; they also bound weakly to BET-1, the anti-μ^a reagent. He wrote in his review of the case, "My conclusion is that O'Toole is correct in claiming that there is an error in the paper; but it is not a flagrant error. The sentence . . . should have said that "the μ^b [antibody] bound strongly to the anti-μ^b [reagent] but also cross-reacted weakly with the anti-μ^a reagent [BET-1]." As all immunologists know, "antibodies don't bind only to something"; they bind to something much more strongly than to other things, but not to one thing exclusively. In Eisen's experienced judgment, "The correction would be too minor to rate a letter [of correction] to the journal [*Cell*] . . . especially because the paper contains a substantial body of other data that is clear and impressive."

Baltimore was satisfied by the Tufts review board findings and by Eisen's decision and recommendation. He told Eisen that he would inform everyone who was working on similar projects about the BET-1 specificity error but would not submit a correction to *Cell*. Regarding the conflict of interpretation, he knew peer review would show which view was correct.

The immunology mechanisms in question were extremely complicated. In such situations, data can be interpreted in a number of ways. Either theory was plausible, as Eisen understood: "I do not think that I or anyone else present at the meeting felt that Margot O'Toole's disagreements were frivolous. They are indeed based on pretty carefully thought out ideas of the limitations of the analytical methods." Such disagreements are common in science.

Baltimore suggested that O'Toole write a letter to *Cell* or another scientific journal voicing her analysis and her different opinion. Every issue of *Science* and *Nature* includes correspondence about the implications or flaws of other people's experiments. Baltimore told her that if she did write such a letter, he would write a response, which is also a common form of scientific discourse. By voicing her opinion in a major scientific journal, O'Toole would have made a valuable contribution. However, she declined to write a letter. She said she was dropping the issue.

In fact, she continued the dispute in a different and, to say the least, unconventional way. O'Toole photocopied from Moema Reis's lab notebook the seventeen pages of data that she considered fraudulent and, as she later told one reporter, analyzed them over and over again, looking for clues. She talked with a former graduate student from Imanishi-Kari's lab, Charles Maplethorpe, who had been in the lab at the same time as O'Toole. He and Imanishi-Kari had had epic screaming matches, and he had sworn to another colleague that he would "get her somehow." He suggested names of people who could help O'Toole: a couple of guys at NIH whom he had contacted might be of use.

Walter Stewart and Ned Feder were known as the "fraudbusters." They did research on snails at the NIH in the 1970s and 1980s, but had produced only one paper in fifteen years. They turned to probing the scientific work of others, to considerably more acclaim. The *Wall Street Journal* wrote of their exploits: "Their first contribution, on a celebrated case of fraud by John Darsee at Harvard Medical School, focused not on the crime, which had been acknowledged, but on the carelessness of Dr. Darsee's co-authors, who had failed to detect internal inconsistencies in papers that carried their names. This contribution was highly original and valuable: It did not destroy any reputations, and it no doubt helped raise standards." O'Toole sent Feder and Stewart the seventeen pages, which they reviewed for a few weeks. Then they produced an informal report (the NIH did not warrant their activities) agreeing with O'Toole, effectively accusing Imanishi-Kari of fraud. They had reviewed only these pages out of the many hundreds of pages of raw data generated by Imanishi-Kari's lab.

In December, Feder and Stewart wrote to Baltimore and Imanishi-Kari and asked for permission to visit their laboratories and examine their notebooks. Baltimore and Imanishi-Kari refused. The National Academy of Sciences publication *On Being a Scientist* summarized the etiquette of sharing data: "The sharing of data and other research tools is subject to certain constraints. Individuals requesting such information need to have demonstrated an ability to develop conclusions relevant to the field of inquiry from raw data." Stewart and Feder had no such qualifications. As Paul Berg summarized, "They became a real nuisance, and they were arrogant as hell. If somebody had come into my lab and said, 'I want your notebooks,' I'd have just booted 'em out."

Stewart and Feder persisted. They circulated their report to various members of the scientific community. To put pressure on Imanishi-Kari, they wrote inflammatory public statements and gave lectures about the fraudulence in the Weaver paper. O'Toole's complaints began to snowball.

THE WAR ON AIDS

By 1985 AIDS was spreading at an incredible rate, yet the president and the federal government were silent on the matter. One million people worldwide were believed to be infected, and approximately twenty thousand cases had been diagnosed. It was estimated that HIV would kill 99 percent of those it infected. In October 1985, the Institute of Medicine, which is the biomedical branch of the National Academy of Sciences, devoted its annual meeting to the subject. They did not make recommendations about how to combat the disease, but they did suggest that it should be a national priority. Near the end of 1985, Baltimore was approached by the academy's Walter Rosenblith, a former provost of MIT. Rosenblith explained that the academy was considering a study on AIDS, and they wanted to know if he was interested in directing it.

Baltimore didn't really feel that he could take on another commitment. Directing the Whitehead Institute, running his expanding lab, and visiting his mother were all extremely taxing. He didn't know the AIDS virus well and had no intention of working on it. But he felt obligated:

> We had a public health emergency in 1986. We had no idea where it was going to go—whether it was going to encompass the whole country or stay within a hardcore group. And we were faced with a brand new challenge. A virus disease with that kind of lethality had

virtually never been seen before. The flu epidemic of 1918 was that way, but it wasn't an ongoing problem. In modern Europe, after World War II, there was no other disease like it. So it seemed to me that we should be responding to it with an immediacy and an organizational perspective that was like what we had done in World War II to get the atomic bomb.

Baltimore understood, as did the leaders of the NAS, that they needed to force the national agenda on AIDS. Because the disease was then associated with the gay community, politicians were reluctant to become involved, even though AIDS might be the largest lethal epidemic ever. The fundamentalist Billy Graham declared that "AIDS is a judgment of God."

Early in 1986, the presidents of the NAS and the Institute of Medicine (IOM) decided "to initiate a special effort to assess the extent of the problems arising from AIDS and to propose an appropriate national response." The committee was christened the Committee on a National Strategy for AIDS. The academy put the project on a very fast track, funding it with NAS money and dedicating considerable staff to the project. Baltimore chaired the research panel, and Sheldon Wolff chaired the health care and public health panel. Wolff was a professor at the Tufts University School of Medicine, and one of the doyens of American medicine. He had studied infectious diseases for decades but had not been involved with AIDS studies before.

Baltimore was selected primarily as a public figurehead for the IOM project, but in fact he had made important general contributions to understanding the disease. The little that scientists understood about HIV depended on knowledge about retroviruses, and Baltimore took great personal pride in the fact that his reverse transcriptase discovery had proved valuable in diagnosing HIV infections. Nevertheless, research into vaccines and antiviral drugs were certainly not his professional forte. Baltimore put his panel together with considerable help from Sam Thier, head of the IOM. About the only individual Baltimore chose personally was Howard Temin.

Once the panels were selected, they met frequently for several months. Their report, *Confronting AIDS: Directions for Public Health, Health Care, and Research,* was published by the NAS before the end of 1986. It was the first major report on AIDS in the world and the first book about AIDS available to the public.

The scientific understanding of AIDS in 1986 was slim. Bob Gallo's laboratory at the National Cancer Institute and Luc Montaigne's laboratory at the Pasteur Institute in France had pinned down HIV as the cause of AIDS, and they and others had identified all of its genes.* But HIV had a whole set of genes no one had ever seen before. It was known that HIV infected the immune system and could also infect the central nervous system, causing dementia. But scientists didn't know the average latency period between contracting the infection and the appearance of AIDS symptoms, and they didn't know what percentage of people infected with HIV might eventually develop AIDS. They had no grasp of how efficiently the disease was transmitted. This limited knowledge made it difficult for the research panel members to make predictions about a cure: "The development of acceptably safe and effective antiviral agents for the treatment of HIV infection is likely to be a long, hard job with no certainty of success." However, they did make one hopeful statement about the development of the drug AZT (azidothymidine, which inhibits HIV's reverse transcriptase enzyme). It appeared to possibly slow the virus down.

Later in the report, they dealt with the possibility of a vaccine. To stop the spread of the epidemic, an AIDS vaccine is needed to protect people from becoming infected with the virus. The difficulties of developing a vaccine were not well understood by anyone at the time: not by scientists, not by the public, not by the government. That poor understanding led to highly overoptimistic statements. The secretary of health, education, and welfare stated that, since scientists had determined that AIDS was caused by a retrovirus, a vaccine was "around the corner." Temin and Baltimore maintained serious doubts:

> The development of a vaccine against viruses like HIV has never been seriously attempted, much less achieved. Except for a vaccine used in cats, no vaccine against such viruses [retroviruses] is available. The properties of viruses related to HIV suggest that developing a vaccine will be difficult. . . . Moreover, even if the scientific obstacles were surmounted, legal, social, and ethical factors could delay or limit the availability of a vaccine. For these reasons, the committee does not believe that a vaccine is likely to be developed for at least five years and probably longer.

This prediction was seen by the public and members of the government as very pessimistic, but Baltimore soon changed his prediction to ten years,

*Credit for the discovery of HIV is still disputed.

and probably longer. His concerns focused on the nature of HIV, the nature of vaccines, and the nature of the body's immune defense system.

Once the body mounts an immune response to a virus, it "remembers" the virus and is prepared to thwart future infections by the same virus. A vaccine consists of either a crippled virus or just pieces of the virus. Introducing these into the body gives the immune system the opportunity to recognize the virus and develop antibodies to it without having to fight off a full-scale infection. A vaccine is equivalent to giving the immune system Cliff's Notes on an invader, telling the immune system what to expect and how to pass the test of an actual infection. The Sabin poliovirus vaccine, for example, consists of a live but weakened mutant poliovirus, typically administered to a child in a sugar cube.* When children eat the sugar cubes, the live poliovirus infects their intestines. The weakened poliovirus begins to replicate rapidly, killing cells and spreading in the body. But it isn't aggressive enough to survive for long.** The cells of the immune system find the poliovirus, make antibodies against it, and destroy the invaders. If poliovirus ever reinfects the body, the immune system already knows how to fight the disease, and its arsenal of antipolio antibodies is ready at a moment's notice.

But what if the virus changes? The flu shots administered widely each winter in the United States are good only for a year. This is because the influenza virus mutates every year, so that the immune system can no longer recognize it. The antibodies that grabbed last year's influenza virus like a steel trap paw harmlessly at this year's new strain. The Centers for Disease Control (CDC) in Atlanta continually tracks the appearance of new influenza strains.†† The CDC produces a new vaccine by growing large batches of influenza in chicken eggs and then "killing" the virus with formaldehyde, mangling its RNA genome. This killed-virus vaccine can be injected into the body, where it floats harmlessly until the immune system finds it, destroys it, and remembers it.

Established vaccine strategies didn't look promising for HIV. Scientists' only real knowledge of HIV could be summarized as three strong and discouraging facts: no one had ever developed a vaccine against any retrovirus

---

*The Salk poliovirus vaccine (developed earlier by Jonas Salk) is a killed-virus vaccine.
**Additionally, and importantly, the genetically mutant vaccine poliovirus has "forgotten" how to replicate in nerve cells and therefore cannot cause paralysis.
††Almost all new influenza strains originate in rural China and then spread eastward around the world. It is now believed that the new influenza viruses are actually mutant duck viruses that cross over to humans. In rural China, people live in very close quarters with ducks.

besides feline leukemia; AIDS was fatal in virtually all cases; and HIV attacked the immune system itself. These last two characteristics made an HIV infection quite different from a poliovirus or influenza infection, because most people's immune systems defeat influenza and poliovirus on their own. In those situations, a vaccine simply allows the body to win its battle with influenza or poliovirus faster, and without getting noticeably sick. With HIV, the vaccine would have to create a stronger immune response than an actual infection, because an actual infection led not to immunity but to death. The research panel members were faced with the conundrum of how to make the immune system recognize and defeat a virus that it never wins against. They had no idea what the best approach might be.

Baltimore pushed hard for two recommendations proposed by the committee. One was realized, and the other was not. The first major recommendation was that the federal government should commit $1 billion annually to research on AIDS by 1990. According to Baltimore:

> This was an attempt to force the nation's agenda. Just at the end of the document, I was looking over what we had done, and I said, "You know, everything's fine, but the only way you catch people's attention in this country is to put a number on it." We had to figure out how much money to ask for. A dollar amount. So we calculated, you know, back of the envelope here, there, and everywhere, and came up with a billion-dollar-a-year research program. At the time that seemed just inconceivably high, but we went for it, because that is what we believed in.

They got it. In 1990 the federal government was committing $1 billion a year to AIDS research, and in 1995 the budget was closer to $1.5 billion.

The second recommendation Baltimore pushed for was a highly directed, strongly centralized AIDS research effort. The model of the Manhattan Project appealed to him in its organizational vision. This view was very different from his philosophy in the 1970s, when he fought the organizational efforts of the War on Cancer. The general success of the War on Cancer must have made him hopeful that this sort of effort could be useful. In contrast to the white-elephant Special Virus Cancer Program, which had neither a viral target nor the tools of recombinant DNA and was a dismal failure, Baltimore argued that with the HIV virus discovered and the tools of recombinant DNA available, the AIDS epidemic was "ripe" for a Manhattan Project–style assault. He said: "We seem to be afraid to say that we have identified a national need and we are going to make sure that the best minds put their attention to it. Why not conscript scientists when their skills could avert a disaster? . . . AIDS certainly represents that emergency." He then asked,

> Does a scientist who can help to learn about AIDS, whose skills provide the ability to contribute to the conquest of this modern plague, have the right to continue investigating an arcane problem of bacterial transposons? I hear the answer from my colleagues as soon as I pose the question: "Maybe," they will say, "the answer will come from work on transposons." Quoting back to me things I might have said once, they will go on, "Head-on research is often the least effective way to get an answer. When we deal with the unknown, answers often come from unexpected quarters."
>
> True, true—because I've made such arguments myself they come easily to my mind, and I deeply believe them. But they are not always the right arguments and are not always applicable. Let's remember the Manhattan Project.

Baltimore's earlier philosophy played devil's advocate to his new philosophy and lost. AIDS was a challenge that excited him, and he wanted to create an army of the brightest minds in the country to fight the disease. But Baltimore's centralization idea gained only mild support from the committee, who recommended not a new Manhattan Project but simply the creation of a National Commission on AIDS, which would "monitor the course of the epidemic; encourage federal, state, philanthropic, industrial, and other entities to participate; stimulate the strongest possible efforts of the academic scientific community . . . and report to the American public." They also recommended that the commission be created as a presidential or joint presidential-congressional commission, and that "the President take a strong leadership role in the effort against AIDS and HIV, designating control of AIDS as a major national goal." The president never listened. Reagan refused to come near an issue so closely associated with homosexuals. If AIDS had appeared as a lethally infectious disease of the heterosexual population, the $1 billion research budget would almost certainly have been provided back in 1986. It is possible that the NAS budget recommendation was met mainly in response to the growing understanding, and fear, that the heterosexual population was also at risk.

Baltimore's dream of centralization never materialized, and without it, AIDS research funding crawled through the normal bureaucratic procedures, which were too slow for an emergency response and difficult, if not impossible, to direct. In the United States, most government funding for biology research comes from NIH grants. Scientists fill out grant applications, explaining the topic they wish to study, their strategy, their resources, and their funding needs. The NIH allocates an amount of funding for each field and selects a panel of scientific peers to review all of the grant applications and decide which deserve funding. Since grants are awarded in batches at specific times, and not on a rolling basis, it usually takes a year to review a specific project and provide funding. Also, the granting process does not provide much direction for research in a field, because the choice of projects is driven primarily by what research scientists want to pursue, and only secondarily by what the NIH is willing to fund. Of course, when substantial funds became available for AIDS research, many biologists applied for AIDS research grants, but in an undirected manner. They applied for grants to study the aspects of AIDS research that were interesting to them at the time, not necessarily those that were significant for public health.

After its final report in September 1986, the Committee on a National Strategy for AIDS disbanded, and Baltimore returned full-time to life at the Whitehead. A new interest in AIDS research returned with him, and he devoted a part of his lab to studying AIDS. The more he thought about the social issues of AIDS, the more curious he became about the biology of HIV.

THE TEST YOU WILL FACE

The Imanishi-Kari/O'Toole question continued to bother Baltimore. The fraudbusters paraded around the country denouncing the Weaver paper. Furious, in January 1987 Baltimore demanded an official NIH investigation of the paper. This was an unusual move, perhaps even a unique one, but the NIH agreed, and an Office of Extramural Research investigation began in May.

The NIH was poorly equipped to deal with issues of scientific fraud. Fraud is rare in science; a Hastings Center report estimates only two cases per year. But with the spate of high-profile scientific fraud cases in the early 1980s— Alsabti, Darsee, Spector, and Long—Representative Al Gore decided that the NIH and the scientific community needed to control their fraud problem more rigorously. Science has replaced religion as the fundamental arbiter of truth in the modern world, and even a few cases of fraud were enough to mar the reputation of science. Gore presided over a hearing at which he announced, "I cannot avoid the conclusion that one reason for the persistence of this type of problem is the reluctance of people high in the science field to take these matters very seriously." Philip Handler, president of the National Academy of Sciences, testified before Gore that fraud was very rare in science and always rooted out. Science is self-correcting; that is its beauty and its power. But Handler did continue,

> I will admit with you, sir, the absence of any sense of what due process should be when some suspicion is aroused. We have never adopted standardized procedures of any kind to deal with these isolated events. We have no courts, no understanding among ourselves as to how any one such incident shall be treated.
>
> We have left them, one at a time, as they have occurred, to the best judgement of the institutions within which such events have transpired. And, in the end, word of such misdeeds, which attaches to the name of the individual, invariably destroys him in the career on which he had embarked. We think that suffices—more than suffices.

Gore had good intentions, but scientists didn't want to deal with his concerns.

Handler's statement that scientists had "never adopted standardized procedures" for handling fraud would come back to haunt him, the NIH, and the scientific community. Several NIH investigations, including the Imanishi-Kari investigation, became painful failures because of this deficit.

In January 1988, six months after initiating the preliminary Imanishi-Kari investigation, the NIH Office of Extramural Affairs appointed a panel of three immunologists to review the Weaver paper and Margot O'Toole's objections to it. Two of the panel members had close ties to Baltimore. James Darnell, who was now at Rockefeller University, was Baltimore's friend, and they had just coauthored *Molecular Cell Biology,* a major college textbook. Fred Alt, a professor at Harvard, had recently been a postdoc in Baltimore's lab. These obvious conflicts of interest showed the NIH's ignorance of proper investigative procedures. Baltimore had not been consulted about the choice of panel members: "I just had to believe that they had their reasons." But obviously it couldn't hurt him to have a couple of good friends on the panel.

Two months later, Michigan Representative John Dingell joined the fray. As chair of the Subcommittee on Oversight and Investigations, within the Committee on Energy and Commerce, Dingell was of the opinion that the

NIH, with its $10 billion budget, was not subject to enough congressional oversight. By all accounts, John Dingell was a much less congenial man than Al Gore. Holding hearings on fraud and waste in the federal government was his passion. Congressional representatives have enormous investigative powers that are almost completely discretionary, limited only by the size of their staff. Dingell used these powers as a tool to attract media coverage and to bring his favorite issues to national prominence. He could call on any witnesses he wanted. His subcommittee was described as the "grand jury for the nation." He had exposed rampant fraud in defense contracting, and he deftly unearthed corruption in a Wall Street firm, though one of his aides pursued the case so energetically that he obtained the necessary information illegally. Dingell thought the nation's research scientists might be wasting public funds, and he knew that if fraud was present, the NIH wasn't capable of controlling it, because their investigations were procedural nightmares. But he needed an example, a test case that would illustrate the need for overhauling the scientific self-regulatory system.

The O'Toole case had all the hallmarks of a coup. A lowly female whistle-blower was desperately fighting a fraud committed by Baltimore, the Nobel Prize winner, and his cronies in the university system had tried to silence her. Dingell's aide in charge of the case said, "We were going to whop the thing; kick 'em a little and go back to [Department of] Defense [fraud investigations]. One goddamn hearing and they'd do the right thing." He also observed, "Dingell will characterize [the MIT and Tufts inquiries] as piss-poor."

In April 1988, Dingell held a congressional hearing into the handling of O'Toole's allegations by MIT, Tufts, and the NIH, and he ripped each one apart. Discovering the conflicts of interest in the NIH panel, he declared that the NIH investigation was critically flawed and must be redone. He stated that "we are only seeing the tip of a very unfortunate, dangerous, and important iceberg," and noted forcefully, "There is widespread understanding within the scientific community of the plight of whistle-blowers. This committee has a special affection for whistle-blowers in connection with defense matters and in connection with other matters. That affection will be manifest in our hearings today." One of Dingell's aides was quoted in an interview with the *Boston Globe* accusing Baltimore of fraud. Headlined "Fraud and Misrepresentation," the article included a picture of Baltimore accompanied by the quote: "It's hard to tell if it's error or fraud. At certain times, it appears to be fraud and other times misrepresentation." The Imanishi-Kari/Baltimore affair rumbled into the public and political arenas.

Baltimore was livid. The involvement of the government blew everything out of proportion, and he felt it was patently absurd. On the basis of O'Toole's dissatisfaction and the antics of the "fraudbusters" at the NIH, his integrity was now being challenged at the highest level. His experience during the recombinant DNA controversy made him want to minimize government involvement in scientific regulation. Science had its own avenues to solve these problems, and they were being obviated. Additionally, neither he nor Imanishi-Kari had been invited to the congressional hearing.

Baltimore's response was quick and forceful. He sent out a withering "Dear Colleague" letter to several hundred scientists, attacking Dingell and declaring that congressional involvement was entirely unnecessary and should be stopped. Because Dingell didn't allow the accused to defend themselves, Baltimore called the hearing "a classic kangaroo court." Scientists flooded Dingell's office with mail protesting his actions. Later, Baltimore spoke bitterly of congressional involvement: "As soon as it became political, it got out of the hands of rational people and became a matter for these congressional investigators, who don't care about the truth. They care about the publicity and the *image* they can create of being tough investigators. . . . The whole process becomes uncontrolled once it gets into a venue like that."

Dingell, not surprisingly, responded poorly to this direct attack. Baltimore's vehemence triggered a "thou dost protest too much" response in Dingell. In the words of a subcommittee staffer, "If Baltimore hadn't raised as much of a stink, I don't think Dingell would have remained interested. The scientific community was really very arrogant." Within a month, Dingell subpoenaed Imanishi-Kari's laboratory notebooks. She complied, but it took her a while. Scientific notebooks are not always the sort of well-organized, complete, detailed notebooks people generally imagine. Some scientists keep notes on torn looseleaf paper, paper towels, and Post-It notes. They may bury the data in a drawer or a folder, digging it out to check a detail or write a paper. Imanishi-Kari's data consisted of papers scattered on benchtops, in drawers, yellowing on the windowsills, sometimes taped to lab notebook pages, sometimes jammed into unlabeled manila envelopes. Baltimore noted,

> It was quite remarkable that in that seeming chaos, when a pointed question came and I said, "Let's look at the data and see what the numbers look like and try plotting them out," whatever, as fast as if she had a notebook in front of her, she could find the relevant material and we could go over them and there was never an issue. I might say

that that is not unique in my experience. I've seen other people who can do that. But it's a rare talent.

Once Imanishi-Kari sent her piecemeal notebooks to Dingell, he sent them to the Secret Service for forensic analysis. Neither the NIH Office of Extramural Research nor Imanishi-Kari and Baltimore were notified of the Secret Service involvement.

After Dingell's scolding, the NIH quickly appointed two new panel members, and the panel met with Imanishi-Kari on several occasions to review her data. One panel member later noted, "There remains difficulty in communication and understanding . . . every time we meet with Dr. Imanishi-Kari—as has been pointed out, English is not her first language. Even yesterday, when we spent four hours with Dr. Imanishi-Kari, we really, at several times, had to discuss what she meant when she used particular words. It's a continuing problem that we have." Though she spoke seven languages, her English was often poor. David Baltimore noted that he also sometimes had problems communicating with her. A sample of her NIH interview transcript looked like this:

> My books were not books. My books were—that one spiral notebook and something [data] inside of here [manila folders] books . . . went all over the place, these data. . . . we took all over. We took to the lab, we took to Moema's [Reis's] lab, we went to the [radiation] counter. It shifted. It went sometimes [with Weaver]. . . . So, they were kept in different folders in different things and they were kept all over the place.

The NIH panel finished its inquiry in six months. They believed that there were "significant errors of misstatement and omission" regarding BET-1 that should be corrected. These were the same misstatements previously reported by Eisen. The panel didn't feel that these problems were grave or fraudulent, but, dissenting from Eisen's view, they felt the data required correction. Therefore the panel instructed Baltimore, Weaver, and Imanishi-Kari to submit a letter of correction to *Cell*. The authors did so without complaint, and the correction was published in November 1988. Various outside commentators have suggested in hindsight that if Baltimore had simply submitted a correction at the time of the Eisen review at MIT, the issue would have disappeared. In fact, the earlier decision not to submit a correction would prove little more than a footnote to the controversy that subsequently exploded.

The NIH findings didn't satisfy Dingell. He was convinced that Baltimore was protecting Imanishi-Kari and stonewalling investigations, and that he was getting away with it because he was a Nobel laureate and a powerful biologist. Dingell scheduled a second hearing and summoned Baltimore to testify. The two had six months to prepare for the clash. With the congressional investigation heating up, and Baltimore's peripheral involvement deepening, John Maddox, the editor of *Nature,* and other scientists urged him to make a public statement shedding full responsibility for the study. As Maddox noted some months later in an editorial, their efforts "revealed an angrily defensive person, most offended that work with which he had been associated should be challenged."*

Baltimore's highly respected friend Phillip Sharp tried to help him out. Sharp, then the director of the Center for Cancer Research at MIT, had a reputation as one of the nicest scientists in America. He was a hero in his home state of Kentucky. One of his schoolteachers said, "Heavens, we're so proud of him, coming from our little schools. He did very well in science, but I figured he would be a high school teacher." He later won the 1993 Nobel Prize in medicine. (A cynical MIT researcher privately referred to MIT's trio of Nobelists—Sharp, Baltimore, and Tonegawa—as "the good, the bad, and the ugly.") He sent an influential letter to colleagues attempting to downplay the impersonality and virulence of Baltimore's "Dear Colleague" letter, noting diplomatically:

> It seems obvious that the congressional subcommittee has decided to continue to hassle David and the other authors, and this has serious implications for all of us. . . . It is difficult to fathom the motives behind the subcommittee's current actions. But I believe that to continue what many of us perceive to be a vendetta against honest scientists will cost our society dearly. . . . When such matters are brought before congressional panels, there is a clear danger that calm scientific judgement will be overshadowed.

Irving Weissman later seconded that thought. "It was inappropriate for the government to be making decisions about scientific validity. . . . We were

*In the *Nature* editorial, Maddox refers to himself as a friend of Baltimore's. Baltimore does not concur.

all worried about what would happen if, in fact, the Dingell committee held more sway over the NIH, its appointments, and its functions."

In the months before the hearing, Baltimore hired lawyers in both Boston and Washington, D.C. Going even further into the political arena, Baltimore and his supporters tried to enlist the help of the Republican minority members on Dingell's subcommittee. It seemed a wild about-face from Baltimore's leftist past, but at this point he was willing to take his lawyers' advice and ask for help from anyone who could rescue him.

Everyone in science knew that the hearing was going to be a thunderous clash between Baltimore and Dingell. The week before the 1989 hearing, *Science* ran a lead article titled "Dingell vs. Baltimore." It was like the press before a big Las Vegas boxing match. In a *New York Times* column two days before the hearing, Robert Pollack, a Columbia University dean, wrote, "I fear that the way Dr. Baltimore is being treated means that witch hunts are in the offing."

Scientists everywhere became nervous about the proceedings. They never wanted to discuss scientific fraud, and certainly not in a dangerous forum like this. Paul Berg said Baltimore was "like a red cape in front of a bull." Many scientists were anxious not to upset Dingell because they were afraid of jeopardizing NIH funding. Others were ambivalent toward Baltimore. The NIH panel had cleared him of wrongdoing, but that panel had been stacked in Baltimore's favor, and the accusations of Margot O'Toole sounded serious. Maxine Singer, Baltimore's friend from the days of the recombinant DNA controversy, tried to rally support for him at a big National Academy of Sciences meeting in Washington just days before the congressional hearing. Going from person to person, Singer encouraged them to stay around for a few extra days to support Baltimore. She was surprised by the resistance she found: "The troubling and almost universal response was negative. Some academy members had already assumed Imanishi-Kari's and Baltimore's guilt, even in the absence of the dispassionate evidence scientists are trained to require." On the other hand, Dingell was working on legislation that would impose sweeping regulations on scientific conduct. The scheme sounded draconian, and numerous scientists from across the country responded to that danger by attending the hearing.

Dingell had an ace up his sleeve. He arranged for the Secret Service to spring the forensic analysis of Imanishi-Kari's notebooks on Baltimore and Imanishi-Kari the Tuesday before the hearing. In a series of high-pressure talks, the Secret Service agents announced that they had detected page sequences in Imanishi-Kari's notebooks that were clearly out of order, a number of pages with changed dates, and data printouts that could not possibly be in chronological order. Baltimore turned ashen. He refused to comment on the Secret Service's results until he could sort out the information and confer with Imanishi-Kari. No written report was made, and no notes were provided to Baltimore and Imanishi-Kari before, during, or after the meetings.

The next day, at the hearing, Dingell began by calming scientists' fears that he would cut government funding for basic science. He was not out to crucify the NIH; he liked the NIH. (Almost all representatives do: it is the only federal agency that consistently receives a greater budget increase than the president recommends. One reason for the generosity is the American fear of disease.) Dingell had other fish to fry: "This subcommittee has examined a number of cases of proven misconduct that have not been handled well. The apparent unwillingness on the part of the scientific community to deal promptly and effectively with allegations of misconduct is unfair to both the accuser and the accused." Then he launched into a long assault on the NIH's handling of the Imanishi-Kari case, characterizing the NIH panel's decision as wrong and lauding O'Toole as a seeker of truth who seemed to have "an understanding of wrongdoing which might otherwise be hushed up."

Baltimore was furious at the way Dingell was manipulating events. He later said, "I do not accept insults lightly. John Dingell revels in insulting people. He wants them to squirm and take it. And I would not." In the hearing Baltimore was completely uncooperative, moving quickly to the attack:

> There are many scientists here today in the audience. They are concerned about this investigation and hearing. They are concerned that it could have a chilling effect on science in America. The problem, Mr. Chairman, is that many in the scientific community do not understand what you are doing. Think about it.
>
> I do question, in the most serious way, the manner in which this investigation has been pursued. . . . This is a classic case of verdict first, evidence later. . . . Those of us accused were not given the opportunity to tell our story, nor were we even formally notified of the [first] hearing.

Dingell, honed by years of intense debates and hearings, did not like to be crossed. Baltimore's self-confidence and browbeating did not intimidate Dingell, who proceeded to rip the previous NIH investigation and university hearings to shreds. He gave great credence to the Secret Service data. In addition, Dingell attacked Baltimore for a confidential letter written to Herman Eisen on September 9, 1986. Taken out of context, the letter amounted to a direct admission that the Weaver paper contained fraudulent data: "The evidence that the BET-1 antibody doesn't do as described in the paper is clear. Thereza's statement to you that she knew it all the time is a remarkable admission of guilt. Neither David Weaver nor I had any idea that there was a problem or an ambiguity with the serum. Why Thereza chose to use the data and to mislead both of us and those who read the paper is beyond me." David Baltimore wished he'd never written that letter.

"Mr. Dingell," said Baltimore, "I've gone to great lengths to apologize for that letter, to explain the conditions under which that letter was written. I think by your reading it, you can tell the intensity of feeling that I had at the time I wrote that letter."

"I can indeed, sir."

"That letter was completely inoperative in its significance within a couple of days of its writing."

There had been a grave misunderstanding between Eisen and Imanishi-Kari, Baltimore explained, that hinged on the fact that Imanishi-Kari's English is poor. Eisen thought she told him that BET-1 always failed; she was, in fact, telling him that sometimes bad batches of BET-1 failed and she had to make new batches. When Eisen told Baltimore what he thought he'd heard from Imanishi-Kari, Baltimore was terrified that he had been deceived, and he wrote the letter. Within a week the misunderstanding had been resolved, but Baltimore's letter, which survived, left onlookers with a complicated story to accept. As corroboration, Baltimore noted that there were several other labs using BET-1 successfully, proving that his own statement was wrong.

Dingell attacked him, arguing, "You said this: 'The evidence that the BET-1 antibody doesn't do as described in the paper is clear.' Is that statement true or not true?"

"That statement is not true."

"That statement is not true?"

"That statement is not true today, and was, in fact, not true when I said it, although I was under a misapprehension."

Dingell continued to question Baltimore, but since he did not understand the science, the questioning was frustrating.

Baltimore was by no means finished with his indictment of the sub-committee:

> The Secret Service apparently conducted a nine months forensic analysis of Dr. Imanishi-Kari's laboratory notes. In a charade of helpfulness, they presented a partial oral summary of their findings on Tuesday, April 25. That presentation was designed to terrify without providing any substance. . . .
> I must tell you, Mr. Chairman, I am very troubled about how this situation got so out of hand. I have a very real concern that American science can easily become the victim of this kind of Government inquiry. . . .
> So what is the case against us? That there are legitimate disagreements over the results of our work? This I recognize and encourage. That we were not as perfect as in hindsight we might have been? This, I can see. That scientists keep notes in ways that are sometimes orderly and sometimes not? Of course. That we committed fraud, created data, or misrepresented the facts? This I reject categorically. The subcommittee can point to nothing that supports these allegations.

Most of Dingell's case centered on O'Toole's testimony and Imanishi-Kari's laboratory notes. Imanishi-Kari admitted that the notebooks were a shambles. Having organized them only in response to the congressional inquiry, she had presented the agents with a forensics playground. She defended her work, stating how foolish it would be of her to lie. "If I had fabricated data, it would have misled scientists, wasted their precious resources and retarded their efforts to cure the disease that killed my sister and threatens me." Dingell did not care for her sympathy plea. In fact, perversely, it turned some people against her. Walter Gilbert, a Harvard professor and Baltimore's friend and fellow Nobelist, said that when he heard this remark he decided something was amiss with her research: "It means you are more likely to fake."

Dingell interrogated Imanishi-Kari about her laboratory notebooks. Flustered, she gave answers like, "That's quite possible, sir, in my case. That is all I can answer." Imanishi-Kari was struggling her way through an answer when Dingell cut her off and began his closing speech:

> It was the purpose then and the hope of the Chair that . . . this meeting in which we are all suffering mightily could have been avoided, and that we could thereby perhaps lay to rest the questions that this committee has [posed]. . . . Your response, Dr. Baltimore, was a rather

ringing attack upon this committee and essentially an allegation that you had been charged with fraud, which happens to be untrue, and the fact, or rather, added allegation, which indicated that some of the persons involved in these matters were behaving in a fashion worthy of Hitler and the Holocaust. Now I will tell you that I take umbrage . . . at those statements.

Baltimore tried to interrupt Dingell, but Dingell did not heed him. Summarizing, Dingell said, "You have a distinguished record and reputation, Dr. Baltimore, one which I had felt would enable us to get better information than we have received today. I am not satisfied with any of the statements or any of the information which has been received. The committee is going to pursue these matters further and we thank you for your assistance to us—"

Baltimore angrily and unconventionally interrupted Dingell. "Mr. Dingell, might I respond? Please?"

Annoyed, but unable to ignore him, Dingell replied, "You may."

"Thank you. I was charged with fraud—"

"Not by any occupant of this room," Dingell retorted.

"By Mr. Stockton [Dingell's main aide], quoted in the *Boston Globe*—"

"I'd like to—"

"And I ask to put it in the record."

"I'd like to see the statement."

"You are welcome to it. It is right here. In fact, the *Globe* compositor happened to have headlined 'Fraud and Misrepresentation' and put my picture next to it, quoting Mr. Stockton directly, both in the article and in the box." Unaware of this, Dingell was hurriedly trying to confirm this statement. Baltimore interrupted him, saying, "I would like to continue, if I might, Mr. Chairman."

"Pardon? Say that again?"

"I wonder if I could continue."

"You're recognized."

"I said that a member of your staff compared scientific fraud of which I am accused to the Nazi Holocaust."

Baltimore continued to berate Dingell. Dingell tried to shut him up, but Baltimore would not stand down: "It's as if we presented you with the *Cell* paper and asked you to analyze it on the spot. That would be pretty unfair to do, and that's the position we're in—taking this snappy Secret Service stuff and telling you about—"

Dingell tried again to argue him down and end the session: "You know, after the briefing—"

"—it right off. So, I think—"

"After the briefing, Doctor—" The exchange continued for several more minutes before Dingell, worn down by Baltimore's badgering, made the exasperated announcement, "It is not the intention of the Chair to quibble further. The Chair is simply going to observe that serious questions have been raised today about scientific research."

Afterwards, Martin Flax, chairman of the beleaguered Tufts University pathology department, joyously said of Baltimore, "He did brilliantly. That was Civics 101 for me." Baltimore, worn out, simply said, "I believed that by confronting Chairman Dingell directly, I was acting in the best interest of all scientists. Only time will tell."

Given the evidence condemning the veracity of Imanishi-Kari's notebooks, Baltimore's arrogance perturbed a lot of scientists. To Baltimore's friends, his stance was not arrogance but a courageous assertion of the rights of due process for himself and for Imanishi-Kari; but many scientists were not convinced that either of them was innocent. Because the *Cell* paper's results had not been reproduced by other labs, its accuracy was doubted. Many scientists believed O'Toole would not have gone to the authorities without good reason. Baltimore's letter to Eisen was clearly disconcerting, and then there were the Secret Service data showing that things were out of order. Some of Baltimore's longtime friends turned against him. Walter Gilbert, the Harvard Nobelist, believed Imanishi-Kari was guilty, and he began to write letters and give testimony against Baltimore and her. His stated motivation was to uphold scientific decorum: "This case has less to do with fraud and much more to do with notions of correct behavior," clearly referring to Baltimore's behavior, which he would publicly condemn over the next seven years. Mark Ptashne of Harvard, who also believed that Baltimore was engaged in a cover-up, took Margot O'Toole under his wing.

Baltimore submitted a long essay to the congressional subcommittee that was entered in the *Congressional Record*. No one paid any attention to it, because it wasn't spoken testimony and few people check the *Congressional Record* later, but it contains an interesting segment on the nature of science in a free society:

> The issue we are faced with today is how does one determine whether a given piece of published science is an appropriate reflection of a set of experimental observations. . . .

The extraordinary success of American science comes from giving the individual scientist complete leeway to determine his or her own style of investigation. We say, in effect, "Do it however you think best. The test you will face is not one of the procedures you followed, but rather of the product you provide: the published record of your experiments. The test you will face is the toughest one imaginable: can the published experiments be replicated by others and, even more importantly, do your experiments provide a basis for further scientific development? This is how we ascertain truth." If your experiments are not reproducible or cannot be built upon, the punishment is the most severe one we know: you are no longer believed as a scientist. If you attempt to publish further work, it is treated with increased skepticism. . . . It is a process of self-purification that goes on continually.

After the hearing, Dingell was fuming; he had been beaten in his home court. Even his hometown newspaper wrote a scathing article headlined "Dingell's New Galileo Trial," criticizing him for his overzealous "witch hunt." Stephen Jay Gould made similar statements in the *New York Times*. A reporter playfully asked Dingell what the difference was between μ^b and μ^a, and Dingell's anger flared: "I don't give a damn, and I really don't know, and I don't intend to spend time finding out!" But he was waging a war, not just a battle. Wielding the new forensics evidence produced by the Secret Service, Dingell forced the NIH to investigate the Weaver case again, this time in conjunction with the Secret Service.

Shortly after the hearings, one of Dingell's aides was interviewed about the case. The reporter suggested that "since the scientific community's consciousness had clearly been raised on the issue of fraud, Dingell and Baltimore could make peace and voice their mutual dedication to good scientific research."

"I don't think Dingell would sell out the staff that way," the aide replied.

"Why would it be a sellout?" the interviewer asked.

"Because Baltimore and the rest covered this up."

"You mean his humiliation is a necessary part of your enterprise?"

"Yes," the aide replied, "In science you have to lie to survive."

With all of the public hoopla about scientific fraud, and the NIH's own inability to deal with scientific fraud cases, NIH director James Wyngaarden disassembled the NIH Office of Extramural Research and created a new Office of Scientific Integrity (OSI), within the Office of the Director, to show that scientific integrity was a major concern and would get substantial attention.

In spite of the fraud publicity, Baltimore's scientific reputation remained solid. Still studying poliovirus, Abelson virus, cancer, transcription factors, antibodies, and HIV, he published great research in the late 1980s. His Whitehead lab continued to work on NF-κB, the prominent immunological "transcription factor" that binds DNA and turns on genes, which the lab discovered in the mid-80s. That work would spawn thousands of papers by other labs over the next decade. Following up on Susumu Tonegawa's Nobel Prize–winning discovery of antibody gene shuffling, David Schatz in Baltimore's lab discovered the two genes that were actually responsible for the shuffling, RAG-1 and RAG-2, and that discovery was a major immunology research coup. Discoveries like these reinforced Baltimore's position as perhaps the most influential figure in modern biology. Between 1988 and 1992, Baltimore was listed ninth on *Science*'s top-ten list of "High-Impact Researchers"; but a second look at the list showed that he published almost twice as many papers as anyone else on the list and had been referenced seven thousand times, over 30 percent more often than anyone else on the list for that period. Baltimore's administration at Whitehead was running smoothly, and he was even under consideration for the MIT presidency. A few months after the Dingell hearings ended, a novel opportunity for Baltimore arose: the presidency of Rockefeller University.

Nine

ROCKEFELLER

The credit belongs to the man who is actually in the arena,
whose face is marred by dust and sweat and blood; . . . who errs,
and comes up short again and again . . . who at best knows in the end
the triumph of high achievement, and who at worst, if he fails,
at least fails while daring greatly.

THEODORE ROOSEVELT
Speech in Paris, April 23, 1910

By 1989 ROCKEFELLER UNIVERSITY's president, the indomitable Nobel lau-reate Joshua Lederberg, was approaching the mandatory retirement age of sixty-five. The Rockefeller trustees were hunting for a suitable re-placement. They wanted someone who could restore the university to the grand status it had held early in the century and at the same time tear Rockefeller away from its stagnant organizational structure and hiring prac-tices and reduce the university's spiraling deficit. Impressed with his suc-cess at the Whitehead, they approached Baltimore, who was captivated by the opportunity. He loved New York, and, after his success at the White-head, he was sure that he could manage a scientific institution with a $100 million budget. (When MIT approached him with a potential offer of its presidency he had declined, because MIT would have been a complex challenge; its $1 billion budget was focused mainly on engineering de-partments that Baltimore knew nothing about.) A twelve-story lab build-ing was due to be completed in 1992, and Baltimore could fill it with bi-ologists of his choice. Slots for thirty new full professors were projected over the next fifteen years as current faculty retired, and ten of them would be appointed in the next two years. Given that Rockefeller had only forty-five full professors, the upcoming wave of retirees attested to the age of the faculty.

However, most of the senior faculty opposed Baltimore's appointment, and they opposed the drastic organizational changes proposed by the trustees. Rockefeller's senior professors controlled the university, and they liked it that way. Paul Berg said, "The place was run like a series of fiefdoms." Each senior professor ran an entire department, much as German universities are run, and each also received a hefty chunk of funding from the university's endowment. The junior faculty possessed no administrative clout. When the senior faculty were polled in September 1989 about Baltimore's candidacy, two-thirds of the professors opposed his appointment. Half of those faculty signed a letter of protest. They did not want Baltimore to implement the changes mandated by the trustees, and they did not want a leader whose reputation—and relationship with government funding institutions—was tainted by controversy and fraud. When Baltimore saw the letter, he withdrew his name from consideration. He felt he could not accomplish anything in that environment.

When Baltimore withdrew his name, trustees Richard Furlaud and David Rockefeller immediately flew to Boston to try to change his mind. Richard Furlaud, president of Bristol Meyers–Squibb, was head of the board of trustees, and David Rockefeller was head of the trustees' executive committee. They stubbornly wanted Baltimore, and they promised him that he would have support from the trustees to get things done at Rockefeller. Furlaud recalled, "Mr. Rockefeller said: 'Look, we still think you're the right person to do the job.' And then he accepted." Baltimore later reflected:

> I was enthralled by that opportunity because—first off, I have this sort of silly romantic streak; I love certain institutions. And I really love Rockefeller. It represented kind of the best of American science at a certain time. And it was an institution that was on hard times in terms of its national reputation and its goals.
>
> I thought I could really reformulate the Rockefeller University, and make it part of the modern world. Because it was still mired, still is sort of mired, it the past—in its past, in its very successful past. So, I agreed to do that [accept the presidency]. . . . So Rockefeller was a vision of a new opportunity. I thought I could make a difference.

The day of his acceptance, the *New York Times* early edition ran the headline, "Fraud Suspect Appointed President of Rockefeller." Things were going to be rough.

One day, driving to Woods Hole with Baltimore, Paul Berg kept asking him, "Why do you want to do it?" Baltimore finally gave Berg a straight reply: "He told me that he was bored at the Whitehead. He said he woke up in the morning and he didn't feel that there was any great challenge for him. Everything was running smoothly. It was a done deal. And it was now just 'minding the store,' in a sense. He wanted a new challenge." Administrative jobs used to bore Baltimore, and he preferred the competitive environment of science. But now, having outpaced his scientific competitors for decades, he was looking for something that would replace the waning adrenaline rush of research. He didn't want to give up research—as he said, "I always planned to, and did, have a laboratory at Rockefeller, and continued on work I wanted to do"—but he needed something new in his life.

Alice took a leave of absence from Harvard, and they moved to New York together. President David Baltimore started work on July 1, 1990. Shortly thereafter, Alice became dean for science at New York University (NYU). Baltimore's office at Rockefeller was the staid office originally built for President Detlev Bronk when Baltimore was a Rockefeller graduate student, with the same mahogany paneling, vaulted ceiling, and fifteen-foot-tall window.

Baltimore took charge immediately. He froze salaries to cauterize Rockefeller's leaking fiscal system. To yank the institution out of its doldrums, he placed a new emphasis on molecular biology, especially on neurobiology, which he felt was the new frontier—a field in which he could trace his interest all the way back to his mother's degree in psychology, and a field where Rockefeller scientists had made significant advances. Then Baltimore attacked the "old world" Rockefeller laboratory structure. Vincent Fischetti, a Rockefeller scientist who was stuck as a junior faculty member for twenty years before Baltimore promoted him, told *Science* about the reforms: "I think it's a real plus for trying to maintain really high-quality science at Rockefeller. In the past, it was very rare for a full professor to be promoted from within."

Baltimore also needed to keep the rest of the junior faculty happy until there was room for more promotions. Jim Darnell was instrumental in recruiting twelve junior faculty between 1986 and 1990, and he became their mentor, much as Baltimore had done with the young Whitehead faculty. Darnell helped them write grants and establish themselves on campus. "This was the future of the university as far as I was concerned," he said. But in 1990 Darnell was considering moving to the Salk Institute. Understanding Darnell's camaraderie with the young faculty, Baltimore asked him to stay and help him continue to change Rockefeller, as Baltimore's right-hand man, a provost of sorts. They were good friends, and Darnell agreed. With the help of the trustees, they began planning for a new wave of junior faculty recruiting.

Baltimore found the presidency more tiresome and difficult than he anticipated: "It turned out to be a kind of burden that I really wasn't overly enjoyed or happy with." During his first year at Rockefeller, Baltimore maintained a lab at both the Whitehead Institute and the Rockefeller to allow his MIT students to graduate or move to New York. He was struggling with Rockefeller's senior faculty for control of the university's future; and the Imanishi-Kari scientific fraud controversy was about to explode.

In mid-March 1991, after two years of work, the NIH OSI panel finished their second investigation of Imanishi-Kari and the Weaver paper, and they distributed their confidential report to a number of reviewers. The draft statement described Secret Service proof that Imanishi-Kari falsified her laboratory notebooks, and it proclaimed her guilty of "serious scientific misconduct." The appropriate course of events was clear: reviewers would submit their comments to the panel, the OSI would write a final report, and the OSI panel would inform Imanishi-Kari of the verdict. Then the report would be made public, and Imanishi-Kari would have a month to respond and appeal. But the NIH OSI procedure broke down. Reviewers were required to keep the report confidential, but there was no way to enforce that requirement. At least one of the initial reviewers leaked the draft report to the press, and Walter Gilbert circulated the report to his Harvard faculty friends. News of Imanishi-Kari's guilt spread like the newest influenza.

Journalists called Baltimore with the news. He was stunned. After steadfastly refusing to go along with the investigations, reviews, and demands for a withdrawal of the paper, he was left with no other options. He made a public and formal retraction of the *Cell* paper. On March 21, the *New York Times* ran a front-page article headlined "Crucial Data Were Fabricated in Report Signed by Top Biologist: Nobel Winner Is Asking That Paper Be Retracted." The faculty of Rockefeller was sickened.

The Secret Service data showed that Imanishi-Kari's notebooks had been altered and were definitely not in chronological order. Moreover, the Secret Service had completed a statistical analysis of the numbers used in Imanishi-Kari's handwritten data and concluded that her number use was distinctly nonrandom; she had a "personal number preference," indicating that she had invented the numbers.

After a month of painful consultation with his lawyers and colleagues, Baltimore sent a statement to the NIH, which was published in *Nature* and *Science* in mid-May:

> I wish to state that if Dr. Imanishi-Kari did falsify data or make misrepresentations, I had no knowledge of the misconduct.
>
> The findings do not undermine either the integrity of the work conducted by my postdoctoral fellow, Dr. David Weaver, under my supervision or the reliability of our records. However the OSI was critical of my response to the mounting challenges raised to the work of Dr. Imanishi-Kari, my coauthor.
>
> The completion of the NIH investigation has prompted me to make these comments, which will address OSI's observations about my conduct and will share the lessons I have drawn from this experience about the appropriate response to such allegations and the respect and candor which must characterize the partnership between the scientific community and the federal government.
>
> OSI criticized me for my strong defense of Dr. Imanishi-Kari, particularly at the May 1989 hearings before the congressional subcommittee, and for my failure to reexamine Dr. Imanishi-Kari's data more critically after serious questions had been raised. I wish to state at the outset that my defense of Dr. Imanishi-Kari was not due to any lack of regard for Dr. Margot O'Toole, the postdoctoral fellow who first uncovered certain discrepancies in Imanishi-Kari's research. I have tremendous respect for Dr. Margot O'Toole, personally and as a scientist, and I have consistently maintained that I believe that her analyses were insightful, her expressions of concern were proper and appropriate, and her motives were pure. Rather, my defense of my coauthor was fueled by my respect for Dr. Imanishi-Kari's demonstrated abilities as a scientist, by my belief that the paper's scientific conclusions were sound, and by my trust in the efficacy of the peer review process. . . .
>
> In good conscience I feared a rush to judgement, and I accorded my colleague the benefit of every doubt. I now recognize that I was too willing to accept Dr. Imanishi-Kari's explanations, and to excuse discrepancies as mere sloppiness. Furthermore, I did too little to seek an independent verification of her data and conclusions. I acknowledge that, for too long, I focused narrowly on the question of whether

the paper could stand; what was important to me was that the solid molecular biology data gathered by my laboratory seemed to lend credence to the serological findings. In other words, as a scientist, my concern was always for the science: Is the result correct? Can it be replicated and built upon?

The OSI report raises very serious questions about the veracity of the serological data [Imanishi-Kari's cell experiments]. I am shocked and saddened by the revelations of possible alteration and fabrication of data. These discoveries are deeply troubling not only because of their impact upon our article, which has been retracted in light of these revelations, but because such allegations of fraud undermine public confidence in the entire scientific community. Science must be an objective search for truth. It was my belief in science and faith in my fellow scientists which led me to set my threshold of suspicion so high.

I wish to state unequivocally that I have never condoned falsity by a scientist. I do not believe it could ever be appropriate to represent that a test which was not performed was in fact completed, or that anything other than the actual results were obtained. Fraud in the laboratory is not only wrong from a moral and legal standpoint, but it impedes the progress of science, as it makes the review and retesting of hypotheses and conclusions impossible. Deliberate falsification demeans all members of the scientific community because it under-mines public trust and confidence in our enterprise. . . .

I have learned from this experience that the accountability to ensure the responsible use of public funds rests not only with each individual scientist but with the scientific and academic communities as a whole. Better self-policing and record-keeping will facilitate the government's oversight function and may obviate the need for the repeated hearings and investigations that were needed in this case. . . .

In conclusion, I commend Dr. O'Toole for her courage and her determination, and I regret and apologize to her for my failure to act vigorously enough in my investigation of her doubts. I recognize that I may well have been blinded to the full implications of the mounting evidence by an excess of trust, and I have learned from this experience that one must temper trust with a healthy dose of skepticism. This entire episode has reminded me of the importance of humility in the face of scientific data.

After five years of hearing David Baltimore stubbornly defend Imanishi-Kari and the paper, many in the scientific community were stunned by Baltimore's statement in *Nature* and *Science,* but they were also relieved. His friends figured he must have choked on every word. Along with Baltimore's statement, *Science* published a short piece gauging the state of affairs at Rockefeller University:

> Richard Furlaud, chairman of the board, said that after the trustees' scientific affairs committee had reviewed the entire controversy in a meeting last week, it reaffirmed its support for Baltimore's presidency. "The question of his resignation was never an issue," Furlaud says. While the trustees and administration officials express unwavering support for Baltimore, faculty sentiment is harder to gauge. "I am sure if you were to take a secret ballot—emphasis on secret—a majority would ask for his resignation," says one faculty member who objected to Baltimore's appointment as president a year and a half ago. Such support from the trustees could vanish abruptly if Baltimore becomes mired any more deeply in the controversy.

Baltimore's presidency, unpopular with senior faculty from its inception, was now in great danger. The articles in *Nature* and *Science* were read by nearly everyone at Rockefeller University and most other major research universities. Jim Darnell said several years later, "Reflecting on it from a distance, I have great sympathy for David's plight at this place at the time. There was a strong and vocal contingent of the faculty that had made noises when he first came, and were inimical to the purpose of . . . designing a more open place for the future. . . . Had David been given enough time to sort of outlive some of this [acrimony with the senior faculty], no problems would have existed. But, unfortunately, things blew up within six to eight months of his arrival. So he was never able to establish beachheads with the senior faculty people who were in this contentious crowd." The controversy now jumped into the scientific and public consciousness as the Imanishi-Kari Affair, the Baltimore Saga, or the Baltimore Affair.

Imanishi-Kari had not yet even seen the official charges of which she was found guilty, much less the evidence to support them. Adding to her woes, the U.S. attorney's office, in light of the NIH OSI draft report, declared that they planned to prosecute her in federal court for fraudulent use of government funds. In newspapers, however, Imanishi-Kari was hardly mentioned; all attention focused on Baltimore. An editorial in the *New York*

Times titled "A Scientific Watergate?" discussed David Baltimore's prominence and possible cover-up. Various papers accused him of stonewalling a federal investigation. An editorial in the *Washington Post* discussed "the scientific fraud of David Baltimore." John Maddox, the editor of *Nature,* wrote a column for the *New York Times* titled "Dr. Baltimore's Experiment in Hubris." Ironically, the *Wall Street Journal,* bastion of the staunchly capitalist ideals Baltimore had once lambasted, was perhaps the only newspaper friendly to him. One of its editorials stated that the *Wall Street Journal* "condemns news coverage of the David Baltimore scientific 'fraud' case and wonders whether the *New York Times* and other newspapers will ever see fit to print all sides of the story," noting the grave lack of due process in the investigations.

The May 16 issue of *Nature* contained a reply by Margot O'Toole to Baltimore's statement, in which she harshly criticized the conduct of Baltimore, Eisen, Wortis, Huber, and others. She stated, "I consider it a disgrace that Drs. Weaver and Baltimore did not immediately retract the paper in 1986 when they learned of the discrepancies between what was actually observed and what was actually published." She later asserted, "In fact, as each piece of evidence is uncovered, someone usually has had to change his or her account to make it fit the evidence, but I have never had to do so. That my account has proved consistent with all the evidence that has come to light is no accident. I have been telling the truth all along."

In fact, even in that statement O'Toole was revising history. In her original complaints brought to MIT, she had simply stated that the BET-1 reagent was unreliable and that she believed in an alternative scientific theory to explain the Weaver paper results. She never asserted that the data were altered or fabricated. The BET-1 concerns in her memo were addressed, and the other concerns were declared differences of opinion. But the general scientific community readership did not know this history, and after the NIH OSI verdict, O'Toole's version of the story carried a lot of weight: the NIH draft report called her actions "heroic in many respects." O'Toole's embellished version was a bitter pill to swallow for the other players in the drama.

Her account could not go unanswered. Two weeks later, David Baltimore and Herman Eisen wrote replies to O'Toole's letter, which were published back-to-back in *Nature.* By this point, *Nature* had dedicated a special section of the magazine, "The Imanishi-Kari Affair," to the controversy. Baltimore's letter, headlined "Baltimore Declares O'Toole Mistaken" by *Nature*'s staff, began: "Doctor Margot O'Toole's recent comments on the draft report of the National Institutes of Health Office of Scientific Integrity create a misleading impression and therefore require a response. The issues she raises have all previously been answered, often several times, but because many are not familiar with the details, I feel that it is necessary to demonstrate publicly that her charges lack substance." Baltimore then proceeded to explain, in three long pages, how O'Toole's comments were lies, exaggerations, or concerns that had been addressed years earlier. He stated time and again that there had been no reason to retract the paper earlier, as no major problems had been identified. Any minor problems identified had been fixed, as requested. Among the many statements that he refuted was O'Toole's claim that "[Baltimore] told me that he would personally oppose any effort I made to get the paper corrected." But, as she admitted elsewhere, including in congressional testimony, Baltimore had actually suggested she write a letter to *Cell* or *Nature,* explaining her theory, and that he would write a reply. Baltimore concluded:

> While Dr. O'Toole has now directly attacked my honesty and integrity, none of my previous remarks nor any of the remarks in this statement were intended to criticize her personally, impugn her abilities as a scientist or question her motives. Rather, I have made this statement in the hope that any assessment of the validity of her comments will be a measured one, based upon a consideration of all of the facts and the entire record of this controversy.

However, the scientific community was just coming to grips with his mea culpa of three weeks before, and they were completely confused by this rebuttal. Was Baltimore now claiming to have been right all along? Clearly someone must be lying. Who was it? The whole procedure was bizarre; this was not the way papers were normally proved right or wrong in science. People were tempted to believe the worst of Baltimore, especially given the Secret Service data and the NIH's report on Imanishi-Kari.

Herman Eisen, too, was determined to refute O'Toole's defamatory remarks: "Doctor Margot O'Toole makes a series of assertions that effectively charge me and many others with dishonest and irresponsible behaviour. These assertions cannot go unchallenged. In what follows, I address several of her more extreme statements, those that from personal knowledge I know to be inaccurate or grossly to misrepresent the true events." He then addressed O'Toole's newly published version of events point by point. She claimed that at the original MIT inquiry meetings "Dr. Imanishi-Kari again admitted that a large series of the published experiments had not even been performed." Eisen declared O'Toole's statements outright lies.

In addition to challenging O'Toole's account of the science, Eisen discussed her treatment at MIT. Representative Dingell had made it sound in the congressional hearings as though O'Toole had lost her job. His aides had repeatedly told newspapers that O'Toole had essentially been fired for insubordination. According to Eisen, this was simply a lie. O'Toole wrote in her *Nature* letter: "I lost my job as a result of raising questions. This is essentially true, but the facts are a little complicated. It is more accurate to say I lost my career because I would not go along with Dr. Imanishi-Kari's pressure to misrepresent my own results. I was left unemployed, and subjected to five years of slander and libel." Eisen responded to this, reasserting points made several times in the past:

> It had been asserted that Dr. O'Toole lost her job at MIT because she challenged the Weaver *et al.* paper. She now says that "this charge is essentially true, but the facts were a little complicated." In fact, they are not. Dr. O'Toole was appointed to a postdoctoral fellowship in June of 1985 with the understanding the position would terminate on 31 May 1986. She was ineligible for more than one year of support from the NIH training grant that provided her stipend on account of previous years of support. Moreover, it was known in 1985 that Dr. Imanishi-Kari was due to move from MIT to Tufts in June 1986.

He summarized:

> Thus it is not inappropriate to ask: who misled whom? It is ironic and sad that, instead of recognizing that she bears some responsibility for creating a misleading situation, Dr. O'Toole now characterizes the initial inquiry at MIT as a "cover-up." Given her choice of words, I also find it remarkable that those of us who were involved in the inquiry are accused of slander and libel.

In the same issue of *Nature,* also in the "Imanishi-Kari Affair" section, appeared part of Imanishi-Kari's reply to the NIH charges. It included a striking condemnation of OSI's inability to understand and sort through the immunology data:

> You have no idea how upsetting it is to find that after five years of controversy and two years of OSI review, an investigation still gets the

most fundamental part of the story—the question of the BET-1 reagent—all wrong. It is demoralizing to find that, after all this time, there is still such a basic misunderstanding of the reagent first questioned by Dr. O'Toole five years ago.

The draft report states that "the BET-1 reagent was key to the reliability and accuracy of the results . . . [it] played a crucial role in the detection of the transgene. A failure of BET-1 to react with appropriate specificity would open the possibility that Dr. Imanishi-Kari was in many cases detecting transgene, rather than endogenous, genes."

Unfortunately this gets the BET-1 story completely backwards. BET-1 is a monoclonal reagent raised against the μ^a allotype. It recognizes the transgene, μ^a. A lack of specificity of BET-1 would lead to recognition of μ^b (endogenous).

This was exactly the same issue that Herman Eisen had resolved five years earlier at MIT. Unfortunately, Imanishi-Kari's statements just generated more confusion. The scientific public did not know what to believe; they didn't know what μ^a and μ^b were, much less their importance for the experiment; but they were not inclined to believe Imanishi-Kari over the Secret Service data and the two-year OSI study.

Two weeks later, in what was beginning to seem more like a soap opera than real life, another series of letters appeared in *Nature*. These were the replies of the members of the Tufts University inquiry panel, who were upset by O'Toole's account of their inquiry. They too responded to her criticisms of them point by point. In addition, each of them made personal comments refuting O'Toole's claims. Henry Wortis wrote: "I was Margot O'Toole's thesis adviser and maintained a sustained friendship with her. . . . In the end I disagreed with her assessment of the science. Different opinions are neither slanders nor libels, and I find it especially painful to hear my opinions so characterized by my first graduate student." Afterwards, Robert Woodland wrote a stinging summation: "I find offensive her statement that I falsely reported what I had seen during the data analysis. It is telling that the one constant to emerge from this unhappy episode is that anyone who has disagreed with Dr. O'Toole's analysis of the scientific issues has been accused of either incompetence or deceit." He was well aware that his statement was being read by a distrusting audience, and he noted at the end, "Unfortunately, it is unlikely that the acrimony in this case will be soon reduced to a level where the facts can emerge."

On the next page was a letter from Imanishi-Kari responding to O'Toole's letter. On the page after that, Margot O'Toole responded to Herman Eisen's response to her from two weeks earlier. In this letter, O'Toole made several sophisticated but inaccurate references to testimony at the 1989 congressional hearings, her original memo at MIT, and Eisen's MIT report. Her manipulation of actual statements was difficult, if not impossible, to refute without looking at the actual congressional testimonies and memos. She wrote: "[Eisen] now again denies that I had indicated in June 1986 that some experiments had not been done, asserting that I made no suggestion that 'reported results were based on nonexistent . . . data.' But my June 1986 memo (1989 hearings, pages 307–310) said that some of the experiments had not been done, and this memo was in Dr. Eisen's files until it was surrendered to investigators."

Eisen did in fact assert in the congressional hearing that O'Toole made no suggestion that "reported results were based on nonexistent . . . data"; and O'Toole's 1986 memo was in fact in Eisen's possession until it was subpoenaed with the rest of the documents regarding the Weaver paper; and O'Toole's memo was in fact reprinted on pages 307–310 of the 1989 hearings transcript; but O'Toole's 1986 memo did *not* state "that some of the experiments had not been done." She very clearly made four points in her 1986 memo. The first was that BET-1 did not work as well as Imanishi-Kari claimed; and the remaining points were that she disagreed with Weaver, Baltimore, and Imanishi-Kari's interpretations of the published data. There was not even the hint of a claim that experiments had not been done. O'Toole continued in her letter to *Nature:* "Dr. Eisen disputes my account of [additional events]. . . . This denial must be viewed in light of his statement that my memo did not inform him of experiments that were not done." Indeed it must, but in this web of accusation and counter-accusation, the readers of *Nature* could not know that it was O'Toole, not Eisen, who was changing the facts.

More turmoil was brewing. The NIH OSI had just published its definition of scientific misconduct, and over two thousand scientists wrote to the NIH denouncing its vagueness. In an "Open Letter on OSI's Methods," 143 concerned scientists stated their objections, published just below O'Toole's letter in *Nature.* The open letter stated:

> As scientists we are deeply concerned by the way in which the charges against Dr. Thereza Imanishi-Kari . . . have been handled. . . . The need for formal, thorough and fair investigations of possible scientific fraud is clear. However, it is apparent that the procedures followed by

the OSI have serious shortcomings, and have not permitted Imanishi-Kari the opportunity to defend herself by a public examination of the evidence against her. Whether or not she is guilty as charged, the precedents which have been set in this case are dangerous.

The NIH had more problems than letter-writing scientists, and powerful John Dingell was at the center of the storm. The press began referring to him as "the formidable congressional watchdog of the NIH." Dingell was dissecting the scientific community. He held six months of hearings and investigations into universities misusing federal funds. The hearings revealed that a number of major research universities overcharged the government for their overhead costs. Stanford University was found guilty of charging the federal government for flowers for a wedding reception, among other, well-publicized improprieties. This embarrassment forced the resignation of Stanford's president, Donald Kennedy, in the first week of August 1991.

Dingell's second target was the NIH itself, and particularly the OSI. After holding two years of continuous hearings on the Imanishi-Kari case and other OSI cases, he still did not feel that the NIH was handling its affairs properly. He stated at one of his hearings, "It is not the business of the subcommittee to supervise the daily workings of the NIH. But if we have to do it, we will." These revelations of poor internal management at the NIH were extensively covered by the media.

Bernadine Healy had just been appointed director of the NIH in April 1991 when the Imanishi-Kari draft report was leaked and the scientific fraud case exploded in the press. Furious about the leak and unhappy with OSI's handling of the Imanishi-Kari case, Healy requested an FBI investigation. She wanted to institute major changes in the OSI, clarifying its mission, speeding up its procedures, and maintaining due process by allowing scientists to face their accusers and know the charges against them. Her proposals echoed the concerns of many scientists. Healy stated: "There is a lesson for science in the play *Amadeus*. . . . [Mozart, the creative genius,] magical and brilliant, [was also] difficult, childish, nasty, and unconventional. [His rival Salieri was] talented in a workmanlike way and popular at court. . . . If medicine is to succeed, the Mozarts must be allowed to flourish."

Healy's first step in rebuilding the OSI was to remove Suzanne Hadley, OSI's deputy director. In Healy's opinion, Hadley had bungled the Imanishi-Kari investigation by allowing the press leak, by not providing Imanishi-Kari with due process, and by becoming all too friendly with Margot O'Toole. This was a strong gambit on Healy's part, because Hadley had been leading the Imanishi-Kari investigation for over two years. Dingell was not happy; Healy's move seemed to him yet another instance of the NIH's terrible management. He immediately called for a hearing in which he dismantled Healy's plans to reform the OSI.

Meanwhile, at Rockefeller University, faculty dissatisfaction was festering. The continuous "public blood-letting" of the Imanishi-Kari affair demoralized the Rockefeller professors. Many were upset with Baltimore's decision to slug it out in the press with Margot O'Toole and anyone else who criticized him. Faculty meetings became debates about the Weaver paper, with David Baltimore against the faculty. Darnell said, "What I was hearing from faculty people as I went out [was]: 'Why doesn't he take responsibility and clear it up?' David was asked this by faculty members." In addition, Darnell said, "There were a couple of meetings held here where a subject was to be discussed with the senior faculty. And in those meetings, David came along with members of the board of trustees. Which many people in the faculty didn't think was necessarily reasonable—he should have handled the faculty by himself. But, at any rate, he was asked in those meetings, 'Why don't you do that?' And his response to them was the same as his response to the public at large; that he thought the questioned part of the work was not his, it was his collaborator's, and it was up to her to get it straightened out."

Darnell continued, "The fallacy there, I think I felt it at the time, and I'm sure others did (and on reflection, it's probably right that I felt this at the time), that a guy who was in the position he was in—that is to say, an already world-famous scientist, and in a sensitive position because of being president here—he might better have devoted the time and energy of some technicians or some people to actually try to get the mice to do the crosses again, to get the cells again. Do the damn experiment again. Had that have happened, I think it would have defused the issue. But he had a legitimate point, that it wasn't his doing, it was hers. And that's just the way he chose to handle it." Rockefeller professors were disappointed that Baltimore was not putting the University's needs before his own.

Darnell said, in Baltimore's defense, "David said to me a number of times, privately, that to take the time to do [the experiment again] wasn't reasonable. Why should he go back and repeat something that was not in his line of business? He's not a serologist [like Imanishi-Kari]. And all that's true. One can certainly look at the events of those times through his eyes and see why, reasonably, he did what he did. But that left him sort of in a pickle with a large number of people in the scientific community."

The atmosphere at Rockefeller was electrified after Paul Doty, professor emeritus of biology at Harvard, wrote a letter to *Nature* indicting Baltimore for his "egregious departure from the usual standards of carrying out and reporting research." Doty stated that the work was "so sloppy as to insult the scientific method." Doty asked the scientific community as a whole to "examine the case of the *Cell* paper . . . and to assess the extent to which this standard [of scientific ethics] has been met or compromised." He was calling for a referendum. Baltimore could not let such a comment pass. Damn the mea culpa. He replied with a savage letter in *Nature* attacking Doty's commentary and making what many scientists interpreted as an un-retraction of the *Cell* paper. Baltimore wrote that "the data have proved more durable than the data in most papers." He was referring specifically to the experiments by his postdoc, David Weaver. Indeed, scientists such as Alan Stall, an immunologist at Columbia, supported Baltimore's claim, noting that Weaver's results were "very striking" and had provided a basis for further research by other labs into the nature of antibody production. But, given Baltimore's mea culpa and Secret Service investigation, defending the data seemed absurd to most scientists.

Baltimore's impassioned response was more than the Rockefeller establishment could bear. Günter Blobel, a senior Rockefeller scientist (and later the 1999 Nobel laureate in medicine), said at the time, "Many of those who were not opposed to Baltimore have been swayed by his extreme mishandling of the situation." Several major professors, including the Nobel laureate Gerald Edelman and his fellow neuroscientist Bruce Cunningham, resigned and moved their laboratories to other institutions. *Science* magazine claimed that "it was at this point, according to a senior faculty member, that the trustees asked Torsten Wiesel, de facto head of the faculty, to survey sentiment once again among Rockefeller's 44 tenured professors. Wiesel conducted a secret straw poll in early October, according to several faculty sources, and communicated the results to the board in writing: About 70% no longer supported Baltimore's presidency."

Baltimore rallied his friends and supporters on the faculty, particularly the junior faculty members, encouraging them to express their support for him to the trustees. They did, and Baltimore's presidency was safe again for a while. However, his end-run around the senior faculty further alienated them. In Paul Berg's opinion, Baltimore couldn't bring himself to reach out to the senior faculty. He kept his faculty friends near, but didn't work with the other faculty. Berg said, "He really found that very difficult. He kept saying, 'They won't listen, they won't listen.'" Darnell agreed: "Paul's right, I suppose. If David had chosen to try to establish better relationships, and stronger relationships, with half a dozen people on campus, he might have done himself a favor."

Things looked dark for Baltimore. Darnell recalled, "David and I talked about [the situation] a few times, once it became closer to the disaster that finally happened. He had said to me on an occasion just a couple weeks before [the end] that it was clear that he was going to be asked for his resignation. We were having dinner at a place called Wilkinson's, a seafood restaurant. He asked me, was I his friend. And I said, 'David, we've known each other for many years, of course I'm you're friend. I always will be.' Then we talked about whether he would be asked for his resignation. He never said to me, 'Do you think I should resign?' I never said to him, 'I think you should resign,' but . . . the handwriting was surely on the wall."

Darnell continued, "I had held on for as long as I could. I was being besieged by large numbers of the senior faculty to get out. And I had heard from people from around the country, and a lot of them thought that the University was being damaged. And so I did it. . . . I went to David Rockefeller and told him that, in spite of David's great gifts—and in spite of the fact that, *had* he been able to get through this without so much public clamor, I thought he'd be a great president—that I thought the whole thing had come to the point where he probably was going to have to resign. I thought that the University was suffering."

David Rockefeller told Paul Berg about Darnell's defection, and Berg called Darnell. Berg confirmed that Darnell had lost faith in Baltimore. Disgusted, Berg also left the conversation with the understanding that Darnell was trying to become Rockefeller's next president. Darnell recalled the conversation differently: "Paul Berg called me and asked me about these things. And I may have said something to the effect that what I thought was important was that the programs that were changing the university stay in place. And to Paul—who has been a longtime friend of mine and now who has decided I shouldn't be his friend—I probably said to Paul something to the effect of, 'I could and would do the job if it came to that.' But that's very different, you know? I was talking to a friend of twenty-five years." Darnell continued, "It is absolutely incorrect and wrong to think that I was snooping around with the board of trustees trying to get rid of David so that I could become president. That's wrong."

Berg told Baltimore that Darnell had betrayed him. Deeply upset, Baltimore went to Darnell. The two argued to an impasse that Darnell had felt approaching for months as the faculty situation had deteriorated. As Darnell recalled, "I said, 'Well, I think perhaps I should resign.' And David said, in a somewhat angry voice to me, 'Yeah, I think you should if that's the way you feel.' And two days later, I did." Darnell added, "I was deeply disturbed by all of this. I felt that this was the worst year of my life. And still do."

Darnell did not resign quietly, though. Torn between his friend and his university, he chose the university. In his resignation letter, he stated:

> It is in the best interest of the University that David Baltimore resign as president. . . . I would like to note that while some Board members have expressed apprehension that the campus might be 'worse off' or 'in chaos' if David resigns, I believe nothing could be further from the truth. . . . If Torsten Wiesel were chosen as interim president, and he and the Board wished me to continue as Vice President for Academic Affairs, I would do so. And in my sincerest opinion the anxiety that is presently rife on campus would vanish overnight.

Baltimore's longtime friend and former mentor, and one of his last strong supporters in the senior faculty, had abandoned him. The board did not ask for Baltimore's resignation, but they did not need to. He conceded defeat and resigned. The board of trustees accepted both Darnell's and Baltimore's resignations on December 3, 1991.

Paul Berg publicly summarized the faculty's three main concerns: "One, the continuing ball-in-play on the *Cell* paper, and all of the negative publicity and the uncertainty about when it would end. That came through clearly. The second was whether Baltimore was so severely wounded that he would be incapable of recruiting new faculty to Rockefeller. The third thing was whether all of the hubbub of the *Cell* controversy, and the public aspects of it, would also poison his ability to raise money." But Berg then immediately resigned, disenchanted with the university: "I was really outraged by the way people on the board behaved, because I didn't think they gave him a fair shake. And I didn't see why I should spend my time working for those characters who were so destructive."

Baltimore gave his own summary of the situation: "I was a threat to the old-line Rockefeller faculty. They used that [Imanishi-Kari affair] as a tool to bludgeon me with, and ultimately to get me out of office. So it had a huge effect, because it provided an opening. Leverage. So to that extent it's probably true that I shouldn't have gone to Rockefeller and allowed that to happen. I didn't see fully at all what was going on; or I would have pulled back." Curiously, Baltimore seemed to think that the struggle may have been resolving itself, right up until he resigned, and even afterward: "I would have come to a much more comfortable relationship with it if I had stayed a little longer, but I never found a real equilibrium—too much was going on." Several years later, looking back at his switch from the Whitehead Institute to Rockefeller, he finally said, "Well, that was probably actually a mistake, to tell you the truth." He added, "But I thought, I thought I could make a difference. . . . And I must say, actually, I *did* make a difference. And the place is a different place for the time that I was there—which didn't turn out to be as long as I expected."

The obvious choice for Baltimore's replacement was Torsten Wiesel, de facto head of the senior faculty, and Darnell's recommendation for president. With Baltimore out of the job and Wiesel in, Darnell was reappointed vice president and was able to regain his role as father to the junior faculty. Baltimore still refuses to speak to the man who betrayed him. Darnell remains sad about the decision he felt forced to make. Darnell said in 1998, "The fact that David has reemerged as a certified leader takes the sting out of it, I hope, to some considerable degree. I would greatly value a reestablishment of friendship with David, but I'm not sure that's possible. He doesn't see things in this rather simple way that I do. But, so be it."

POST-PRESIDENCY

Before submitting his official letter, Baltimore had resigned as president by cell phone, speaking with Richard Furlaud while driving to his sanctuary in Woods Hole, on Cape Cod. What happened that afternoon at Rockefeller is telling. Furlaud called former MIT provost Rosenblith and told him of Baltimore's resignation. Rosenblith then picked up the phone and called both Maurice Fox, head of the MIT biology department, and Phillip Sharp. Rosenblith explained the events of the past weeks at Rockefeller and encouraged Fox and Sharp to give Baltimore the option of returning to MIT. Shortly after Baltimore's resignation was made public the following day, Charles Vest, president of MIT, called Baltimore, gave his condolences, and told Baltimore that he would always be welcome at MIT. Baltimore greatly appreciated the support. It was the second time that MIT had offered him a fresh start during troubled times, and some months later he formally accepted.

Things were looking dark for Imanishi-Kari; her professional appointments were put on hold, and all of her grant applications were left in limbo.

Several months later, she finally received the Secret Service forensic data that allegedly proved her guilty of fraud. She knew she wasn't guilty, but she couldn't understand the data, and she enlisted the help of the forensic scientist Albert Lyter. Lyter had pioneered the development of the statistical techniques that the Secret Service had used to analyze Imanishi-Kari's notebooks. He spent a full year checking the Secret Service's results and discovered flaws permeating the analyses. On July 14, 1992, because of Lyter's conclusions, the U.S. attorney's office dropped all charges against Thereza Imanishi-Kari. Nevertheless, the NIH OSI investigation was still open.

As soon as Lyter's analysis was complete, Baltimore declared, "I feel vindicated," and announced that he would un-retract the *Cell* paper—an unprecedented move. "So far as I can tell, the paper is a valid contribution to scientific discourse. The only thing that ever bothered me was that the Secret Service had evidence that purported to show criminal conduct, that [Imanishi-Kari] had somehow attempted to consciously fabricate data. It's now clear from the analysis of the Secret Service information that they have no such evidence."

At the behest of John Dingell, the NIH OSI was disbanded and rebuilt as the Office of Research Integrity (ORI) in the Department of Health and Human Services, further delaying any conclusion of Imanishi-Kari's case. The NIH was no longer in control. The ORI launched the third federal investigation of the Imanishi-Kari case. In the face of this bedlam, after conferring with his lawyers and the other authors of the paper, Baltimore then decided not to retract the retraction. He would wait until things calmed down.

Baltimore's handling of the Imanishi-Kari controversy continued to polarize the scientific community. Most scientists were dazed by the complexity of the affair and could be sure only that the situation was a gargantuan mess. There were vocal supporters of Baltimore's actions, such as microbiologist Bernard Davis at Harvard, Phillip Sharp at MIT, and Maxine Singer at the Carnegie Institute; and there were vocal critics, such as Walter Gilbert, Mark Ptashne, and Paul Doty of Harvard, all of whom published their opinions in major magazines and newspapers. Bernard Davis, who had not formed a good impression of Baltimore when they first met at Harvard in 1967, became one of Baltimore's strongest allies. In 1992 Davis was seventy-six years old and crippled by prostate cancer, but he was passionately working on a manuscript describing the machinations of the Imanishi-Kari affair. He continued to write, even while bedridden, until his death on January 14, 1994. The manuscript remained incomplete.

Howard Temin also died in 1994. Baltimore wrote a moving homage to Temin, in which he reflected on the life of a kindred spirit: "Howard's death at such a young age removes from us one of the treasures of modern science. . . . It is important to remember that he who toils alone may become the revolutionary, that insight goes further than logic, and that a life lived in uncompromising reach for personal goals is the greatest legacy an individual can leave to the world."

Baltimore remained at Rockefeller for two more years as a professor, concentrating on research. He continued to make major contributions to cancer research, AIDS research, immunology, and virology, and his status as one of the most referenced scientists in the world reflected that importance. Irving Weissman observed, "The group that he had at the Rockefeller were making groundbreaking discoveries at about the same rate his lab always has." In 1994 he returned to MIT, leaving the chaos of Rockefeller behind him.

Ten

Baltimore's return to the MIT biology department was heralded as a homecoming. Some MIT researchers wondered why he didn't return to the Whitehead. That had been an option, but the biology department made him a lucrative offer, funded through a multimillion-dollar donation by Ivan Cottrell, a wealthy Rochester dentist. The Whitehead Institute was still just across the street, and Baltimore ate his lunch in the Whitehead cafeteria almost every day. Phillip Sharp had just won the 1993 Nobel Prize in medicine and was now head of the department, which he moved to the new Building 68, on the north side of campus, comfortably situated between old Building 16, the Center for Cancer Research, and the Whitehead. The new biology building had cost over $60 million. Baltimore was given the north end of the third floor, which, with twenty full lab benches and half a dozen associated rooms, was the largest lab space he had ever occupied. Since he no longer shouldered administrative responsibilities, he spent a lot more time in his lab. But that wasn't enough; he needed to explore new possibilities. "I don't know that I relax much. . . . [I] have taken a particular interest in trying to understand and consult in biotechnology. . . . It's partly because I have some time, and I find it interesting. Something to do. Always looking for something new and different."

His wife, Alice, still served as dean for science at NYU and commuted between New York and Boston. Their daughter Teak was now in college, studying psychology and theater at Yale University. Baltimore noted, "She said she never wanted anything to do with what her parents do." He smiled, "We'll see. There's still time."

Elsewhere, looking for another crusade, Walter Stewart and Ned Feder had broadened their "fraudbuster" investigations. They wrote a computer program that compared scientific papers for plagiarism. The effort was doomed to fail because plagiarism in science rarely involves copying words; it involves stealing ideas. Unable to find any plagiarism in scientific articles, Stewart and Feder then used their software to analyze the prominent biography of Abraham Lincoln by Stephen Oates, who had previously been charged with (and cleared of) plagiarism. All of this was done in their laboratory at the NIH, supported by the NIH's Institute of Diabetes and Digestive and Kidney Diseases.

The program churned out reams of analysis that Stewart and Feder compiled into a 1,400-page document claiming that Oates's biography was rife with plagiarism. A committee of historians reviewed the accusations and summarily dismissed the charges. None of the charges amounted to even a plagiarized sentence. When Feder and Stewart's activities became publicly known, the NIH locked them out of their laboratory and seized their files. In May 1993, the NIH permanently closed their lab. The director of the National Institute of Diabetes stated, "The essential reason the office was closed is that their work progressively moved outside this institute's mission, authority, and responsibility. . . . This is not appropriate, nor do they have the authority to do that in this institute." Stewart immediately began a hunger strike. No one paid any attention beyond an occasional mocking remark in the press. Dingell and his staff rapidly distanced themselves from Stewart's antics. Thirty-three days later, Stewart ended his fast, noting that he had reached a stage where malnutrition could cause permanent physical damage. He declared victory. No one has determined what he was victorious over.

Despite the downfall of Stewart and Feder, Imanishi-Kari's problems were far from over. In winter 1994, after two more years of slow investigation, the ORI issued a new report stating that Imanishi-Kari had fabricated data in the Weaver paper. No one was surprised that the ORI stuck by the OSI's original conclusions. The numerous federal investigations had taken over eight years. In that time, the investigative office was revamped no fewer than three times. Each incarnation of the office carried out between one and four different inquiries and investigations. And Imanishi-Kari still had not been given the opportunity to respond. The affair had become a tragicomedy of accusations, failed procedures, and outright stubbornness by everyone involved.

Imanishi-Kari planned to appeal and finally get her day in court. Joseph Onek, a lawyer who had won a similar case the previous year, agreed to take Imanishi-Kari's case pro bono. (Baltimore had already paid over $100,000 of Imanishi-Kari's legal fees out of his own pocket.) The appeals process was expected to take all of 1995.

Imanishi-Kari's professorial position at Tufts had been revoked, but she was allowed to stay on staff as a temporary research associate until the appeals verdict was decided. She published a series of scientific papers building on the results of the Weaver paper, notably one paper in the *Journal of Immunology* in 1993, which extended some of her observations. Several other authors published studies that confirmed some of the original paper's results.

The Department of Health and Human Services appeals board hearings took until April 1996, exactly ten years after the initial publication of the Weaver paper in *Cell*. The panel consisted of two permanent members, Judith Ballard and Cecilia Sparks Ford, and an independent virologist, Julius Younger. The panel amassed over 6,500 pages of hearings transcript, 70 laboratory notebooks, the entire collection of Secret Service evidence, Imanishi-Kari's supporting documents, and the ORI's obsessive list of thousands of "findings of facts and conclusions of law." The format of the hearings was similar to that of a trial, with witnesses and cross-examinations. Walter Gilbert was the ORI's star scientific witness testifying to Imanishi-Kari's fraud. The appeals panel deliberated for a month and then released their decision on June 21, 1996: not guilty. The federal juggernaut ground to a halt.

The appeals panel demolished the ORI's findings: "The Panel found that much of what ORI presented was irrelevant, had limited probative value, was internally inconsistent, lacked reliability or foundation, was not credible or corroborated, or was based on unwarranted assumptions." The panel cleared Imanishi-Kari's name in their opening comments: "Because the history of this case involved a direct attack on Dr. Imanishi-Kari's honesty, we evaluated her statements carefully, and relied primarily on evidence in the record other than her testimony. . . . The credibility of her testimony before us was bolstered, however, when much of the evidence in the record, and in particular, some of the document examination evidence, corroborated her statements and directly contradicted representations made by ORI." They continued, "ORI's description of the forensics findings were not always dependable. For example, as described by the ORI, one type of Secret Service analysis seemed to provide support (albeit limited) for ORI's position on two important issues. . . . The actual results, however, were not as described and were consistent with (indeed, arguably substantiated) Dr. Imanishi-Kari's version of events (which was also corroborated by other evidence.)"

Regarding the Secret Service analysis of Imanishi-Kari's laboratory notebooks, the panel felt that "at most, these [forensics] analyses identified some possible anomalies." Most of the allegedly fabricated data were not used in the *Cell* paper, nor in any other scientific paper: "For example, the 'January Fusion' controversy [regarding recent ORI complaints about hybridoma cell fusions made in January 1986] . . . centers on the data from transgenic fusions not used for any purpose whatsoever." The Secret Service and the ORI could ascribe no motive for Imanishi-Kari to fabricate such useless data, and most of their examples of "fraud" centered on unpublished data, falsification of which made no sense. The ORI's logic baffled the appeals panel: "ORI's attempts at establishing a possible motive for fabrication or falsification [of some data] requires very convoluted reasoning. . . . On the whole, most of the alterations for which no reasonable motivation was adduced looked much more like the marks of untidy 'real life,' than like suspicious efforts at some intentional laundering." In particular, the panel found that the infamous seventeen pages of data that obsessed O'Toole, Feder, and Stewart contained nothing fraudulent or unseemly.

The ORI had hoped that some of their evidence would hold up under cross-examination. When the Secret Service evidence first came to light at the congressional hearings, and when the OSI declared Imanishi-Kari guilty in 1991 based on the Secret Service data, two types of evidence had seemed particularly incriminating. In one case, the Secret Service inspected the pages in Imanishi-Kari's notebooks and declared that they were out of order, on the basis of the pages involved, the ink used, and the color of the radiation counter printouts (green versus yellow paper) that were taped to various notebook pages (Imanishi-Kari's data involved radiation counts of radioactively labeled antibodies). On the surface, this evidence seemed damning. But the appeals panel concluded that the Secret Service dating techniques didn't work even on laboratory notebooks whose veracity was unchallenged, including Margot O'Toole's. The controversy about green paper versus yellow paper arose from inspection of the notebooks of Charles Maplethorpe, Imanishi-Kari's disgruntled postdoc. His notebooks, it turned out, were incorrectly dated. In addition, the Secret Service and ORI made strenuous efforts to show that identical paper types and ink types in the notebooks bore very different dates. The ORI claimed that these "exact matches" in paper and ink proved that Imanishi-Kari was creating data ex post facto. The appeals panel concluded that the matches simply indicated that Imanishi-Kari used ballpoint pens and notepaper from the same manufacturers about fifteen months apart—a mundane explanation to anyone who works with institutional office supplies.

The Secret Service agents had even used infrared technology to analyze writing on certain pages, looking for numbers that had been changed. Those infrared searches only corroborated Imanishi-Kari's story, but the ORI came up with convoluted explanations to assert her guilt (which were rebuked by the appeals panel and witnesses). Secret Service agent Hargett admitted, "[We] didn't know what researchers' laboratory notebooks were to look like, quite frankly." The Secret Service had never before attempted document analysis of this sort; they had no real context to work with. They had been dragged into the affair by Dingell's office. The appeals panel became even more skeptical of the Secret Service work when it became clear that Dingell's aides had met with them and told them what data were "good" and what were suspicious.

The Secret Service had also attempted statistical analyses of Imanishi-Kari's data. In many places, Imanishi-Kari did not tape the original radiation counter printouts into her notebook but wrote the data in by hand. After studying the handwritten numbers, the Secret Service declared that she used certain numbers far too frequently and that this pattern strongly suggested that she was inventing the data. This evidence swayed many scientists when it was first published in a *Science* article in 1991, along with the OSI verdict. However, the appeals panel concluded that the analysis was meaningless. The forensics analysis nonsensically demonstrated that she used different numbers more or less frequently on different days, even though their whole premise was that she had consistent "personal number preferences." Secret Service analysis of other researchers' undisputed notebooks yielded similar useless results.

Ironically, the panel also noted that the ORI's statistician, Dr. Dahlberg, who accused Imanishi-Kari of data selection, engaged in data selection and interpretation of his own. Under intensive investigation, Imanishi-Kari's data selection technique was corroborated by other immunologists who analyzed the data. Dahlberg's own data selection technique held up less well; he had strayed from what other statisticians noted were "more accurate" techniques.

The panel dealt yet again with disagreement over BET-1, noting pointedly that even according to O'Toole's notebooks BET-1 worked quite well, conflicting with her assertion that BET-1 "never, ever, ever worked" for her. And they incredulously noted ORI's complete misunderstanding of the science of BET-1 after so many years of investigation.

The panel took serious issue with stories told by O'Toole and Maplethorpe. Maplethorpe testified that he overheard a conversation among Imanishi-Kari, Weaver, and a student working in the laboratory in June 1985 in which Imanishi-Kari admitted the failures of BET-1. Maplethorpe claimed to have a clear recollection of this overheard conversation because he had tape-recorded it. Maplethorpe was never able to produce this supposed tape or the student alleged to have taken part in the conversation. His story became even more doubtful when others testified that Maplethorpe had vowed to "get" Imanishi-Kari somehow.

O'Toole was in similar straits. She claimed at the hearings that she had "a tape recording of assertions to the contrary" regarding the Tufts inquiry panel's statements that Imanishi-Kari showed them her data. O'Toole also failed to produce this interesting tape or explain why it wasn't available. The panel diplomatically stated, "After hearing Dr. O'Toole and the other witnesses testify and examining all of her statements over the years, we question the accuracy of Dr. O'Toole's memory and her increasing commitment to a partisan stand." In the panel's opinion, "While we share others' concern that a 'whistleblower' be protected from adverse consequences, we are also concerned about the implications of involving a whistleblower too heavily in an investigation. Such involvement can compromise both the ability of the investigators to maintain objectivity and the ability of the whistleblower to avoid becoming too vested in the outcome. We think that happened here."

Man Alive, a play written by O'Toole's father in Ireland many years before, presaged key aspects of her behavior in the Baltimore affair. The main character, Tim O'Malley, rebels against the large bureaucratic power company he works for, pledging, "As long as I stay I'll be a thorn in their backside, and every time they sit on anyone again they'll think of me."

When the acquittal was announced, Imanishi-Kari could hardly believe it. She spent most of the evening on the phone to her family in Brazil, and then she stayed up until 4 A.M. reading the two-hundred-page appeals board decision. She woke up again at 7 A.M. feeling fresh. Within a year she became a tenured professor at Tufts. Reflecting on the experience two years later, she said, "I don't get upset about much of anything anymore."

Though Imanishi-Kari was exonerated, the affair had been deeply damaging. Donald Kennedy, the Stanford president ousted by Dingell, commented that the appeals board decision marked "the end of the sorriest chapter in American science that I can think of. . . . A lot of people owe David an apology." Paul Berg said, "It's a sad fact that his exoneration comes only after he took such a beating. The abuse he took at Rockefeller, the way he was manhandled and basically forced to resign, I hope they hang their heads in shame." Bernadine Healy, former head of the NIH, said, "There was a lot of cruelty and abusive behavior tolerated in the name of rooting out fraud," when, actually, "the fraud, the abuse, the dishonesty, was in the process."

Many people pontificated on what Baltimore could have done differently to resolve the controversy. Perhaps the most astute observations were made by Irving Weissman, who was both friend and colleague to Baltimore throughout this tumultuous period: "What could David have done different? I think that he could have taken the responsibility himself, although he is not a cellular immunologist, to fund or to do [Imanishi-Kari's experiments again] in his lab, or find funding for an independent lab to test the experiment again. That's the one step that he didn't take that—it's easy [to say] in retrospect—I urged him, and others I think urged him, to do. That's the only step that I can see where you might have gone one step further than he did. And I know that people think that he was arrogant for not doing that, and arrogant for not following it to the *n* degree. But, in a way, he was fulfilling, as far as he could, the bargain with Thereza and her laboratory, that he wasn't second-guessing her—he was looking at the data as presented."

Baltimore has not changed his style. He does not run his lab any more tightly than he used to: "I think that would be destructive of the scientific atmosphere. I believe that science is based on trust, and that you *must* trust people. There's no way to get enough information to be a policeman. And even if there was, that process of trying to be a policeman would undercut the whole creative aspect of science."

How did the Baltimore affair turn into the most publicized and most divisive scientific fraud controversy ever, when no fraud occurred? Blaming O'Toole is a simple answer, but her role is easy to overstate. O'Toole clearly believed, at least early on, that she was searching out the truth. She began her quest in earnest and made some prescient insights about alternative scientific explanations for the results of the Weaver paper. It is unfortunate that she never published them. Of greater concern is how one postdoc's misguided accusations captured the imagination of the U.S. Congress, the Secret Service, the scientific community, and the media. Clearly the affair unfolded in an atmosphere of great distrust of scientists, both by other scientists and by outsiders. Various observers blamed the controversy on Dingell and his aides, the lack of due process at the NIH, scientists with a vendetta against Baltimore, or the media's quest for sensation.

Imanishi-Kari was the victim of a character assassination by Dingell's aides. A staffer for another representative defended Dingell himself as an earnest and honorable man, but said that Dingell's aides "went after 'The Big Story' as opposed to the truth." Dingell's team ruined careers to advance their own, and then they moved on to new jobs, their relative obscurity absolving them from responsibility.

However powerful, Dingell and his aides couldn't have gone so far on their own. The scientific community contributed to the problems. Philip Handler had readily admitted to Al Gore that scientists had no sense of due process in possible fraud cases. The NIH investigations proved that point time and time again. The name "Office of Scientific Integrity" was actually recommended as an Orwellian joke by the lawyer Robert Charrow. Later, Charrow noted, "While scientists may be very good at doing science, they are not very good at doing law." Bernadine Healy said, "It had become obvious that this was a totally polluted system where these [ORI] scientists got behind closed doors and worked out their venom, taking down their colleagues. It was a star chamber, a hideous travesty of justice."

Even with the obvious lack of fairness and due process in the federal investigations, there had been as many scientists declaring Baltimore guilty as there were defending him. Maxine Singer was mortified by her colleagues' actions: "Sadly and inexplicably, the scientific community itself contributed to the unfolding of this tragedy. . . . Soon after [the Dingell hearings], it became evident that a group of important scientists was actually conspiring to read Baltimore out of the community." Among them was the legendary Jim Watson, the discoverer of the DNA double helix. Watson spent considerable time and effort arranging private meetings with major scientists and administrators to encourage them to help him evict David Baltimore from science. He sweepingly declared that Baltimore's Nobel Prize should be revoked, he should be expelled from the National Academy of

Science, and he should be banned from federal research for life. Paul Berg said later, "Watson was vicious, was *vicious*." What drove a brilliant man to take such a position on paper-thin evidence? No one knows. Most are too scared of Watson even to talk about it. As one participant in the drama said, "There was no reason for this. Watson was mean. Some people are just nasty—you wouldn't want them to babysit your children—and he took pleasure in this."

As an extremely competitive man, Baltimore had made many enemies. And those enemies attacked when they smelled blood. As Irving Weissman noted, "There were scientists on the East Coast, his old friends, who picked up the issue for reasons I still don't understand, and who just made it clear to me I'm glad to be a West Coast scientist; because we fight with each other on data, but they go for your heart and soul."

Mark Ptashne, Walter Gilbert, John Edsall, and Paul Doty of Harvard became known to some as the "Harvard Cabal" or the "Harvard Mafia" for their zeal in pursuing the case against Baltimore. Years prior to the Imanishi-Kari affair, Ptashne was on friendly terms with Baltimore; they had fought side by side in the recombinant DNA controversy. And Gilbert and Baltimore had been good enough friends to sail together in the South Pacific. But for some reason both Ptashne and Gilbert turned on him. Ptashne wrote letters to *Nature* attacking the paper, took O'Toole under his wing, encouraged his Harvard colleagues to speak out against Baltimore, and approached members of the Rockefeller board of trustees to recommend that they get rid of Baltimore. Gilbert became the prime scientific witness against Baltimore and Imanishi-Kari in the ORI appeals board hearings. Even now, Gilbert doesn't accept Imanishi-Kari's innocence. Baltimore has refused to speak to Gilbert for years.*

Why did the Harvard Mafia and Jim Watson turn on Baltimore? The most gracious explanation of their actions is that they held an irreducible faith in the Secret Service. Such faith would by no means be entirely misplaced. After all, the Secret Service exhibits extraordinary skill at tracking down counterfeiters of U.S. currency and various other frauds. But this explanation doesn't seem to hold up. Gilbert, a man whom Phillip Sharp once called "the brightest man I ever met," considered Imanishi-Kari guilty of fraud even after the Secret Service data was clearly discredited.

*Imanishi-Kari's comments about Gilbert after all of this were quite measured. She considered the appeals board hearings a "great human experience" and says that what she learned from Gilbert's testimonial was that even the "crème de la crème of science" could have "such bad judgment."

Maxine Singer and others saw the vindictiveness as self-preservation: "The self-serving reason given for all of this was concern that unless the scientific community was seen as policing itself, the flow of federal research funds would be in jeopardy." Clearly that undercurrent was present in both public and private discussions. John Cairns of Harvard wrote, in a letter published in *Nature* and sent to the president of the National Academy of Sciences, "Simply at the mundane level of money, I could imagine fund-raising for the Academy becoming much harder if Congress is left with the image of the Academy as the organization that sided with Baltimore right or wrong, through thick and thin, to the bitter end."

But the Harvard Mafia seemed motivated by additional, less tangible concerns. Some scientists and writers blamed professional jealousy. A postdoc at Harvard at the time commented on Mark Ptashne's strong opposition to Baltimore and his support of Margot O'Toole: "Publicly Mark said it was about the science, but members of the lab saw it as an obvious chance for Mark to bash one of his biggest competitors." He continued, "I like Mark, but, if push came to shove and Mark was cornered [in a difficult situation], he would be ruthless. If it took a couple of grad students and postdocs being sunk to the bottom of the Charles River, metaphorically speaking, to save his own hide, Mark would do it."

Perhaps Baltimore's rapid establishment of the Whitehead Institute as the premier biomedical research facility in Cambridge, almost in Harvard's own 350-year-old backyard, rubbed the Harvard professors the wrong way. In fact, in 1984 Gilbert was asked to leave Biogen, the $100 million company that he had helped found. When Baltimore heard about this, he floated the idea that Gilbert could join the Whitehead Institute. But the Whitehead faculty didn't like the idea, and Baltimore didn't offer Gilbert a position. This professional slight may have offended Gilbert. For other players in the drama, academic rivalry probably only intensified deeper conflicts.

Some colleagues have suggested that perhaps Watson and Gilbert turned against Baltimore because he initially opposed the Human Genome Project, of which they were two of the country's biggest proponents. They proposed to sequence the entire human genome, all three billion letters of information. At the time it was an enormous undertaking, because sequencing a mere two hundred letters of DNA then took one person a full day. But Watson and Gilbert saw the project as biology's equivalent of the Apollo space program. It was a chance for the nation to look into the very nature of being human. Baltimore staunchly opposed the project for several reasons. He was concerned that the proposed sequencing strategy was flawed;

that the Human Genome Project would take funding away from other areas of biology; and that it would take money away from biologists with small labs and give the money to a few large labs that robotically churned out sequence information. Throughout 1986 and 1987, Gilbert and Baltimore engaged in a public war of hyperbole. Gilbert proclaimed that "the total human sequence is the holy grail of human genetics." Baltimore sarcastically remarked, "The idea [of a human genome project] is gathering momentum. I shiver at the thought." But, in a replay of his position on the War on Cancer, Baltimore changed his mind when the project organizers agreed to improve their sequencing strategy,* and Watson, Gilbert, and others convinced him that special federal funding would be allocated for the Human Genome Project without affecting funding for other biology research.

Once the program was under way, perhaps Watson and Gilbert were concerned that the Imanishi-Kari affair jeopardized the Human Genome Project funding by tarnishing Congress's view of science. In Paul Berg's opinion, "The most benevolent thing I could even attribute to Jim [Watson's motivations] was that he thought the whole [Baltimore Affair] thing was hurting science, and that it was his responsibility to try to defend the good image of science—to call attention to how science had to cleanse itself." (Having said this, Berg expressed doubt that it was Watson's real reason.) The high visibility of the case, both in the press and in Congress, impugned the trustworthiness of scientists and the ability of science to regulate itself. Walter Gilbert said, "Everyone could have walked away after making a public retraction. . . . I'll never know why David defended the paper down the line like that. There was no reason to defend the paper like that." There are two ways to interpret this statement. One is that Gilbert believed that the paper was fraudulent; the other, which may have weighed equally or more heavily with Gilbert, is that Baltimore's behavior contradicted Gilbert's notions of scientific conduct. Gilbert said elsewhere that "this case has less to do with fraud and much more to do with notions of correct behavior." Baltimore fought too hard for Gilbert's liking. Baltimore's aggressiveness also upset Paul Doty and others who wished he had taken a more staid approach. Doty was extremely concerned that Baltimore had violated what he referred to as the "Feynman principle" of scientific conduct. In his infamous referendum letter on Baltimore in *Nature,* Doty wrote,

*Gilbert's orginal proposal was to sequence the genome randomly. Baltimore, among others, was convinced that this approach was hopeless and that the Human Genome Project would need to do genetic mapping before engaging in full-scale sequencing of the genome. This approach won widespread backing.

"The late Richard Feynman captured the spirit when he wrote, 'It's a kind of scientific integrity (that is at stake), a principle of scientific thought that corresponds to a kind of utter honesty—a kind of leaning over backwards . . . (to) report everything that you think might make (an experiment) invalid.'" Baltimore would certainly note that the redundancy of the molecular biology and hybridoma work in the Weaver paper evidenced a "kind of leaning over backwards."

More interesting, however, is the continuation of Feynman's remarks, a passage that was not included in Doty's letter: "We've learned from experience that the truth will come out. Other experimenters will repeat your experiment and find out whether you were wrong or right. Nature's phenomena will agree or they'll disagree with your theory. And although you may gain some temporary fame and excitement, you will not gain a good reputation as a scientist if you haven't tried to be very careful in this kind of work." These sentiments were remarkably akin to those that Baltimore expressed so passionately in his written testimony at the Dingell hearing:

> The test you will face is the toughest one imaginable: can the published experiments be replicated by others, and, even more importantly, do your experiments provide a basis for further scientific development? This is how we ascertain truth. If your experiments are not reproducible or cannot be built upon, the punishment is the most severe one we know: you are no longer believed as a scientist.

Part of this sentiment offended Doty and Ptashne. It seemed to abrogate a fundamental obligation, suggesting that Baltimore would, in Doty's words, "leave to others the responsibility of establishing the validity of what you have published." The conceptual difference is a fine one. It was not Baltimore's belief that the obligation lay with other people to prove or disprove his results. He clearly felt that he had proved his conclusions, but the ultimate test of scientific truth is indeed peer review and verification.

Baltimore's opinion on the decade-long Imanishi-Kari affair is straightforward: "I think that the . . . [immunological] community knows that the paper is largely correct." Irving Weissman took a larger view of the science of the network theory: "What do I think? I think [the Weaver paper] was a promising contribution, not the first and not the last, to the field of idiotype [networks] and immune response, and that idiotypes and immune response largely are a footnote to immunology history. Not central, not determinative. Hardly important at all. But nobody knew that in the early 1980s." The science of network theory is still unresolved, and Imanishi-Kari continues her studies.

In spring 1995, MIT bestowed its highest professorial honor on David Baltimore, naming him institute professor. There are more Nobel Prize winners at MIT than institute professors. The title made him a professor of the entire university, not just of the biology department, freeing him of various administrative responsibilities and constraints. The letters of recommendation submitted on his behalf serve as poignant reflections on Baltimore's career. One scientist said, "Baltimore is the premier biomedical scientist of his time and has had a lasting impact on virtually every realm of modern biology." Another colleague commented, "It is not an exaggeration to say that one could write a pretty decent history of the last 25 years in biology by reviewing Dr. Baltimore's contributions."

From time to time Baltimore managed to relax. That summer, as usual, he went out to Montana to spend a week at his Cutthroat Ranch. He took his nephew along with him, and they spent their days fly-fishing. Even in Montana, though, he had a fax machine so that he could edit papers from his lab in the evenings. Later in 1995 he visited his old classmate, Francis Ford Coppola, at his Napa Valley winery. In August, David and Alice threw their annual clambake at their house in Woods Hole on Cape Cod. They dug a huge hole in their back yard at noon and baked clams, lobsters, and corn for a hundred people until sunset.

Besides fishing, Baltimore loved sailing. He kept a classic 1926 varnished wood sailboat at the marina in Woods Hole. One weekend, in a story that becomes a metaphor of Baltimore's life, Paul Berg had made plans to go sailing with David and Alice, but strong winds and rough seas were giving Berg second thoughts about the outing. Baltimore waved away the weather, and the three set out, with Baltimore at the helm. The winds of Woods Hole are famous for confounding even the best sailors, but Baltimore sent his vessel racing through the heavy swells, into the thick of it. A surprise wind started driving them into the treacherous rocks. One of the great tricks and thrills of sailing is the invisibility of wind: if a sailor pushes his senses he can "see" the wind in distant puffs of ripples racing across the water's surface or in the drift of the spray off the whitecaps. Yelling commands to Alice and Paul, who knew little about sailing, Baltimore managed to swing the sailboat just past the shoals, with Berg leaning over the side and pushing off the rocks, and rode the boat into harbor.

AIDS VACCINE

Are viruses good for anything? I don't think so. If you subtracted them from the world, where would we be? I think we'd be better off.

DAVID BALTIMORE, QUOTED IN PAUL RADETSKY,

THE INVISIBLE INVADERS

AIDS fatalities continued to rise, killing over four hundred thousand Americans by 1997. Nearly one million Americans were infected with HIV. In Zimbabwe, HIV had reduced the average life expectancy from sixty-five years to a terrifying thirty-eight years. In other African countries the situation was similar, and beyond Africa the levels of HIV infection were increasing rapidly. In January 1997, Baltimore agreed to head the NIH's AIDS Vaccine Research Committee. He might have done so years earlier but for the fraud scandal and Dingell's power in Congress. Larry Kramer, founder of the AIDS activist group ACT UP, said that in his search for someone to head up a national AIDS vaccine effort in the late 1980s, Baltimore's name "kept coming up no matter where you looked." Baltimore "was the only person—and I mean that—who seemed to have the unalloyed respect of everybody," Kramer said, "They might not have liked his personality, they might not have liked where he parted his hair, or one thing or another. But nobody had anything but praise and admiration for his brains and his ability to get things done. Now that's unheard-of in this world."

The short history of the AIDS vaccine effort was this: sixteen years, no vaccine, and no good prospects. Vaccines are incredibly powerful at preventing sickness and saving lives, and in the opinion of the World Health Organization the only thing that can stop the AIDS pandemic is a highly effective vaccine. Baltimore's job was, and is, to coordinate industry, government, and academic AIDS vaccine efforts. AIDS vaccine leadership had been sorely lacking. Companies were reluctant to work on AIDS vaccine development because few believed that it was possible or profitable. And academic scientists didn't want to work on an AIDS vaccine because vaccine research was not popular and HIV posed very difficult problems.

Vaccines work in complicated ways that no one fully understands. Most scientists consider designing a vaccine more like treasure hunting or playing the lottery than real science. A researcher can work for ten years developing a vaccine that passes every conceivable laboratory test but completely fails when tested in people. Because of the capricious nature of the work, many of the brightest biologists preferred to continue working on interesting, basic science virology and immunology problems that gave clear answers. In Irving Weissman's opinion, "We spent a shitload of money on [failed AIDS vaccine trials], but you didn't have the thought leaders in the field [of immunology] evaluating or acting on, or even involved in, research. . . . We're paying for that." One of Baltimore's mandates was to recruit brilliant immunologists and virologists to AIDS vaccine research. The field was in desperate need of fresh ideas.

Vaccine development has always been an empirical science based on two approaches. The first approach looks at the immune system of people who have survived the disease and developed an immunity to the virus. The hepatitis B vaccine was developed this way by Maurice Hilleman and his colleagues at Merck Pharmaceuticals.* Hepatitis B normally causes an acute infection of the liver, which lasts for a painful month before the immune system manages to kill off the swarms of virus. Once the virus has been cleared from the body, it is possible to detect antibodies to hepatitis B in a patient's blood. In particular, antibodies against a specific part of hepatitis B, the protein known as surface antigen, are present. Hepatitis B surface antigen antibodies grab hepatitis B virus floating in the bloodstream and prevent the virus from infecting new cells. Less commonly, the immune system can fail to clear hepatitis B, and then the virus ravages the liver for decades. In those people the immune system never develops protective anti-surface-antigen antibodies. So, for hepatitis B, antibodies against surface antigen were a "correlate of immunity": if patients had the antibodies, they were immune; if they didn't, they weren't. This correlate of immunity was further substantiated by showing that intravenously injected antibodies from someone immune to hepatitis B could protect a nonimmune person from infection. This gave Hilleman a clear goal: develop a vaccine that stimulated the body to produce antibodies against hepatitis B surface antigen.

---

*Maurice Hilleman is credited with the development of vaccines for measles, mumps, and hepatitis A and B, all done at Merck.

His group purified virus-free clumps of the surface antigen protein from the blood of patients chronically infected with hepatitis B and then injected that purified protein clump into uninfected people. The vaccinated people developed antibodies against hepatitis B surface antigen. Since then, it has been shown that Hilleman's hepatitis B vaccine is highly effective at preventing infection, and several Asian countries have instituted programs to immunize all of their children in the hope of eradicating this serious liver disease.*

Unfortunately, HIV completely negates this approach to vaccine development, because no one develops immunity to HIV. There are no survivors, there are no correlates of immunity, there is no immunity.** The HIV infection ends only at death.

The second classic approach to vaccine development is to use an animal disease model. The Salk vaccine against polio was developed using an animal model. Viruses infect human cells and tissues in selective ways. For example, poliovirus first infects cells in the intestines and tonsils and then muscle, nerve cells, and brain tissue. It does not infect liver or kidney cells. Also, viruses differ in the promiscuity with which they infect animals. Poliovirus causes poliomyelitis in chimpanzees, rhesus monkeys, cynomolgus monkeys, and humans; but it does not infect dogs or mice. Jonas Salk exploited this observation to develop a polio vaccine by running vaccine trials in monkeys. No one knew how to develop a polio vaccine, so he tried everything he could think of. His laboratory killed thousands of monkeys in their experiments, and they finally came up with a killed-virus poliovirus vaccine that could protect monkeys from a lethal dose of polio. To produce

*After the first hepatitis B vaccine was developed, an improved version was created using recombinant DNA technology. The gene for hepatitis B surface antigen was inserted into a special strain of yeast. That yeast, grown in massive vats at Merck, produces huge quantities of pure hepatitis B protein without producing the rest of the virus, making the vaccine safer and more economical to produce.

**I refer only to HIV-1 (type 1 HIV) throughout the book. The related virus HIV-2, which is common in some regions of Africa but virtually never seen in the United States and Europe, is lethal in only a minority of cases. All of the major vaccine efforts are directed against HIV-1.

More than 95 percent of the people infected with HIV-1 die from AIDS within ten years. Currently, there are two groups of long-term HIV-1 survivors, but they do not survive because their immune systems have managed to beat the virus. One subgroup of long-term survivors has been infected by a mutated HIV-1 virus that permanently infects them but is too weak to lead to AIDS. The second subgroup is taking the powerful anti-HIV drug cocktails that suppress the virus but do not cure the infection. A third, separate, small group of people actually cannot be infected with HIV because they have inherited fascinating genetic mutations that make HIV unable to enter their cells.

the Salk vaccine in industrial volumes, two hundred thousand monkeys were ordered by vaccine production labs in 1955 alone. Their sacrifice led to a poliovirus vaccine that saves an estimated six hundred thousand human lives per year.*

No good animal model exists for HIV. Besides humans, HIV infects only chimpanzees, but HIV does not cause AIDS in chimpanzees. Additionally, research using chimpanzees is incredibly expensive: laboratory chimpanzees cost $70,000 apiece, including the initial purchase and lifelong care of the infected animal. Without a good animal model, and without having any idea about the correlates of immunity, many immunologists, vaccinologists, and virologists have considered HIV vaccine work too difficult a challenge.

This is not to say that no scientists were working on HIV. In 1997 the national HIV research budget was almost $1.5 billion, and thousands of biologists studied HIV. Most scientists studied the virus life cycle or specific proteins, much as Baltimore studied poliovirus. In fact, it was through such test-tube studies of HIV that pharmaceutical companies developed the drugs that block HIV replication. Their general strategy was to look at the HIV proteins, analyze their function, design (or find) drugs that inhibited the proteins in vitro,** test the drugs in cell culture to make sure that they actually stopped HIV replication, and then test the drugs in people. Because drugs fight the virus directly, cell culture work is a reasonable model for HIV replication and a drug's ability to stop it. Vaccine research, however, isn't possible in cell culture because a vaccine is not designed to destroy the virus directly. It is designed to teach and stimulate the body's immune system to destroy the virus. Assessing vaccines requires a living organism.

For the pharmaceutical industry, vaccines are very difficult and expensive to develop, and an AIDS vaccine might not be profitable in the United States. Companies cited surveys that suggested that very few people will take an AIDS vaccine voluntarily, because most don't believe that they are at risk. And why would a company make a product that won't sell? When companies claimed that they were racing for a vaccine, they were in fact racing for drugs.

---

*Albert Sabin developed the live attenuated (mutant) poliovirus vaccine a couple of years later, also by running vaccine trials in monkeys. The live Sabin polio vaccine is now the more widely used, and it is the primary tool in the current worldwide effort to eradicate poliomyelitis, organized by the World Health Organization and heavily funded by Rotary International.

**Most of these drugs acted against HIV reverse transcriptase, and so the biochemical techniques used to test their efficacy in vitro were derived from the Nobel Prize–winning techniques Baltimore developed in the early 1970s to measure reverse transcriptase activity.

The development of drugs that inhibit HIV was, of course, a major accomplishment. The AIDS "cocktails" currently prescribed usually contain two drugs that inhibit HIV reverse transcriptase and one drug that inhibits the HIV protease, an enzyme that cuts other proteins. But even the multidrug cocktails are helping only 50 percent of AIDS patients who take them, and none of those patients are cured. If an AIDS patient stops taking the drugs, the suppressed HIV infection flares up again. And there are already HIV strains resistant to all three drugs in the cocktail. Most important, no one in AIDS-ravaged third world countries can possibly afford the anti-HIV drugs, even if the price ($15,000 for a year's supply) is heavily discounted: Uganda's 1997 health care expenditures totaled $14 per person, and Kenya's totaled $17. Only a vaccine can help those countries.

What are the chances of developing an AIDS vaccine? Irving Weissman said in 1997, "Even if we hit something really good—and we don't have anything good right now—the time scale for trials before it would be used with people would be at least five years, *at least*. A realistic estimate is, if we *really* go after it powerfully, somewhere between five and fifteen years. There is always the chance that the virus will outwit us—I don't believe that."

Baltimore has said that he will give the AIDS vaccine effort ten years, until 2006. If there is no good candidate vaccine by then, it is hopeless, and he will give up the project. In the meantime, he has tried to jump-start vaccine development on a number of fronts. He has visited pharmaceutical companies and encouraged them to work harder—a big change for a man who once called them disgusting monopolies. He organized a national series of brainstorming workshops, inviting the most brilliant biologists he knew to present new ideas about how to defeat the disease. And, unable to organize a truly centralized AIDS vaccine program like the Manhattan Project, he orchestrated a new "fast track" for federal AIDS research grants, allowing AIDS funds to be rapidly directed to promising new areas of study. He now more or less waits for a promising candidate vaccine to appear.

Scientists have spent over a decade working on alternative laboratory animal models for HIV infection, including HIV infection of special "humanized" mice (mice that have had their mouse immune system replaced by a human immune system, which can be infected with HIV), infection of monkeys with simian immunodeficiency virus (SIV, the monkey virus closely related to HIV), and infection of chimpanzees with pathogenic SIV/HIV hybrid viruses (SHIV). The most important result to come from this large body of work is that multiple laboratories have been able to protect monkeys against deadly strains of SIV. Correlates of immunity for HIV have remained fairly elusive, but progress is being made. Scientists have now shown that anti-SIV antibodies exist that, when injected intravenously, can protect monkeys from SIV infection. Other scientists have shown that they can protect monkeys in non-antibody-dependent ways (cellular immune responses, generally referred to as cytotoxic T cells and helper T cells). It remains a substantial challenge to integrate these results and obtain specific data about potential HIV correlates of immunity and how to stimulate them with a vaccine, but it at least appears possible that immune responses exist that could protect humans from HIV.

Several of these SIV, HIV, and SHIV vaccine experiments have produced results promising enough to justify experiments in humans. For example, based on SIV work in monkeys, a group led by Andrew McMichael at Oxford University and a group led by Robert Johnston at the University of North Carolina are producing candidate HIV vaccines to test in Africa starting in 2001 or 2002. These two candidate vaccines make use of a new technology, viral vectors, that uses variants of current vaccines to fight HIV. The viral vector not only expresses its natural viral proteins but also expresses some HIV proteins. The idea is to add a piece of HIV to the normal vaccine and then make the immune system learn to become immune to that piece of HIV at the same time that it is developing immunity to the normal vaccine virus. Viral vectors take advantage of the fact that these vaccines already generate an excellent immune response in humans. McMichael's group is working with a vaccinia vector based on the smallpox vaccine, and Johnston's group is studying a VEE vector based on the Venezuelan equine encephalitis vaccine. When these and related vectors were tested in small groups of monkeys, they protected 25 to 45 percent of the monkeys from a lethal dose of SIV. Only time will tell if these or other AIDS vaccine candidates are effective in humans. If the history of other vaccines is any indication, it will take several attempts in humans before a truly effective vaccine is identified— if ever.

Eleven

You cannot deny history, you must accommodate it.

DAVID BALTIMORE
1998

IN A MOVE THAT SURPRISED even his close friends, Baltimore accepted the presidency of Caltech, the California Institute of Technology, effective fall 1997. Paul Berg said incredulously, "I was *sure* he was not going to take it. . . . He kept telling me about how much he would miss Boston, how much he liked Boston, and how MIT was pulling out all stops to keep him." But Baltimore made the move wholeheartedly. Why? Perhaps it was just the draw of sexagenarians to the sun, but Baltimore spun it as, "If it was not a challenge, why do it?" He elaborated, "The experiment is that here I am, a functioning scientist, taking over the reins of a university. I will be, I believe, the only functioning scientist who is running a major university in the United States." The appeal of the challenge of Caltech certainly had something to do with his failure at Rockefeller. Berg speculated, "It can't not have influenced him, to a certain extent, to feeling, 'Well, I blew it once, but I'm not going to blow it again. I mean, I'm going to show everybody that I can do this.'"

Caltech was not concerned about Baltimore's past problems. They wanted Baltimore because he had the four qualities they were looking for: he was a biologist, he had good people skills, he had leadership experience, and he was well-connected in Washington.

We end with Baltimore's Caltech inauguration and his sixtieth birthday party, the weekend of March 8, 1998. The weather was, as it always is in

Pasadena, seventy-nine degrees and sunny. In his inauguration speech, Baltimore talked about his history:

I have said a lot about what I have learned about Caltech, but little about myself. Let me end on a more personal note. I deeply believe in the power, beauty, and comfort that comes from a rational outlook on the world. In my younger years, I hankered after a world in which rationality would conquer emotion and bring peace. It was reinforced in my early schooling—remember that I was in school in the post–World War II era, when the country was still basking in the glory of having defeated the irrationality of the Nazis and when the science and technology that had won the war for us were seen as the key to the future. Even the philosophy that then opposed America's, the Communist philosophy, seemed to come from a rational analysis of society and seemed a humane alternative to America's capitalist society, which was so hard on those who were unable to cope with its demands.

When you grow up with a worldview like that, there is a central aspect of society that makes no sense: politics. For years, I simply could not comprehend what the word meant. When people said that in making decisions, you need to consider both the rational elements of an issue and the political ones, I did not understand what they meant—why wasn't rationality enough? So my whole life since I left my parents' nest has been an education in irrationality. I've had to learn that you cannot deny the passions of people, you must accommodate them; that you cannot deny history, you must accommodate it. I think this is a perspective that all scientists who are willing to work within the larger society have to learn, and it is what sometimes limits the effectiveness of scientists when they do venture outside of their laboratories and institutions.

Shortly thereafter he donned the Caltech presidential garb, the hood of the physicist Robert Millikan.

The previous day had mixed heavy science and much lighter fare in a whirlwind of well-wishers, former students, and longtime colleagues laden with birthday gifts and tall tales. Robert Weinberg, whose laboratory in MIT's Center for Cancer Research and the Whitehead had held joint group meetings with Baltimore's lab for twenty years, had organized a Festschrift— a Germanesque banquet and academic symposium—in his honor. Baltimore hardly looked sixty; he could easily have been forty-five. Alice said lovingly, "He has aged well." Eleven former members of Baltimore's laboratory gave scientific talks ranging from John Rose's novel use of VSV as a predator of HIV to Stephen Harrison's whimsical "Some Structures Interesting to David." A grand banquet followed. Harold Varmus, the Nobel Prize–winning head of the National Institutes of Health, contributed this story to the birthday festivities: Harold and a well-respected friend of his attending this very banquet backpacked together on several occasions. In the middle of the night on one trip, a bear ambled into their campsite, looking for food. To get rid of the bear, this well-respected friend, a North Long Islander as it happened, tossed various "pharmacological agents" out of his tent to relax the bear, which the bear ate and then went bonkers, climbing up and down a tree like a huge wind-up toy. Varmus's solution, that of a South Long Islander, was to quietly pack up everything in the campsite while the bear was distracted and make for a midnight river crossing. As more banquet drinks poured into plastic cups and down throats, and the warm Pasadena night wore on, conversations about HIV and VSV and poliovirus and B-cells and NF-κB and retroviruses and cancer overflowed with "I remember when" stories about labmates, volleyball games, infamous quotations, food truck lunches, late-night drinking, and endless experiments that became lives.

ACKNOWLEDGMENTS

In writing this biography I depended on a wide variety of primary and secondary sources. I conducted a series of interviews with David Baltimore between 1994 and 1998. I am indebted to a number of other people for participating in interviews, including Paul Berg, Thereza Imanishi-Kari, James Darnell, Irving Weissman, Robert Baltimore, Maurice Fox, Marc Girard, Michael Bishop, Detmar Finke, Inder Verma, Peter Temin, Charlie Weiner, Alice Huang, Phillip Sharp, Keith Yamamoto, Stephen Goff, Chris Kaiser, Robert Weinberg, Gil Harman, Raul Andino, Volker Vogt, and a number of informal or confidential sources.

The MIT Archives hold a wealth of material. The Recombinant DNA History Collection, held at the MIT Archives and put together by Charlie Weiner and Rae Goodell, is an extraordinary resource. The collection contains three substantial interviews with David Baltimore, conducted by Charlie Weiner and Rae Goodell on May 13 and July 22, 1975, and May 3, 1977. The collection also contains transcripts of dozens of other interviews and boxes of clippings, photographs, timelines, letters, and other documents that informed my research. David Baltimore's personal archives are also kept in the MIT Archives, and these too were invaluable.

A wonderful collection of photographs from the Asilomar conference was available from the National Academy of Sciences archives. Material provided by the Jackson Laboratory Archives, the University of Wisconsin—

Madison Archives, and the Cold Spring Harbor Archives was also helpful. Government documents were essential, particularly the several thousand pages of the *Congressional Record* pertaining to the Dingell hearings, and the Department of Health and Human Services Appeals Board report.

I personally visited David Baltimore's laboratory in Building 68 at MIT, the old Building 16, the Whitehead Institute, the Center for Cancer Research, Rockefeller University, the Salk Institute, Swarthmore College, Stanford University, the Asilomar Conference Grounds, and Caltech.

Alan Lightman, Kenneth Manning, Don Fehr, Alice Huang, David Baltimore, Sondra Schlesinger, Raul Andino, Alan Frankel, and Maurice Fox read the manuscript critically at various stages. I thank them for their time, effort, and sage advice; any failings of the book that remain, factual or otherwise, are entirely my own responsibility. Any corrections or comments are welcome at Ahead@shanecrotty.com.

I am deeply grateful to my writing mentors, Alan Lightman and Kenneth Manning, for encouraging this project into existence, and to my editors Holly Hodder, Erika Büky, and Howard Boyer for expertly guiding it the rest of the way. Additional useful discussion on writing and other subjects came from Barbara Goldoftas, Dave Custer, Rosalind Williams, Eugene Skolnikoff, Laura Crotty, and Anna Hazel Crotty. Finally, the skills and multifaceted advice of Jane Gelfman were indispensable to me, for seeing things when I did not.

NOTES

PROLOGUE

2 *"The AIDS epidemic has rolled back":* Edmund White, *States of Desire: Travels in Gay America* (New York: Dutton, 1991), 342.

But now, through his involvement with the AIDS committee: Interview with David Baltimore, January 13, 1995.

He currently has one graduate student studying HIV: G. Nabel and D. Baltimore, "An Inducible Transcription Factor Activates Expression of Human Immunodeficiency Virus in T cells," *Nature* 326 (1987): 711–713.

"My life is dedicated": Frank Magill, ed., *The Nobel Prize Winners: Physiology or Medicine, Volume 3: 1969–1990* (Pasadena: Salem Press, 1991).

"In my view cancer": David Baltimore, "The Impact of the Discovery of Oncogenes on Cancer Will Come Slowly," *Cancer* 59 (1987): 1985–1986.

5 *Vials full of poliovirus RNA:* For examples of projects in the Baltimore lab, see N. C. Andrews and D. Baltimore, "Purification of a Terminal Uridylyl Transferase Which Acts as Host Factor in the In Vitro Poliovirus Replicase Reaction," *PNAS* 83 (1986): 221–225; P. Sarnow, H. D. Bernstein, and D. Baltimore, "A Poliovirus Temperature-Sensitive RNA Synthesis Mutant Located in a Noncoding Region of the Genome," *PNAS* 83 (1986): 571–575; K. Kirkegaard and D. Baltimore, "The Mechanism of RNA Recombination in Poliovirus," *Cell* 47 (1986): 433–443; R. Sen and D. Baltimore, "Multiple Nuclear Factors Interact with the Immunoglobulin Enhancer Sequences," *Cell* 47 (1986): 921–928; and M. Lenardo, J. Pierce, and D. Baltimore, "Pro-

tein Binding Sites in Ig Gene Enhancers Determine Transcriptional Activity and Inducibility," *Science* 236 (1987): 1573–1577.

5 *Brilliant, eloquent, and personable:* S. E. Luria, *A Slot Machine, A Broken Test Tube: An Autobiography* (New York: Harper and Row, 1984); interviews with Paul Berg, Inder Verma, and confidential sources.

"He has the best killer instincts": Conversations with confidential sources.

6 *"It is not an exaggeration":* Confidential letter of recommendation quoted in MIT *Tech Talk,* June 5, 1995.

One fellow Nobel Prize winner: See Bernadine Healy, "The Dangers of Trial by Dingell," *New York Times,* July 3 1996; Maxine Singer, "Assault on Science," *Washington Post,* June 26, 1996.

"I know what I believe": Interview with David Baltimore, January 13, 1995.

ONE: GREAT NECK, LONG ISLAND

Baltimore's birthdate is not specifically mentioned in the text. He was born on March 7, 1938, in New York Hospital in Manhattan.

7 *He was one of those students:* Interview with Robert Baltimore, July 22, 1996.

8 *A Shimmy Bird starts dancing:* Rube Goldberg, *The Best of Rube Goldberg* (Englewood Cliffs, N.J.: Prentice-Hall, 1979).

9 *He recalls having "a kind of knee-jerk reaction":* Charlie Weiner interview with David Baltimore, May 13, 1975, MIT Archives, Recombinant DNA History Collection.

He was accepted, and in early summer: Interview with David Baltimore, March 23, 1994; interview with Robert Baltimore; Charlie Weiner interview with David Baltimore.

Shortly thereafter, at age eighteen, he published: Theodore Ingalls, Frederick Avis, Francis Curley, and H. M. Temin, "Genetic Determinants of Hypoxia-Induced Congential Anomalies," *Journal of Heredity* 44 (1953): 185–193.

"Will be one of the future giants": Halcyon, Swarthmore College yearbook, 1955.

11 *Months later, the mouse with the skin graft:* Willys Silvers and Elizabeth Russell, "An Experimental Approach to Action of Genes at the Agouti Locus in the Mouse," *Journal of Experimental Zoology* 130 (1955): 199–220; Willys Silvers, "Genes and the Pigment Cells of Mammals," *Science* 134 (1961): 368–373.

David didn't like killing mice: Interview with roommate Gil Harman, May 11, 1998. He and David shared an apartment in Cambridge during their first year of graduate school.

12 *"[I] venerated him":* David Baltimore, "In Memoriam: Howard Temin, the Fierce Scholar," *Cell* 76 (1994): 967–968.

He encouraged young scientists: Baltimore, "Thinking about Howard Temin," *Genes and Development* 9 (1995): 1303–1306.

13 *"That was it":* Interview with David Baltimore, March 23, 1994.

They are friends to this day: Interview with David Baltimore, January 15, 1997; interview with Keith Yamamoto, November 12, 1996.

David loved it: Interview with David Baltimore, January 13, 1995.

"They're greedy?": This and subsequent quotations from Jean Giraudoux, *The Madwoman of Chaillot* (La folle Chaillot), trans. Maurice Valency (New York: Random House, 1947), 135, 29–30, 131.

14 *Swarthmore's academic reputation: Saturday Evening Post,* 1956, cited by Richard Walton, *Swarthmore College: An Informal History* (Swarthmore: Swarthmore, 1986).

He enrolled at Swarthmore: Information on David's decision to attend Swarthmore comes from David Baltimore, "Milestones in Biological Research: Discovery of the Reverse Transcriptase," *FASEB Journal* 9 (1995): 1–4; Charlie Weiner interview with David Baltimore; author interview with David Baltimore, March 23, 1994.

TWO: SWARTHMORE

Most of the material in this chapter comes from my interviews and Charlie Weiner's interviews with David Baltimore. Descriptions of the Swarthmore campus are based on personal observations, historical documents, and, particularly, the wonderful Swarthmore College Scott Arboretum brochures. Descriptions of Cold Spring Harbor Laboratories (CHSL) are from my visit there and from the photographs published in the Cold Spring Harbor Symposium on Quantitative Biology series. The history of molecular biology has been pieced together from a large number of sources, but several excellent general references are listed here:

James Watson, Nancy Hopkins, Jeff Roberts, Joan Steitz, and Alan Weiner, *Molecular Biology of the Gene,* 4th ed. (Menlo Park: Benjamin/Cummings, 1987).

James Darnell, Harvey Lodish, and David Baltimore, *Molecular Cell Biology,* 2nd ed. (New York: Scientific American Books, 1995).

Bruce Alberts et al., *Molecular Biology of the Cell,* 3rd ed. (New York: Garland, 1994).

William Purves, Gordon Orians, and Craig Heller, *Life: The Science of Biology,* 3rd ed. (Sunderland, Mass.: Sinauer, 1994).

Horace Judson, *The Eighth Day of Creation* (New York: Simon and Schuster, 1979).

16 *In 1996 the graffiti in the men's bathroom:* Personal observation. A close friend checked the women's bathroom and found nothing.

In David's junior year, Swarthmore protested: Interview with Gil Harman; Richard J. Walton, *Swarthmore College: An Informal History* (Swarthmore: Swarthmore College, 1986).

17 *"Women were just as important":* Interview with Detmar Finke, April 15, 1998.

"We didn't sit around": Ibid.

17 *"College in the fifties":* Interview with Gil Harman, May 11, 1998.

Baltimore got a C in organic chemistry: David Baltimore's Swarthmore College transcript.

In his freshman year David also dabbled: Halcyon, Swarthmore College yearbook, 1960.

18 *Racial integration issues:* Interview with Detmar Finke; interview with Peter Temin, May 18, 1998.

"The spirit of Swarthmore": Halcyon, Swarthmore College yearbook, 1959.

"He came to me and he said": Interview with Detmar Finke.

"David has always been arrogant": Ibid.

19 *"There was a group of men":* Ibid.

20 *He planned to return to Mt. Sinai:* Interview with David Baltimore, July 23, 1996.

"It was sort of a dump": Interview with David Baltimore, May 1998.

Detmar's recollection: Interview with Detmar Finke.

"David and I used to have": Ibid.

21 *"Temin's academic feats":* David Baltimore, "In Memoriam: Howard Temin, the Fierce Scholar," *Cell* 76 (1994): 967–968.

"Most students quiver": Ibid.

"Howard was individual": Interview with Peter Temin.

"At Swarthmore the teaching of biology": Interview with David Baltimore, March 23, 1994.

25 *Avery and his colleagues:* My account of the proof of DNA as the molecule of heredity draws from conversations with several senior molecular biologists and from the following sources: Judson, *Eighth Day of Creation;* Anthony Griffiths, Jeffrey Miller, David Suzuki, Richard Lewontin, and William Gelbart, *An Introduction to Genetic Analysis,* 5th ed. (New York: W. H. Freeman, 1993), chapter 11, "The Structure of DNA"; Purves et al., *Life: The Science of Biology,* chapter 11, "Nucleic Acids as the Genetic Material"; James Watson, Michael Gilman, Jan Witkowski, and Mark Zoller, *Recombinant DNA,* 2nd ed. (San Francisco: W. H. Freeman, 1992), chapter 2, "DNA Is the Primary Genetic Material."

27 *"I was sick and tired of reading about bacteriophages":* Charlie Weiner interview with David Baltimore, May 13, 1975, MIT Archives, Recombinant DNA History Collection.

28 *When he asked about getting bacteria:* Interview with David Baltimore, January 20, 1995.

One of the great experimenters of phage genetics: My account of George Streisinger's science and personality draws from three sources: Franklin W. Stahl, "George Streisinger," obituary, *Genetics* 109 (1985): 1–2; Salvador Luria, *A Slot Machine, A Broken Test Tube: An Autobiography* (New York: Harper and Row, 1984), 131; interview with Maurice Fox, January 5, 2000.

28 *Pleased by Baltimore's interest, Streisinger:* David Baltimore, "Milestones in Biological Research: Discovery of the Reverse Transcriptase," *FASEB Journal* 9 (1995): 1–4; Charlie Weiner interview with David Baltimore.

30 *Nothing much came of the data:* Charlie Weiner interview with David Baltimore; author interview with David Baltimore, March 23, 1994.

   Streisinger showed Baltimore: Charlie Weiner interview with David Baltimore.

   "I think during the summer": Quoted in Judson, *Eighth Day of Creation,* 44.

31 *It was obvious to Baltimore:* Interview with David Baltimore, March 23, 1994; Charlie Weiner interview with David Baltimore.

   "He was an extraordinary man": Interview with David Baltimore, March 23, 1994.

THREE: APPRENTICESHIPS

32 *The rigid educational attitude of MIT:* Charlie Weiner interview with David Baltimore, May 13, 1975, MIT Archives, Recombinant DNA History Collection; author interview with David Baltimore, November 7, 1995.

33 *"Baltimore was a pain in the ass":* Interview with confidential source.

   "I can't attend your lectures": Salvador Luria, *A Slot Machine, A Broken Test Tube: An Autobiography* (New York: Harper and Row, 1984), 136.

   "Humility is not a state of mind": Peter Medawar, *The Art of the Soluble* (London: Methuen, 1967) 110.

34 *A key part of the Central Dogma:* For additional information on different systems of genetic information storage and expression, see James Watson, Nancy Hopkins, Jeff Roberts, Joan Steitz, and Alan Weiner, *Molecular Biology of the Gene,* 4th ed. (Menlo Park: Benjamin/Cummings, 1987).

35 *Levinthal was happy to have him:* Interview with David Baltimore, March 23, 1994.

   In 1957 James Killian . . . 532 Beacon Street: The address of the MIT Alpha Theta chapter of the Sigma Chi Fraternity. I lived there too.

37 *"Among scientists are collectors":* Peter Medawar, *Pluto's Republic* (Oxford: Oxford University Press, 1982), 116.

38 *Versions of this legend differ:* I originally heard this story from Chris Kaiser at MIT. I have since heard it corroborated by several other professors, one of whom knew personally of the initial incident that founded the legend.

   Apart from the "star experiment": David churned through so much scientific coursework during his first year that he took his biophysics preliminary exams that May instead of waiting until his second year.

39 *"A virus is a piece of bad news":* Quoted in Peter Radetsky, *The Invisible Invaders* (Boston: Little, Brown, 1991), 8.

   "I love to teach about viruses": Interview with David Baltimore, January 20, 1995.

40 *Biologists were rapidly determining:* D. Baltimore, "Polio Is Not Dead," in *Perspectives in Virology,* vol. 7, ed. Morris Pollard (New York: Harper and Row, 1971), 1–14. First given as Baltimore's Gustave Stern Award honorary address, 1971.

He felt a debt to Luria: David Baltimore, "Milestones in Biological Research: Discovery of the Reverse Transcriptase," *FASEB Journal* 9 (1995): 1–4.

By the end of the summer a new professor: Charlie Weiner interview with David Baltimore, May 13, 1975.

41 *"I was convinced":* Interview with David Baltimore, March 23, 1994; Charlie Weiner interview with David Baltimore.

Darnell didn't think he could use Baltimore: Interview with David Baltimore, March 23, 1994.

"That's all I really wanted": Ibid.

42 *"So I lost my chance":* Interview with Jim Darnell, May 19, 1998.

The graduate program would be stripped: Interview with David Baltimore, July 23, 1996.

"All you had to do was work": Interview with David Baltimore, March 23, 1994.

43 *"I'd go to the movies":* Ibid.

"Did I have the right": David Baltimore, "On Doing Science in the Modern World," *Tanner Lectures on Human Values,* vol. 13, ed. Sterling McMurrin (Cambridge: Cambridge University Press, 1992), 275.

"When he had closed the door": Sinclair Lewis, *Arrowsmith* (New York: Harcourt Brace Jovanovich, 1972), 303.

44 *"That epiphanal time":* Baltimore, "On Doing Science in the Modern World," 275.

The work went reasonably well: David Baltimore, "Viruses, Polymerases, and Cancer," 1975 Nobel lecture, reprinted in *Science* 192 (1976): 632–636.

RNA synthesis normally wasn't observed: R. M. Franklin and J. Rosner, "Localization of RNA Synthesis in Mengovirus Infected L-Cells," *Biochimica & Biophysica Acta* 55 (1962): 240.

Mengo, which was easy to work with: Interview with David Baltimore, March 23, 1994.

46 *The best-known human tumor cell line:* J. Michael Bishop, "Cancer: The Rise of the Genetic Paradigm," address given at the Keystone Symposium "Oncogenes: Twenty Years Later," January 5, 1995.

48 *Slipping the mass into a new tube:* The experiment is described in D. Baltimore and R. Franklin, "The Effects of Mengo Virus Infection on the Activity of the DNA-Dependent RNA Polymerase of L-Cells," *PNAS* 48 (1962): 1383–1390. Details of Baltimore's lab techniques come from my interviews with David Baltimore.

49 *The only thing to do was repeat:* The experiments and detail of this scene are real, and Baltimore almost certainly failed at this experiment several times before getting the conditions right, but his bungling it in this specific way (with radiation counts that were too low), though highly plausible, is of my own invention. The main reasons

for mentioning this failure are to highlight the reality that experimental failure is an everyday occurence even for the most talented of scientists and to show the nature of experimental troubleshooting. Details of the experiment are from Baltimore and Franklin, "Effects of Mengo Virus Infection." Details of Baltimore's lab techniques come from my interviews with him.

50 *Baltimore saw Dulbecco as "one of the great grandfathers":* Interview with David Baltimore, March 23, 1994.

Dulbecco was so fascinated by the work: See *Cold Spring Harbor Symposium of Quantitative Biology 1962* (Cold Spring Harbor: CSH Press, 1962).

They were so diverse: Ibid.

51 *"It was clear that this was a guy":* Interview with Paul Berg, June 24, 1997.

52 *Ed Simon, co-instructor:* E. Simon, "Evidence for the Nonparticipation of DNA in Viral RNA Synthesis," *Virology* 13 (1961): 105–118.

53 *The first RNA bacteriophage:* See Norton Zinder, *RNA Phages* (Cold Spring Harbor: CSH Press, 1975); interview with Maurice Fox, July 15, 1996.

This was an important discovery: S. Cooper and N. D. Zinder, "The Growth of a Bacteriophage: The Role of DNA Synthesis," *Virology* 18 (1962): 405; R. H. Doi and S. Spiegelman, "Homology Test between the Nucleic Acid of an RNA Virus and the DNA in the Host Cell," *Science* 138 (1962): 270; and S. Spiegelman, "Information Transfer from the Genome," *FASEB Federation Proceedings* 22 (January–February 1963): 36–54.

54 *Nevertheless, his Rockefeller lab was full of excellent scientists:* Interview with David Baltimore, November 7, 1995.

55 *The first paper was published:* D. Baltimore and R. M. Franklin, "Preliminary Data on a Virus-Specific Enzyme System Responsible for the Synthesis of Viral RNA," *Biochemical and Biophysical Research Communications* 9 (1962): 388–392.

"Baltimore and Franklin have recently reported": C. Weissmann, L. Smith, and S. Ochoa, "Induction by an RNA Phage of an Enzyme Catalyzing Incorporation of Nucleotides into Ribonucleic Acid," *PNAS* 49 (1963): 407–414.

Baltimore and Franklin proved that an RNA replicase: D. Baltimore and R. Franklin, "A New Ribonucleic Acid Polymerase Appearing after Mengovirus Infection of L-Cells," *Journal of Biological Chemistry* 238 (1963): 3395–3400. A poliovirus polymerase was finally purified in 1974: see R. Lundquist, E. Ehrenfeld, and J. Maizel, "Isolation of a Viral Peptide Associated with the Poliovirus Replication Complex," *PNAS* 71 (1974): 4774–4777, and B. Flanegan and D. Baltimore, "A Poliovirus-Specific Primer Dependent RNA Polymerase Able to Copy Poly A," *PNAS* 74 (1977): 3677–3680.

"The way to do significant science": Baltimore, "Milestones in Biological Research."

56 *A single poliovirus that infects:* D. Spector and D. Baltimore, "The Molecular Biology of Poliovirus," *Scientific American,* May 1975, 24–32. See also Watson et al., *Molecular Biology of the Gene,* 911.

57 *By doing this experiment at a variety of time points:* D. Baltimore and R. Franklin, "Effects of Puromycin and P-Fluorophenylalanine on Mengo Virus Ribonucleic Acid and Protein Synthesis," *Biochimica & Biophysica Acta* 76 (1963): 431–441.

"Everything started breaking": Charlie Weiner interview with David Baltimore.

That was a rate of almost one per week: References were counted from the Science Citation Index for the periods 1960–1964 and 1965–1969.The three papers were Baltimore and Franklin, "Effect of Mengovirus Infection"; D. Baltimore, R. M. Franklin, H. J. Eggers, and I. Tamm, "Poliovirus-Induced RNA Polymerase and the Effects of Virus-Specific Inhibitors on its Production," *PNAS* 49 (1963): 843–849 ; and Baltimore and Franklin, "A New Ribonucleic Acid Polymerase."

58 *Seven years later Hewish won a Nobel Prize:* Committee on Science, Engineering, and Public Policy, National Academy of Sciences, National Academy of Engineering, Institute of Medicine, *On Being a Scientist,* 2nd ed. (Washington, D.C.: National Academy Press, 1995).

Flabbergasted, but left without many options: Interview with David Baltimore, March 23, 1994.

Though no one keeps records of these kinds of feats: Such a claim will always be argued, because the data aren't clean or easy to get hold of. Baltimore finished all of his Ph.D. work in two years and nine months, and though Rockefeller didn't hand over the diploma immediately, Baltimore was holding a paid postdoctoral position at MIT. Surely there are other such cases, and they are exceptional.

59 *And so here was someone Girard thought:* Interview with Marc Girard, February 20, 1998.

"No more than a couple of nights": Interview with Jim Darnell.

Darnell not only encouraged Baltimore: David Baltimore, "In Vitro Synthesis of Viral RNA by the Poliovirus RNA Polymerase," *PNAS* 51 (1964): 450–456. The paper acknowledges Darnell's advice and the use of his laboratory.

Darnell helped Baltimore to begin thinking: Charlie Weiner interview with David Baltimore.

"I thought it would be the perfect place": Interview with David Baltimore, March 23, 1994.

60 *"David was by no means the most technically adept":* Interview with Jim Darnell.

From this training with Darnell: D. Baltimore, Y. Becker, and J. E. Darnell, "Virus-Specific Double-Stranded RNA in Polio-Virus Infected Cells," *Science* 143 (1964): 1034–1036.

61 *And it had been proposed:* J. Hogle et al., "Three-Dimensional Structure of Poliovirus," *Science* 229 (1985): 1358–1365 .

Baltimore arranged to work for two years: Charlie Weiner interview with David Baltimore.

62 *Periodically retreating, Baltimore sought refuge:* J. Darnell, S. Penman, and D. Balti-

more, "Molecular Events in the Synthesis of Poliovirus," in *Perspectives in Virology*, vol. 4, ed. Morris Pollard (New York: Harper and Row, 1965), 16–33; J. Darnell, M. Girard, D. Baltimore, D. Summers, and J. Maizel, "The Synthesis and Translation of Poliovirus RNA," *Molecular Biology of Viruses*, ed. J. S. Colter and W. Paranchych (New York: Academic Press, 1967), 375–400.

63 *Though he would always consider the discovery his own:* See U. Maitra, A. Novogrodsky, D. Baltimore, and J. Hurwitz, "The Identification of Nucleoside Triphosphate Ends on RNA Formed in the Ribonucleic Polymerase Reaction," *Biochemical and Biophysical Research Communications* 18 (1965): 801–811; interview with David Baltimore, November 7, 1995.

During David's free time at Einstein: Interview with David Baltimore, 13 January 1995. Sandra Woodward graduated from Swarthmore in 1963.

In February 1965, Dulbecco called Baltimore: Charlie Weiner interview with David Baltimore.

FOUR: SALK INSTITUTE

65 *Baltimore's experiments and techniques flowed:* Charlie Weiner interview with David Baltimore, May 13, 1975, MIT Archives, Recombinant DNA History Collection.

66 *"She was very messy":* Interview with Marc Girard, February 20, 1998.

Huang's postdoctoral project: See D. Baltimore and A. S. Huang, "Isopycnic Separation of Sub-cellular Components from Poliovirus Infected and Normal HeLa Cells," *Science* 162 (1968): 572–574; D. Baltimore, M. F. Jacobson, J. Asso, and A. S. Huang, "The Formation of Poliovirus Proteins," *Cold Spring Harbor Symposium on Quantitative Biology*, vol. 34 (Cold Spring Harbor: CSH Press, 1969), 741–746; D. Baltimore and A. S. Huang, "Interaction of HeLa Cell Proteins with RNA," *Journal of Molecular Biology* 47 (1970): 263–273; A. S. Huang and D. Baltimore, "Initiation of Polyribosome Formation in Poliovirus-Infected HeLa Cells," *Journal of Molecular Biology* 47 (1970): 275–291.

"I . . . found a kind of know-nothing-ism": Charlie Weiner interview with David Baltimore.

Historically, however, a number of scientists: "Microbiology: Hazardous Profession Faces New Uncertainties," *Science* 182 (1973): 566.

67 *And before the polio vaccine:* R. M. Pike, "Laboratory-Associated Infections: Summary and Analysis of 3,921 Cases," *Health Laboratory Science* 13 (1976): 105–114.

"Those guys are crazy": Conversations with scientists who work next to a poliovirus lab, 1997.

Baltimore was ecstatic: See M. Jacobson and D. Baltimore, "Polypeptide Cleavage in the Formation of Poliovirus Proteins," *PNAS* 61 (1968): 741–746; Charlie Weiner interview with David Baltimore.

The polyprotein's novelty: Charlie Weiner interview with David Baltimore.

67 *"Any pursuit so far beyond present knowledge":* David Baltimore, "Milestones in Biological Research: Discovery of the Reverse Transcriptase," *FASEB Journal* 9 (1995): 1–4.

"I really was an anticapitalist": Interview with David Baltimore, January 20, 1995.

68 *In addition, she was chair of the "Open Letter Committee":* San Diego Coordinating Council for Social Action, *Gadfly*, September 1966. MIT Archives, David Baltimore Collection.

"Mr. President: STOP the BOMBING": New York Times, January 15 and 22, 1967.

"On January 29 in Boston": Newsweek, February 5, 1967.

69 *"In terms of my power":* Charlie Weiner interview with David Baltimore.

He wanted a more egalitarian power structure: Ibid.

70 *"I went there and I talked to him":* Ibid.

"I can't remember what he did": Interview with David Baltimore, March 23, 1994.

"That was enough for me": Ibid.

Baltimore accepted the offer: Letter from Irwin Sizer to David Baltimore, April 17, 1967; letter from David Baltimore to Irwin Sizer, May 10, 1967. MIT Archives, David Baltimore Collection.

Baltimore found them a rental house: Interview with Jim Darnell, May 19, 1998.

71 *"I live in the future":* Interview with David Baltimore, January 20, 1995.

FIVE: MIT

The general state of affairs at MIT between 1969 and 1972 was pieced together from my interviews with Charlie Weiner and David Baltimore. Additional material was gathered from material in the David Baltimore Collection in the MIT Archives and MIT campus newspapers.

72 *Eight months later, they were married:* Interview with David Baltimore, March 23, 1994; address from New University Conference Group mailing list, 1969. MIT Archives, David Baltimore Collection.

A photograph of Associate Professor Baltimore: Photograph from MIT Archives, David Baltimore Collection, 80–2, box 7.

73 *"I thought it would be fun":* Interview with David Baltimore, March 23, 1994.

"We support the new student movement": NUC manifesto, MIT Archives, David Baltimore Collection.

74 *"Different people had different views":* Interview with David Baltimore, January 20, 1995.

Beyond administrative politicking . . . "to help the students": Ibid.

Baltimore . . . regarding "the relevance of radical ideas": Letter to Members of the MIT NUC from Ethan Signer (for the steering Committee), October 1, 1968. MIT Archives, David Baltimore Collection.

74 *"We have hoped that the university"*: NUC manifesto.

75 *The NUC declared March 4:* Letter to Members of the MIT NUC from Ethan Signer.

76 *"No one imagined that this class of viruses"*: Interview with David Baltimore, March 23, 1994.

With some help from Martha Stampfer: D. Baltimore, A. Huang, and M. Stampfer, "RNA Synthesis of VSV, II: An RNA Polymerase in the Virion," *PNAS* 66 (1970): 572–576.

The obvious candidates: Ibid.

The influenza polymerase was discovered: The influenza polymerase was a somewhat more complex polymerase. See D. H. L. Bishop, J. F. Obijeski, and R. W. Simpson, "Transcription of the Influenza Ribonucleic Acid Genome by a Virion Polymerase," *Journal of Virology* 8 (1971): 66–80.

Temin called it his provirus theory: "A Two-Way Street for Genetics," *Science News* 98 (1970): 54.

Michael Bishop, a virologist: J. Michael Bishop, Program in Biological Sciences Pizza talk, UCSF, May 22, 1997.

77 *"Teaching is very important"*: Interview with David Baltimore, March 23, 1994.

Temin had already revolutionized: A good summary of paradigm shifts in retrovirology can be found in Peter Vogt, "A Historical Introduction to the General Properties of Retroviruses," in *Retroviruses,* ed. John Coffin, Stephen Hughes, and Harold Varmus (Cold Spring Harbor: CSH Press, 1997).

"It was a throwaway experiment": Interview with David Baltimore, March 23, 1994.

78 *MIT's faculty held a meeting:* MIT *Tech* (student newspaper), May 5 and 6, 1970.

Not only did they cancel classes: Charlie Weiner interview with David Baltimore, May 13, 1975, MIT Archives, Recombinant DNA History Collection.

"Howard, there's DNA polymerase": Reconstructed from Charlie Weiner interview with David Baltimore and "The War on Cancer: A Progress Report," *Newsweek,* February 22, 1971, 84–90.

In fact, Temin thought Baltimore: "War on Cancer," 84–90.

Nature was so excited: Charlie Weiner interview with David Baltimore. The papers were David Baltimore, "RNA-Dependent DNA Polymerase in Virions of RNA Tumor Viruses," *Nature* 226 (1970): 1209–1211, and Howard Temin and S. Mizutani, "RNA-Dependent DNA Polymerase in Virions of Rous Sarcoma Virus," *Nature* 226 (1970): 1211–1213.

An unusual rumor (promoted by Baltimore's detractors in the Imanishi-Kari affair) has spread in the scientific community about the discovery of reverse transcriptase. It alleges that Baltimore stole the discovery of reverse transcriptase from Temin by hearing about Temin's announcement in Houston, rapidly repeating the experiment on his own, and submitting a paper. The rumor is completely unfounded and flawed with chronological impossibilities. First of all, Baltimore wasn't in direct contact with anyone who went to the meeting. Second, Baltimore could not possibly have obtained the retroviruses, done the experiments, written a paper, and submitted it in the few days between Temin's announcement and the date Baltimore's manuscript arrived at *Nature*. In actuality it took him an incredibly fast five weeks to do the work and write it up, and the intellectual and experimental pathway he followed from VSV polymerase to his independent discovery of the retrovirus polymerase (reverse transcriptase) was clear. Additionally, the rumor has been denounced by both David Baltimore and Howard Temin. Bernadine Healy asked Temin about the rumor in the early 1990s, and she summarized: "Temin is a man of impeccable honesty and courage. And he was distraught about this rumor and the attacks made on distingushed scientists. The rumor was absolutely untrue" (interview with Bernadine Healy, June 23, 2000). The rumor has persisted, in large part, because it spread so widely during the Imanishi-Kari affair. For more information, see Daniel Kevles, *The Baltimore Case* (New York: Norton, 1998), 256.

79 *"Howard's whole life":* "War on Cancer," 86.

First, Temin was not a biochemist: Vogt, "Historical Introduction."

Medical care saved fewer: "War on Cancer," 84–90.

80 *The program was showered:* There is no authoritative source on the SVCP. However, Robert Weinberg's book *Racing to the Beginning of the Road* (New York: W. H. Freeman, 1998) does an excellent job of putting the SVCP in its historical context.

81 *He found that the enzyme activity:* "War on Cancer," 86–88.

Members of the NIH: Ibid., 90.

"When I discovered the reverse transcriptase": Interview with David Baltimore, January 20, 1995.

"My life is dedicated to increasing knowledge": Quoted in Frank Magill, ed., *The Nobel Prize Winners: Physiology or Medicine, Volume 3: 1969–1990* (Pasadena: Salem Press, 1991).

82 *"Despite the picture of almost unrelieved gloom":* "War on Cancer," 84.

"Although much progress has been made": House Committee on Interstate and Foreign Commerce, Subcommittee on Public Health and Environment, statement by David Baltimore regarding S.1820, Conquest of Cancer Act, September 1971. MIT Archives, David Baltimore Collection.

"In this circumstance, to maintain progress": Ibid.

83 *He insisted that "cancer research is progressing slowly":* Letter from David Baltimore to Rep. Paul Rogers, September 15, 1971. MIT Archives, David Baltimore Collection. He sent copies to several other representatives.

Involvement in politics: Interview with David Baltimore, January 20, 1995.

84 *At the May national meeting . . . "monopoly situations":* The quotes and comments in this paragraph were pieced together from articles from several newspapers printed on May 5, 1971, all citing an Associated Press newsbit: the *Rochester Tribune Post* (New York), the *Washington Post,* and the *Press Enterprise* (Riverside, California).

84 *"I must say I was* extremely *naïve then":* Interview with David Baltimore, January 20, 1995.

85 *That gift, in combination with major grants:* The benefactor was the Seeley G. Mudd Fund. See "MIT Cancer Center Correspondence and Review Committee Notes, 1971–1973, " MIT Archives, David Baltimore Collection, 80–2, box 11.

   "First of all, it worked out much better": Interview with David Baltimore, January 13, 1995.

   "It was not an efficient program": Ibid.

86 *"I know what I believe":* Ibid.

   It was not surprising: See, for example, Salvador Luria, *A Slot Machine, A Broken Test Tube: An Autobiography* (New York: Harper and Row, 1984), 136; "How Investigation of a Lab Fraud Grew into a Cause Célèbre," *New York Times,* March 26, 1991; John Maddox, "Greek Tragedy Moves on One Act," *Nature* 350 (1991): 269. Also confidential conversations with numerous biologists.

SIX: RECOMBINANT DNA

Susan Wright's *Molecular Politics* (Chicago: University of Chicago Press, 1994) is a good history of the regulation of recombinant DNA. Most of the statements from Rae Goodell's interview with Paul Berg in 1975 were confirmed in my interview with Berg in 1997.

88 *Berg was initially concerned:* Rae Goodell interview with Paul Berg, May 17, 1975, MIT Archives, Recombinant DNA History Collection.

   They simply hoped SV40 was as harmless: Interview with Paul Berg, June 24, 1997.

89 *In 1969, Hamilton Smith:* T. Kelly and H. Smith, "A Restriction Enzyme from *Hemophilus influenzae,* I: Purification and General Properties," and "A Restriction Enzyme from *Hemophilus influenzae,* II: Base Sequence of the Recognition Site," *Journal of Molecular Biology* 51 (1970): 379–409. This discovery was technically the discovery of the first sequence-specific restriction enzyme. Matt Meselson had previously discovered a non-sequence-specific restriction enzyme in *E. coli,* which cut any unmethylated DNA.

   Paul Berg, who knew Herbert Boyer: Rae Goodell interview with Paul Berg.

90 *And they would hold together:* They made their recombinant DNA molecule by taking a lambda construct, which already contained a set of *E. coli* galactose metabolism genes, linearizing it, and using terminal transferase to add a string of thymidines to the ends. Then they took the circular SV40 genome, cut it with the EcoRI restriction enzyme provided by Boyer (it only cut once in SV40), and used terminal transferase to add a string of adenosines to the ends. The populations of molecules were mixed, and hybrids were formed via complementary cohesive ends. Berg's lab did not use ligase to create covalent bonds; they depended on the complementarity alone, which required them to work at low temperatures.

   One of the students, Janet Mertz: Bacteria don't particularly like to take up foreign DNA:

researchers have to somehow induce them to do so. Mertz was optimizing a method using calcium salt that is still the most popular bacterial transformation technique.

90 *Other members of the workshop:* Rae Goodell interview with Paul Berg.

When Pollack suggested that Berg cancel: Ibid.

91 *"He was absolutely dumbfounded":* William Bennett, "Science That Frightens Scientists," *Atlantic Monthly,* February 1977, 43–62.

"The Berg experiment scares the pants off": Nicolas Wade, "Microbiology: Hazardous Profession Faces New Uncertainties," *Science* 182 (1973): 566.

Berg discussed the problem with Joshua Lederberg: Rae Goodell interview with Paul Berg.

"This specific issue of biohazards": Charlie Weiner interview with David Baltimore, May 13, 1975, MIT Archives, Recombinant DNA History Collection.

"The more and more I talked": Rae Goodell interview with Paul Berg.

Berg and Baltimore decided they would hold a conference: Charlie Weiner interview with David Baltimore, and supplementary note added by Baltimore, July 1977. See also Rae Goodell interview with Paul Berg.

92 *A photo taken of Baltimore:* MIT *Tech* 93, no. 9.

He threw parties: Interview with Inder Verma, June 25, 1997.

He reverse-transcribed rabbit hemoglobin: I. M. Verma, G. F. Temple, H. Fan, and D. Baltimore, "In Vitro Synthesis of DNA Complementary to Rabbit Reticulocyte 10S RNA," *Nature New Biology* 235 (1972): 163–167. Several other groups completed similar experiments simultaneously in the labs of Sol Spiegelman, Ed Skolnick, and Phil Leder. See also D. Baltimore, I. M. Verma, H. Fan, and G. Temple, "Synthesis by Reverse Transcriptase of DNA Complementary to Globin Messenger RNA," in *Viral Replication and Cancer,* ed. J. L. Melnick, S. Ochoa, and J. Oro (Barcelona: Editorial Labor, 1973), 153–170.

93 *But he was unable to pull the students away:* Interview with Paul Berg.

"Introns are junk DNA": Sydney Brenner, talk given at UCSF, Department of Biochemistry and Biophysics, 1998.

94 *"It just seemed like an issue":* Ibid.

"We considered there would be a second meeting": Charlie Weiner interview with David Baltimore.

95 *A tumor grew on his palm:* Wade, "Microbiology."

"I have no doubt that if you gave enough": Ibid.

"Blood is pouring from all apertures": Laurie Garrett, *The Coming Plague* (New York: Farrar, Straus, and Giroux, 1994), 55.

"What came out of it": Rae Goodell interview with Paul Berg. See also Paul Berg et al., *Biohazards in Biological Research* (Cold Spring Harbor: CSH Press, 1973).

96 *The technique was so straightforward:* S. Cohen, A. Chang, H. Boyer, and R. Helling,

"Construction of Biologically Functional Bacterial Plasmids In Vitro," *PNAS* 70 (1973): 3240–3244.

96 *The Russians ignored the treaty:* For the history of biological weapons development in the United States, see Keith Yamamoto and Charles Pillar, *Gene Wars* (New York: Morrow, 1988). For information on the Russian biological warfare program, see Ken Alibek, *Biohazard* (New York: Random House, 1999).

97 *"We are writing to you":* Maxine Singer et al., "Letter Regarding the Safety of Recombinant DNA," *Science* 181 (1973): 1114. (Letter dated July 17, 1973.)

Immediately after the publication: Maxine Singer had referred them to Paul Berg because she knew he had thought about the problem for years.

He refused to make a statement: Rae Goodell interview with Paul Berg.

He recruited seven prominent molecular biologists: Letter from Paul Berg to Hans L. Kornberg, June 18, 1974.

They wrote that their results "now suggest": A. Chang and S. Cohen, "Genome Construction between Bacterial Species In Vitro: Replication and Expression of Staphylococcus Plasmid Genes in *Escherichia coli*," *PNAS* 71 (1974): 1030–1034.

98 *The frog gene was stably inherited:* J. Morrow, S. Cohen, A. Chang, H. Boyer, H. Goodman, and R. Helling, "Replication and Transcription of Eukaryotic DNA in Escherichia coli," *PNAS* 71 (1974): 1743–1747. The frog gene was rDNA, ribosomal DNA, coding for rRNA. The gene product was an RNA; this particular gene had no protein product.

All seven of the other invited professors: Stanley Cohen, Herbert Boyer, Ron Davis, and Dave Hogness were not present but later asked to sign the Berg Committee letter (Rae Goodell interview with Paul Berg). Hermann Lewis did not sign the letter.

99 *"I thought it was most ingenious":* Charlie Weiner interview with Hermann Lewis, July 30, 1975.

"No" was the unanimous response: Rae Goodell interview with Paul Berg.

"Well, if we had any guts": Ibid.

Experiments they blacklisted: The Cohen-Boyer frog gene results were published in May, while the committee was still drafting the moratorium letter, but that experiment did not fall under the proposed restrictions in any case.

100 *This move was a big leap:* David Baltimore, "When Does Molecular Biology Become More of a Hazard Than a Promise?" lecture at MIT, November 6, 1974 (MIT Archives, David Baltimore Collection).

The moratorium letter went through four major revisions: The letter was drafted primarily by Roblin.

By all accounts, the audience: Charlie Weiner interviews with Theodore Friedman (October 21, 1977) and David Baltimore, MIT Archives, Recombinant DNA History Collection; Rae Goodell interview with Paul Berg.

100 *The committee finished the statement:* P. Berg, D. Baltimore, et al., "Potential Bio-hazards of Recombinant DNA Molecules," *Nature* 250 (1974): 175; *Science* 185 (1974): 303; *PNAS* 71 (1974): 2593–2594; Baltimore, "When Does Molecular Biology Become More of a Hazard Than a Promise?"

Baltimore was there to answer questions: Charlie Weiner interview with David Baltimore.

"What I hope is that the dangers": Baltimore, "When Does Molecular Biology Become More of a Hazard Than a Promise?"

101 *"Yes, it does":* David Baltimore, "Hazards in Molecular Biology: A Report on the Asilomar Conference," lecture to the Tech Studies Seminar, MIT, April 15, 1975. MIT Archives, David Baltimore Collection.

"We can always argue": Ibid.

102 *"My wife and I have thought":* Letter from David Baltimore to Niels Jerne, December 12, 1974. MIT Archives, David Baltimore Collection.

"I would never accuse Berg": Charlie Weiner interview with Hermann Lewis.

They felt that it was imperative: Charlie Weiner, "Historical Perspectives on the Recombinant DNA Controversy," in *Recombinant DNA and Genetic Experimentation,* ed. Joan Morgan and W. J. Whelan (New York: Pergamon Press, 1979), 281–287.

103 *"The big question involved":* Baltimore, "When Does Molecular Biology Become More of a Hazard Than a Promise?"

"Although we've had enormous successes": "The DNA Debate: Science against Itself," *Newsmark,* CBS News, October 29, 1974.

104 *The NAS had provided them:* NAS-NRC, Assembly of Life Sciences, "Proposal for Conference," August 21, 1974. MIT Archives, Recombinant DNA History Collection, box 17, f. 215.

"A secret international meeting": Michael Rogers, "The Pandora's Box Congress," *Rolling Stone,* June 19, 1975.

They would have to select the reporters: NAS-NRC, "Proposal for Conference."

"The response of the biological community": Baltimore, "When Does Molecular Biology Become More of a Hazard Than a Promise?" 12–13.

105 *The organizing committee would spend:* Assorted documents on the International Conference on Recombinant DNA in the MIT Archives, Recombinant DNA History Collection, box 17, f. 221.

"Here we are, sitting in a chapel": Rogers, "Pandora's Box Congress."

106 *"It's hard to know":* Rae Goodell interview with Paul Berg, 101, modified per my correspondence with Paul Berg, May 1, 1998.

Some of the younger scientists confided: Rogers, "Pandora's Box Congress."

"He's a bit too downbeat": Rae Goodell interview with Graham Chedd (*New Scientist* reporter), August 14, 1975. MIT Archives, Recombinant DNA History Collection.

106 *"He always used to bring"*: Rae Goodell interview with Stu Auerbach, July 28, 1975. MIT Archives, Recombinant DNA History Collection.

"A nice, quiet, boring person": Rogers, "Pandora's Box Congress."

"Nature does not need to be legislated": Ibid.

One conference photo shows Baltimore: The scenes described are recreated from a series of NAS photos in the MIT Archives, Recombinant DNA History Collection, box 17, f. 236.

107 *"I think you* fucked *the plasmid group!"*: Charlie Weiner interviews with Stanley Falkow, May 20, 1976, and February 26, 1977. MIT Archives, Recombinant DNA History Collection.

"We can't even measure *the fucking risks!"*: Rogers, "Pandora's Box Congress."

"Jim, you could be sued": Rae Goodell interview with Paul Berg, 97–98, modified per my correspondence with Paul Berg, August 8, 1998.

"Is the 'war' over?": See NAS photos in MIT Archives, Recombinant DNA History Collection, Box 17, f. 236.

108 *Sometimes she would stroll outside:* Ibid. See also Rae Goodell interview with Paul Berg.

At beer hour battles were won and lost: Rae Goodell interview with Paul Berg.

It became painfully apparent: Ibid.

The other was to "keep the Feds out": Bennett, "Science That Frightens Scientists."

"In the United States the government": Baltimore, "When Does Molecular Biology Become More of a Hazard Than a Promise?"

109 *"Yes," replied the lawyer:* Quoted in Rogers, "Pandora's Box Congress."

"It is your responsibility": Rae Goodell interview with Paul Berg.

"He reminded the scientists": Rae Goodell interview with Stu Auerbach.

110 *"Frankly, most of us who work"*: Rae Goodell interview with Paul Berg.

"One, we should": Ibid.

"We thought we would be voted down": Quoted in Bennett, "Science That Frightens Scientists."

111 *It passed with a show of hands:* Baltimore, "Hazards in Molecular Biology," cites "about three dissenters." Bennett, "Science That Frightens Scientists," states that there were five.

Surprised and happy: The Asilomar statement was finished five months later, after several more rounds of drafting by the organizing committee and the NAS, and then published in *Science* in June. See P. Berg, D. Baltimore, S. Brenner, R. Roblin III, and M. Singer, "Asilomar Conference on Recombinant DNA Molecules," *Science* 190 (1975): 401–402. Twelve months later, the tenets developed at Asilomar became the NIH's official guidelines on recombinant DNA safety, and every American biologist, university, and company worked from them.

111 *"It was the beginning of the industrial application"*: Interview with David Baltimore, January 20, 1995.

"The whole Asilomar process": Ibid.

112 *Exacerbating public fears: New York Times,* January 18, 1970.

"Scientists to Resume Risky Work": *Boston Globe,* February 28, 1975, 1.

Before the Asilomar conference: MIT Archives, David Baltimore Collection, 80–2, box 2.

In 1972, Baltimore had given a lecture: Technology and Culture Lecture Series, MIT, December 7, 1972. MIT Archives, David Baltimore Collection, box 10.

113 *The discussion:* Baltimore, "When Does Molecular Biology Become More of a Hazard Than a Promise?"

"Those people were around here": Interview with David Baltimore, January 20, 1995.

King said that letting biologists decide: Bennett, "Science That Frightens Scientists."

SEVEN: NOBEL GOLD

114 *They lived in the on-campus Rockefeller faculty housing:* Interview with David Baltimore, March 24, 1994.

"It was very, very interesting:" Ibid.; interview with David Baltimore, January 20, 1995.

115 *When David finally made it back:* Interview with David Baltimore, November 7, 1995.

Although it was too early: Interview with David Baltimore, March 24, 1994.

Alice rushed to the nearest phone: New York Times, October 17, 1975, 1, 12. Also interview with David Baltimore, November 7, 1995.

116 *As a result, his father:* Interview with David Baltimore, March 23, 1994.

The Nobel Committee awarded . . . for their "discoveries": MIT Tech, October 17, 1975.

By nine that morning: Interview with David Baltimore, November 7, 1995. See also *New York Times,* October 17, 1975.

Before flying to MIT: Interview with David Baltimore, November 7, 1995. See also Charlie Weiner interview with David Baltimore, May 3, 1977.

Bob decided to stay behind: Interview with Robert Baltimore, July 22, 1996.

At MIT, a news conference: All of the quotes and comments for this scene come from film footage of David Baltimore's Nobel Prize press conference, MIT Archives, Recombinant DNA History Collection.

117 *"I'll tell you the same thing"*: Quoted in Natalie Angier, *Natural Obsessions* (New York: Houghton-Mifflin, 1988).

118 *"Listen, buddy"*: Quoted in James Gleick, *Genius* (New York: Vintage, 1993), 378.

119 *His tax-free quarter of the $143,000:* Charlie Weiner interview with David Baltimore.

Time *magazine applauded the laureates:* "Nobelmen of 1975," *Time,* October 27, 1975.

119 *For years after the announcement:* See MIT Archives, David Baltimore Collection.

120 *All the proceedings and winners:* Blake Morrison, "So You Want to Win a Nobel Prize," *New York Times Magazine,* October 1, 1995, 62–65.

"I spent much more time there with David": Interview with Peter Temin, May 18, 1998.

Baltimore talked about "bringing molecular biology": "David Baltimore, 1975," in *The Nobel Prize Winners: Physiology or Medicine, Volume 3: 1969–1990,* ed. Frank Magill (Pasadena: Salem Press, 1991), 1201–1211.

Temin's lecture was titled: "Howard Temin, 1975," ibid., 1225–1234.

Dulbecco, a writer as well as a scientist: "Renato Dulbecco, 1975," ibid., 1213–1224.

121 *"It's interesting, both Howard Temin and I":* Interview with David Baltimore, January 20, 1995.

It even appeared in Temin's . . . obituary: See "Dr. H. M. Temin, 59, Dies; Cancer Research Laureate," *New York Times,* February 11, 1994.

122 *"It's about time the scientists":* Quoted in Arthur Lubow, "Playing God with DNA," *New Times,* January 7, 1977.

Scientists from the two universities: Rae S. Goodell, "Public Involvement in the DNA Controversy: The Case of Cambridge, Massachusetts," *Science, Technology, and Human Values,* spring 1979, 36–43.

Science *described the Cambridge City Council hearings:* Barbara Culliton, "Recombinant DNA Bills Derailed: Congress Still Trying to Pass a Law," *Science* 199 (1978): 274; cited in Goodell, "Public Involvement."

"Just what the hell do you think": Quoted in William Bennett, "Science That Frightens Scientists," *Atlantic Monthly,* February 1977, 43–62.

"I have learned enough about recombinant DNA molecules": Quoted in Lubow, "Playing God with DNA."

"In today's edition": NIH Guidelines for Research Involving Recombinant DNA Molecules (Washington, D.C.: National Institutes of Health, 1977).

123 *"The recombinant DNA debates":* Interview with David Baltimore, January 20, 1995.

Senator Edward Kennedy held the first congressional hearings: Senate Committee on Labor and Public Welfare, Subcommittee on Health, and the Committee on the Judiciary, Subcommittee on Administrative Practice and Procedure, "Oversight Hearing on Implementation of NIH Guidelines Governing Recombinant DNA Research," September 22, 1976 (hereafter Kennedy Committee hearings).

In 1884, Louis Pasteur's neighbors: Lubow, "Playing God with DNA."

"I think that we had a responsibility to do it": Charlie Weiner, "Historical Perspectives on the Recombinant DNA Controversy," in *Recombinant DNA and Genetic Experimentation,* ed. Joan Morgan and W. J. Whelan (New York: Pergamon Press, 1979).

Protesters disrupted a National Academy of Sciences meeting: J. Watson and J. Tooze, *The DNA Story* (San Francisco: W. H. Freeman, 1981).

124 *At that hearing, the members:* Kennedy Committee hearings and Charlie Weiner interview with David Baltimore, May 13, 1975, MIT Archives, Recombinant DNA History Collection.

"It needs emphasis that wise exploration": Senate Committee on Human Resources, Subcommittee on Health and Scientific Research, "Recombinant DNA Regulation Act, 1977: Hearing on S. 1217," April 6, 1977.

Later the same lawyer: Ibid., 291, 292.

Jeremy Rifkin and . . . Michael Dukakis: Ibid., 191, 30.

Scientists at the hearing responded: Ibid., 119.

"I can't believe that I was here": Ibid.

125 *Several other recombinant DNA regulatory bills:* House Committee on Interstate and Foreign Commerce, Subcommittee on Health and the Environment, "Recombinant DNA Research Act of 1977," March 15–17, 1977; House Committee on Science and Technology, Subcommittee on Science, Research, and Technology, "Recombinant DNA Act," April 11, 1978; and Senate Committee on Commerce, Science, and Transportation, Subcommittee on Science, Technology, and Space, "Regulation of Recombinant DNA Research," November 2, 8, and 10, 1977.

He showed them a chart: Senate, "Regulation of Recombinant DNA Research," November 2, 8, and 10, 1977.

The citizen panel recommended a moratorium: Goodell, "Public Involvement."

Baltimore even wrote an article: David Baltimore, "Recombinant DNA," *TV Guide,* March 12–18, 1977.

126 *"There were times there":* Interview with David Baltimore, January 20, 1995.

With this in mind, Baltimore joined: Interviews with David Baltimore. See also Watson and Tooze, *DNA Story,* 251–263.

"It was a learning process": Interview with David Baltimore. January 20, 1995.

127 *"What this all boils down to":* Alvin P. Sanoff, "Can Genetic Science Backfire?" *U.S. News & World Report,* 28 March 1983, 52–53.

In Baltimore's opinion . . . "a certain fear": Senate Subcommittee on Health and Scientific Research, testimony by David Baltimore, September 22, 1976.

128 *"In the long run, his influence":* Interview with Paul Berg, June 24, 1997.

Dozens of his students: The NAS members are Owen Witte, Robert Weinberg, Inder Verma, and Fred Alt.

"The model was clear": Interview with Inder Verma, June 25, 1997.

129 *The most obvious choice:* Interview with David Baltimore, January 20, 1995.

"It's interesting, I never really thought": Ibid.

130 *After a lot of work, Baltimore's lab:* Interview with David Baltimore, November 7, 1995.

131 *In autumn 1974, Scher succeeded:* C. Scher and R. Siegler, "Direct Transformation of 3T3 Cells by Abelson Murine Leukaemia Virus," *Nature* 253 (1975): 729–731, and N.

Rosenberg, D. Baltimore, and C. Scher, "*In Vitro* Transformation of Lymphoid Cells by Abelson Murine Leukemia Virus," *PNAS* 72 (1975): 1932–1936.

131 *"He has an almost uncanny ability":* Tim Beardsley, "A Troubled Homecoming," *Scientific American,* January 1992.

POLIOVIRUS: AN INTERLUDE

133 *This is all of the information necessary to create poliovirus:* I have taken the liberty of expressing this information as a DNA sequence, since that was the information that was actually collected, and doing so simplifies matters. Poliovirus's genetic information, as has been explained earlier, is coded as RNA. Therefore, in an actual poliovirus particle, all of the Ts of the DNA would instead be the Us of RNA.

EIGHT: WHITEHEAD INSTITUTE

139 *"It's easier to make $100 million":* Quoted in "Patron of Science," *Nature* 355 (1992): 574; see also interview with David Baltimore, November 7, 1995, and MIT *Tech,* September 29, 1981.

140 *Whitehead agreed to the conditions:* "Patron of Science"; interviews with David Baltimore, March 23, 1994, and January 23, 1995.

141 *"It was a consciously very simple, conservative goal":* Interview with David Baltimore, March 23, 1994.

Baltimore brought these issues to Jack Whitehead: MIT *Tech,* September 18 and November 20, 1981.

142 *"I remember getting my first grant application":* Quoted in Robert Lee Hotz, "Reversal of Fortune," *Los Angeles Times Magazine,* September 28, 1997.

Under Baltimore's stewardship: "Patron of Science."

The MIT biology department ranked second: "Edwin C. Whitehead," obituary, *New York Times,* February 4, 1992; Institute for Scientific Information, *Science Citation Index, 1992* (Philadelphia: Institute for Scientific Information, 1993), CD-ROM.

The disease "induces slow and irreversible destruction": Committee on a National Strategy for AIDS, Institute of Medicine, *Confronting AIDS: Directions for Public Health, Health Care, and Research* (Washington, D.C.: National Academy Press, 1986).

"As a virologist": Interview with David Baltimore, January 13, 1995.

143 *"The nice thing about being in charge":* Ibid.

144 Src *was discovered:* D. Stehelin, R. V. Guntaka, H. E. Varmus, and J. M. Bishop, "Purification of DNA Complementary to Nucleotide Sequences Required for Neoplastic Transformation of Fibroblasts by Avian Sarcoma Viruses," *Journal of Molecular Biology* 10 (1976): 349–365; D. Spector, H. Varmus, and J. M. Bishop, "Nucleotide Sequences Related to the Transforming Gene of Avian Sarcoma Virus Are Present in DNA of Uninfected Vertebrates," *PNAS* 75 (1978): 4102–4106. A good review of the history of cancer research is J. Michael Bishop, "The Inherited Character of Cancer: A Historical Survey," *Cancer Cells,* August–September 1990.

144 *In 1980, Owen Witte:* I have oversimplified the name of the *abl* cancer gene. The proper name for it is *v-abl,* because it came from a virus. The human version is named *c-abl,* for cellular *abl.* See O. N. Witte, A. Dasgupta, and D. Baltimore, "The Abelson Murine Leukemia Virus Protein Is Phosphorylated *In Vitro* to Form Phosphotyrosine," *Nature* 283 (1980): 826–831.

Simultaneously and independently, Tony Hunter: T. Hunter and B. M. Sefton, "Transforming Gene Product of Rous Sarcoma Virus Phosphorylates Tyrosine," *PNAS* 77 (1980): 1311–1315.

The same part of the cancer-causing mutant: These sequences are from three papers published at the same time, regarding a point mutation found in *ras* in the T24 bladder carcinoma cell line, reviewed in Bishop, "Inherited Character of Cancer." The papers are C. J. Tabin, S. M. Bradley, C. I. Bargmann, et al., "Mechanism of Activation of a Human Oncogene," *Nature* 300 (1982): 143–149; E. P. Reddy, R. K. Reynolds, E. Santos, and M. Barbacid, "A Point Mutation Is Responsible for the Acquisition of Transforming Properties by the T24 Human Bladder Carcinoma Oncogene," *Nature* 300 (1982): 149–152; and E. Taparowsky, Y. Suard, O. Fasano, K. Shimizu, M. Goldfarb, and M. Wigler, "Activation of the T24 Bladder Carcinoma Transforming Gene Is Linked to a Single Amino Acid Change," *Nature* 300 (1982): 762–765.

146 *"I think all of us":* Quoted in Natalie Angier, *Natural Obsession* (Boston: Houghton-Mifflin, 1988), 15.

"We must, I believe": David Baltimore, "The Impact of the Discovery of Oncogenes on Cancer Mortality Rates Will Come Slowly," *Cancer* 59 (1987): 1985–1986.

"The genetic properties of cancer cells": Ibid.

147 *Some of his most exciting discoveries:* A. Bothwell, M. Paskind, R. C. Schwartz, G. E. Sonenshein, M. Gefter, and D. Baltimore, "Dual Expression of λ Genes in the MOPC-315 Plasmacytoma," *Nature* 290 (1981): 65–67; N. Crawford, A. Fire, M. Samuels, P. A. Sharp, and D. Baltimore, "Inhibition of Transcription Factor Activity by Poliovirus," *Cell* 27 (1981): 555–561; A. Ross, D. Baltimore, and H. N. Eisen, "Phosphotyrosine-Containing Proteins Isolated by Affinity Chromatography with Antibodies to a Synthetic Hapten," *Nature* 294 (1982): 654–656; E. Mather, F. W. Alt, A. L. M. Bothwell, D. Baltimore, and M. E. Koshland, "Expression of J Chain RNA in Cell Lines Representing Different Stages of B Lymphocyte Differentiation," *Cell* 23 (1981): 369–378; S. Goff, C. J. Tabin, J. Y. Wang, R. Weinberg. and D. Baltimore, "Transfection of Fibroblasts by Cloned Abelson Murine Leukemia Virus DNA and Recovery of Transmissible Virus by Recombination with Helper Virus," *Journal of Virology.* 41 (1982): 271–285; P. D'Eustachio, A. Bothwell, T. T. Takaro, D. Baltimore, and F. H. Ruddle. "Chromosomal Location of Structural Genes Encoding Murine Immunoglobulin λ Light Chains," *Journal of Experimental Medicine* 153 (1981): 793–800.

As the result of collaborative work: A. L. M. Bothwell, M. Paskind, M. Reth, T. Imanishi-Kari, K. Rajewsky, and D. Baltimore, "Heavy Chain Variable Region Contribution to the NP^b Family of Antibodies: Somatic Mutation Evident in a γ2a Variable Region," *Cell* 24 (1981): 625–637.

148 *Susumu Tonegawa, a senior member:* N. Hozumi and S. Tonegawa, "Evidence for Somatic Rearrangement of Immunoglobulin Genes Coding for Variable and Constant
Regions," *PNAS* 73 (1976): 3628; C. Brack, M. Hirama, R. Lenhard-Schuller, and S.
Tonegawa, "A Complete Immunologlobulin Gene Is Created by Somatic Recombination," *Cell* 15 (1978): 1–14.

The results of the research were exciting, and Baltimore and Rajewsky continued:
A. L. M. Bothwell, M. Paskind, M. Reth, T. Imanishi-Kari, K. Rajewsky, and D.
Baltimore, "Somatic Variants of Murine λ Light Chains," *Nature* 298 (1982):
380–382.

Baltimore's lab did significant work: F. Alt, G. Yancopoulos, T. Blackwell, C. Wood,
E. Thomas, M. Boss, R. Coffman, N. Rosenberg, S. Tonegawa, and D. Baltimore,
"Ordered Rearrangement of Immunoglobulin Heavy Chain Variable Region Segments," *EMBO Journal* 3 (1984): 1209–1219; F. Alt and D. Baltimore, "Joining of Immunoglobulin Heavy Chain Gene Segments: Implications from a Chromosome with
Evidence of Three D-JH Fusions," *PNAS* 79 (1982): 4118–4122; D. Baltimore, "Somatic Mutation Gains Its Place among the Generators of Diversity," *Cell* 26 (1981):
295–296.

These studies frequently used the tools: F. Alt, N. Rosenberg, S. Lewis, E. Thomas, and
D. Baltimore, "Organization and Reorganization of Immunoglobulin Genes in Abel-
son Murine Leukemia Virus Transformed Cells: Rearrangement of Heavy but Not
Light Chain Genes," *Cell* 27 (1981): 381–390.

"Well, MIT is a very competitive place": Quoted in Daniel Kevles, "The Assault on
David Baltimore," *New Yorker,* May 27, 1996, 96.

149 *She continued to work with the antigen:* Interview with Thereza Imanishi-Kari, May
18, 1998.

He knew that his lab could accomplish: The reagent Imanishi-Kari was developing was
a monoclonal antibody against the T-cell receptor (TCR), which had recently been
cloned by Mark Davis's lab at Stanford.

They smashed glassware and screamed: Confidential interviews with two independent
MIT sources, March 1995 and August 1996.

"Susumu can be very charming": Interview with Thereza Imanishi-Kari.

"I got very upset": Ibid.

150 *He explained their work and suggested:* Interview with David Baltimore, January 13,
1995. See also R. Grosschedl, D. Weaver, D. Baltimore, and F. Costantini, "Introduction of a μ Immunoglobin Gene into the Mouse Germ Line: Specific Expression
in Lymphoid Cells and Synthesis of Functional Antibody," *Cell* 38 (1984): 647–658.

In 1985 they published one well-received paper: D. Weaver, F. Costantini, T. Imanishi-
Kari, and D. Baltimore, "A Transgenic Immunoglobin μ Gene Prevents Rearrangement of Endogenous Genes," *Cell* 42 (1985): 117–127.

. . . and in April 1986 Weaver: D. Weaver, M. Reis, C. Albanese, F. Costantini, D.
Baltimore, and T. Imanishi-Kari, "Altered Repertoire of Endogenous Immunoglob-

ulin Gene Expression in Transgenic Mice Containing a Rearranged μ Heavy Chain Gene," *Cell* 45 (1986): 247–259.

151 *Shortly before . . . Baltimore went on a wilderness fishing trip:* My account of this trip, including the quotations, is based on my interview with Irving Weissman, August 14, 1997.

152 *The history of their personality conflict:* Material regarding the Imanishi-Kari affair is gathered from a wide range of sources: interviews with David Baltimore; testimony before Congress, the NIH, and the Department of Health and Human Services; and the letters that raged back and forth in *Nature.* Regarding Imanishi-Kari's and O'Toole's different recollections of events, see the sentiments expressed by the review panel in Department of Health and Human Services, Research Integrity Adjucations Panel, "Decision No. 1582," June 21, 1996 (the panel's final decision on the case): "The improbable and ominous construction which Dr. O'Toole put on Imanishi-Kari's complaint is typical of the escalating pattern of miscommunication running through the long history of this conflict" (75 n. 111). Extensive details on the Imanishi-Kari case are available in the well-documented history by Daniel Kevles, *The Baltimore Case* (New York: Norton, 1998).

Admittedly O'Toole's project required the greatest finesse: Research Integrity Adjucations Panel, "Decision No. 1582," 65. The panel noted: "We find it more likely in light of this history, that, in retrospect, Dr. O'Toole interpreted encouragement and pressure to publish from Dr. Imanishi-Kari in the most ominous light, i.e., as meaning she should publish at any cost including dishonesty" (ibid., 88).

"Until that moment I was frantic": Quoted in Kevles, *Baltimore Case,* 56. Originally quoted in Kevles, "Assault on David Baltimore."

153 *O'Toole said in interviews:* Statement from Judy Sarasohn, *Science on Trial* (New York: St. Martin's Press, 1993), 5. Sarasohn conducted interviews with O'Toole and Imanishi-Kari.

Also, she was in the process of moving: Ibid., 93; Kevles, "Assault on David Baltimore"; "Six Years of Intrigue," *Nature* 350 (1991): 262.

O'Toole knew that such a mistake: Gathered from a variety of sources, including interview with David Baltimore, January 13, 1995; testimony by Brigitte T. Huber, Robert T. Woodland, and Henry H. Wortis to House Committee on Energy and Commerce, Scientific Fraud Hearings, May 4 and 9, 1989, serial no. 101–64; Brigitte T. Huber, Robert T. Woodland, and Henry H. Wortis, "Opinions from an Inquiry Panel," *Nature* 351 (1991): 514; Sarasohn, *Science on Trial;* and Research Integrity Adjucations Panel, "Decision No. 1582."

In a conversation with a journalist: Sarasohn, *Science on Trial,* 6; Kevles, *Baltimore Case,* 67–68.

Fraud is the most serious allegation: Sarasohn, *Science on Trial,* 7.

154 *His ruse didn't last long:* David Miller, "Plagiarism: The Case of Elias A. K. Alsabti," in *Research Fraud in the Behavioral and Biomedical Sciences,* ed. David Miller and Michael Hersen (New York: Wiley, 1992).

154 *That was the harshest sentence:* See Nicholas Wade and William Broad, *Betrayers of the Truth* (New York: Simon and Schuster, 1982), 13; Eugene Braunwald, "Cardiology: The John Darsee Experience," in Miller and Hersen, *Research Fraud,* 55–79; George Howe Colt, "Too Good to Be True," *Harvard Magazine,* July–August 1983, 22–54.

"It was obvious to me": Quoted in Kevin McKean, "A Scandal in the Laboratory," *Discover,* November 1981, 18–23. I interviewed Volker Vogt in October 1999 and corroborated the details of the incident.

155 *"What this shows":* Quoted in Wade and Broad, *Betrayer,* 72. Another excellent version of the Mark Spector story appears in in Robert Weinberg, *Racing to the Beginning of the Road* (New York: W. H. Freeman, 1998).

"There is no question": Quoted in Wade and Broad, *Betrayers,* 96.

All three were friends: Research Integrity Adjucations Panel, "Decision No. 1582," 8.

156 *Her comments worried Wortis:* Ibid., 88.

By the end of the meeting: For descriptions and comments on this, see Sarasohn, *Science on Trial,* 9, 94; Kevles, *Baltimore Case,* 74–86.

"Baltimore has said": John Maddox, "Greek Tragedy Moves On One Act," *Nature* 350 (1991): 269.

O'Toole did not bring up the charge of fraud: David Baltimore, "Dr. Baltimore Says 'Sorry,'" *Nature* 351 (1991): 94–95 ; Huber, Woodland, and Wortis, "Opinions from an Inquiry Panel."

157 *O'Toole then produced a detailed memo:* Margot O'Toole memo submitted as testimony to House, Scientific Fraud Hearings.

In Eisen's view: Herman Eisen memo to Maury Fox, December 30, 1986, submitted as testimony to House, Scientific Fraud Hearings.

"This allegation concerns": I have manipulated this sentence slightly. It originally reads: "This allegation concerns a monoclonal antibody termed 'BET-1.'" I have eliminated the words "monoclonal antibody" and replaced them with "reagent" because it is much easier to think of BET-1 as a reagent, without going into the specifics of it being a monoclonal antibody. Monoclonal antibodies are a common reagent used by immunologists because they detect one antigen very specifically.

"In all my experiments": O'Toole memo.

Other members of Imanishi-Kari's laboratory: Eisen memo to Fox, December 30, 1986. See also Nicholas Yannoutsos, letter, *Nature* 352 (1991): 102 ; J. Iacomini et al., "Endogenous Immunoglobulin Expression in μ Transgenic Mice," *International Immunology* 3 (1991): 185–196; and T. Imanishi-Kari, C. A. Huang, J. Iacomini, and N. Yannoutsos, "Endogenous Ig Production in μ Transgenic Mice, II: Anti-Ig Reactivity and Apparent Double Allotype Expression," *Journal of Immunology* (IFB) 150 (1993): 3327–3346.

157 *"My conclusion is that O'Toole is correct":* Eisen memo to Fox, December 30, 1986.

As all immunologists know: Research Integrity Adjucations Panel, "Decision No. 1582," 54.

157 *"The correction would be too minor":* Eisen memo to Fox, December 30, 1986.

Regarding the conflict of interpretation: See David Hamilton, "Verdict in Sight in the 'Baltimore Case,'" *Science* 251 (1991): 1168–1172; Baltimore, "Dr. Baltimore Says 'Sorry.'"

158 *"I do not think that I or anyone else":* Herman Eisen memo to Maury Fox, June 17, 1986; see also Eisen memo to Fox, December 30, 1986.

She said she was dropping the issue: House, Scientific Fraud Hearings; Sarasohn, *Science on Trial,* 14–17.

He and Imanishi-Kari had had epic screaming matches: Interview with Thereza Imanishi-Kari; Charles Maplethorpe quoted in Research Integrity Adjucations Panel, "Decision No. 1582," 35. See also Sarasohn, *Science on Trial,* 35.

"Their first contribution": Bernard Davis, "The New Inquisitors," *Wall Street Journal,* April 26, 1993.

159 *"The sharing of data":* Committee on Science, Engineering, and Public Policy, National Academy of Sciences, National Academy of Engineering, Institute of Medicine, *On Being a Scientist* (Washington, D.C.: National Academy Press, 1989).

"They became a real nuisance": Interview with Paul Berg, June 24, 1997.

Rosenblith explained that the academy: See Committee on a National Strategy for AIDS, *Confronting AIDS,* v.

"We had a public health emergency": Interview with David Baltimore, January 13, 1995.

160 *"AIDS is a judgment of God":* Quoted in Laurie Garrett, *The Coming Plague* (New York: Farrar, Straus, and Giroux, 1994), 330. See also Committee on a National Strategy for AIDS, *Confronting AIDS.*

Early in 1986, the presidents . . . decided "to initiate": Committee on a National Strategy for AIDS, *Confronting AIDS,* v.

161 *"The development of acceptably safe":* Ibid., 23–25.

The secretary of health, education, and welfare: This statement is often wrongly attributed to Robert Gallo, who was present at the same press conference (for example, in Garrett, *The Coming Plague,* 333).

"The development of a vaccine": Committee on a National Strategy for AIDS, *Confronting AIDS.*

162 *This killed-virus vaccine:* American Society of Hospital Pharmacists, *Drug Information 1997* (Bethesda: American Society of Health System Pharmacists, 1997), 2598; Arnold Levine, *Viruses* (New York: Scientific American Library, 1992).

Almost all new influenza strains originate in rural China: Arnold Levine, *Viruses* (New York: Scientific American Library, 1992).

163 *"This was an attempt":* Interview with David Baltimore, January 13, 1995.

"We seem to be afraid": David Baltimore, "On Doing Science in the Modern World," *Tanner Lectures on Human Values,* vol. 13 (Cambridge: Cambridge University Press, 1992).

164 *"Does a scientist"*: Ibid.

National Commission on AIDS, which would "monitor the course": Committee on a National Strategy for AIDS, *Confronting AIDS, 32.*

They also recommended . . . "the President take a strong leadership role": Ibid., 33.

165 *This was an unusual move:* House, Scientific Fraud Hearings, "Short Chronology of the Dispute over the *Cell* Paper." See also Christopher Anderson, "The Baltimore Case: A Chronology," *Nature* 351 (1991): 95.

Fraud is rare in science: Patricia Woolf, "Fraud in Science: How Much, How Serious?" Hastings Center Report, vol. 11, no. 5, October 1989; House, Scientific Fraud Hearings. However, many cases of scientific fraud might go unreported, and the actual number could be closer to ten or twenty cases per year. For example, see "Journals Link Up in Fight against Fraud," *Nature* 388 (1997): 415.

166 *"I cannot avoid the conclusion"*: House Committee on Science and Technology, Subcommittee on Investigations on Oversight, "Fraud in Biomedical Research," March 31 and April 1, 1981.

"I will admit with you, sir": House Committee on Science and Technology, "Fraud in Biomedical Research."

"I just had to believe": Quoted in Sarasohn, *Science on Trial,* 58.

167 *He had exposed rampant fraud:* Barbara Culliton, "Dingell vs. Baltimore," *Science* 244 (1989): 412–414.

"We were going to whop the thing": Quoted in Sarasohn, *Science on Trial,* 56. Sarasohn interviewed Peter Stockton, a Dingell aide.

"Dingell will characterize . . . as piss-poor": Quoted in Judy Foreman, "Scientific Fraud," *Boston Globe,* April 10, 1988.

He stated that "we are only seeing the tip": House, Scientific Fraud Hearings, April 12, 1988.

"It's hard to tell": Judy Foreman, "Fraud and Misrepresentation," *Boston Globe,* April 10, 1988.

168 *Baltimore called the hearing "a classic kangaroo court"*: David Baltimore, "Dear Colleague," May 1988, from David Baltimore's personal files.

"As soon as it became political": Interview with David Baltimore, January 13, 1995.

"If Baltimore hadn't raised as much of a stink": Michael Barrett, quoted in Sarasohn, *Science on Trial,* 96.

"It was quite remarkable": Research Integrity Adjucations Panel, "Decision No. 1582," 29, 19.

169 *Neither the NIH Office of Extramural Research:* Anderson, "Baltimore Case"; House, Scientific Fraud Hearings, May 4 and 9, 1989.

"There remains difficulty": House, Scientific Fraud Hearings, May 4 and 9, 1989; Kevles, "Assault on David Baltimore."

169 *"My books were not books":* Research Integrity Adjucations Panel, "Decision No. 1582," 27.

170 *He was convinced that Baltimore was protecting Imanishi-Kari:* See Sarasohn, *Science on Trial.*

As Maddox noted: John Maddox, "Greek Tragedy Moves on One Act," *Nature* 350 (1991): 269.

"Heavens, we're so proud of him": Quoted in Elizabeth Karagianis, "Making the Grade," *Spectrum* (MIT Alumni Office), spring 1996, 16.

"It seems obvious": Phillip Sharp, letter to colleagues, April 18, 1989.

"It was inappropriate for the government": Interview with Irving Weissman.

171 *Going even further into the political arena:* Culliton, "Dingell vs. Baltimore."

"I fear that the way Dr. Baltimore": Robert Pollack, "In Science, Error Isn't Fraud," *New York Times,* May 2, 1989.

Paul Berg said Baltimore was "like a red cape": Quoted in Hotz, "Reversal of Fortune."

"The troubling and almost universal response": Maxine Singer, "Assault on Science," *Washington Post,* June 26, 1996.

The scheme sounded draconian: Miller and Hersen, *Research Fraud,* 40.

172 *No written report was made:* House, Scientific Fraud Hearings, May 4 and 9, 1989. See also Kevles, *Baltimore Case.*

"This subcommittee has examined a number of cases": House, Scientific Fraud Hearings, May 4 and 9, 1989, 1–3.

"I do not accept insults lightly": Quoted in Hotz, "Reversal of Fortune."

"There are many scientists here today": House, Scientific Fraud Hearings, May 4 and 9, 1989, 88–92; Maddox, "Greek Tragedy Moves on One Act."

173 *"The evidence that the BET-1 antibody":* House, Scientific Fraud Hearings, May 4 and 9, 1989, 164.

"Mr. Dingell . . . I've gone to great lengths": Ibid.

"You said this": Ibid., 165.

174 *"The Secret Service":* Ibid., 88–92.

"If I had fabricated data": Quoted in Philip Weiss, "Conduct Unbecoming?" *New York Times Magazine,* October 29, 1989, 40–41;

"It means you are more likely to fake": Quoted in Sarasohn, *Science on Trial,* 167.

"It was the purpose then": House, Scientific Fraud Hearings, May 4 and 9, 1989, 171–174.

175 *"You have a distinguished record":* Ibid. The quotations in the exchange that follows are all from this source.

176 *"He did brilliantly. . . . I believed that":* Quoted in Weiss, "Conduct Unbecoming?"

"This case has less to do with fraud": Sarasohn, *Science on Trial,* 265, 168, 166, and Gilbert testimony before Research Integrity Adjucations Panel, "Decision No. 1582."

176 *"The issue we are faced with":* House, Scientific Fraud Hearings, May 4 and 9, 1989, 101.

177 *Even his hometown newspaper:* "Dingell's New Galileo Trial," *Detroit News,* May 17, 1989.

Stephen Jay Gould: Stephen Jay Gould, "The Perils of Official Hostility to Scientific Error," *New York Times,* July 30, 1989.

"I don't give a damn": Quoted in Weiss, "Conduct Unbecoming?"

The reporter suggested: Suzanne Garment, *Scandal: The Culture of Mistrust in American Politics* (New York: Anchor Books, 1992), 166.

178 *Following up on Susumu Tonegawa's Nobel Prize–winning discovery:* D. Schatz and D. Baltimore, "Stable Expression of Immunoglobulin Gene V(D)J Recombinase Activity by Gene Transfer into 3T3 Fibroblasts," *Cell* 53 (1988): 107–115; D. Schatz, M. Oettinger, and D. Baltimore, "The V(D)J Recombination Activation Gene, RAG-1," *Cell* 59 (1989): 1035–1048; M. A. Oettinger, D. G. Schatz, C. Gorka, and D. Baltimore, "RAG-1 and RAG-2, Adjacent Genes That Synergistically Activate V(D)J Recombination," *Science* 258 (1990): 1517–1523.

Baltimore was listed ninth: "Random Samples," *Science* 261 (1993): 989.

NINE: ROCKEFELLER

179 *Slots for thirty new full professors:* Interview with Paul Berg, June 24, 1997. See also Stephen S. Hall, "David Baltimore's Final Days," *Science* 254 (1991): 1576–1579.

180 *"The place was run like a series of fiefdoms":* Interview with Paul Berg.

He felt he could not accomplish anything: Tim Beardsley, "A Troubled Homecoming," *Scientific American,* January 1992, 33–36; Philip Weiss, "Conduct Unbecoming?" *New York Times Magazine,* October 29, 1989, 40–95.

"Mr. Rockefeller said": Quoted in Hall, "David Baltimore's Final Days."

"I was enthralled by that opportunity": Interview with David Baltimore, April 25, 1994.

The day of his acceptance: Only the early edition ran this title. Later morning editions were toned down.

181 *"He told me that he was bored":* Interview with Paul Berg.

"I always planned to": Interview with David Baltimore, April 25, 1994.

"I think it's a real plus": Quoted in Hall, "David Baltimore's Final Days."

"This was the future": Interview with Jim Darnell, May 28, 1998.

182 *With the help of the trustees:* Ibid.; correspondence from David Baltimore, August 28, 1998.

"It turned out to be a kind of burden": Interview with David Baltimore, March 24, 1994.

The draft statement described Secret Service proof: Philip J. Hilts, "Crucial Data Were Fabricated in Report Signed by Top Biologist: Nobel Winner Is Asking That Paper Be Retracted," *New York Times,* 21 March 1991.

182 *News of Imanishi-Kari's guilt:* "Even Misconduct Trials Should Be Fair," *Nature* 350 (1991): 259; Jock Friedly, "Trial and Error," *Boston Magazine,* January 1997.

On March 21, the New York Times *ran:* Hilts, "Crucial Data Were Fabricated."

183 *"I wish to state":* David Baltimore, "David Baltimore Says 'Sorry,'" *Nature* 351 (1991): 94–95; David Baltimore, "Mea Culpa," *Science* 252 (1991): 769.

185 *"Richard Furlaud, chairman of the board":* David P. Hamilton, "Baltimore Throws in the Towel," *Science* 252 (1991): 768–770.

"Reflecting on it from a distance": Interview with Jim Darnell.

The controversy now jumped: Hilts, "Crucial Data Were Fabricated"; James Maddox, "The End of the Baltimore Saga," *Nature* 351 (1991): 85.

In newspapers, however: Pieces cited, in order, are editorials in *New York Times,* March 26, 1991, and *Washington Post,* March 28, 1991; John Maddox, "Dr. Baltimore's Experiment in Hubris," *New York Times,* March 31, 1991; editorials in *Wall Street Journal*, April 5 and March 29, 1991.

186 *"I consider it a disgrace":* Margot O'Toole, "Margot O'Toole's Record of Events," *Nature* 351 (1991): 180–183.

"In fact, as each piece of evidence": Margot O'Toole, "O'Toole Re-challenges," *Nature* 351 (1991): 692–693.

NIH draft report . . . "heroic in many respects": O'Toole, "Margot O'Toole's Record of Events."

"Doctor Margot O'Toole's recent comments": David Baltimore, "Baltimore Declares O'Toole Mistaken," *Nature* 351 (1991): 341–343.

187 *But, as she admitted elsewhere:* O'Toole, "Margot O'Toole's Record of Events;" Congressional testimony; Appeals Panel verdict.

"While Dr. O'Toole has now directly attacked": Baltimore, "Baltimore Declares O'Toole Mistaken."

"Doctor Margot O'Toole makes a series of assertions": Herman Eisen, "Origins of MIT Inquiry," *Nature* 351 (1991): 343–344.

"Dr. Imanishi-Kari again admitted": Quoted in O'Toole, "Margot O'Toole's Record of Events."

188 *Representative Dingell had made it sound:* Judy Foreman, "Scientific Fraud," *Boston Globe,* April 10, 1988; House Committee on Energy and Commerce, Scientific Fraud Hearings, May 4 and 9, 1989, serial no. 101–64.

"I lost my job as a result": O'Toole, "Margot O'Toole's Record of Events."

"It had been asserted": Eisen, "Origins of MIT Inquiry."

"Thus it is not inappropriate to ask": Ibid.

"You have no idea how upsetting": Thereza Imanishi-Kari, "OSI's Conclusions Wrong," *Nature* 351 (1991): 344–345. I have silently corrected the actual *Nature* arti-

cle, which says "would lead to recognition of μ^a (endogenous)" instead of μ^b. I believe that this is a typographic error on the part of *Nature*. This view is confirmed by an article that appeared two weeks later, "Imanishi-Kari's Riposte," *Nature* 351 (1991): 691–692, in which Imanishi-Kari states, "While BET-1 detects μ^a immunoglobulin (the transgene), it cross-reacts with μ^b (the endogenous . . .)."

189   *"I was Margot O'Toole's thesis adviser":* Henry Wortis, Brigitte Huber, and Robert Woodland, "Opinions from an Inquiry Panel," *Nature* 351 (1991): 514.

     "I find offensive her statement": Ibid.

     On the next page was a letter from Imanishi-Kari: Imanishi-Kari, "Imanishi-Kari's Riposte."

190   *"[Eisen] now again denies":* O'Toole, "O'Toole Re-challenges."

     "Dr. Eisen disputes my account": Ibid.

     "As scientists we are deeply concerned": "An Open Letter on OSI's Methods," *Nature* 351 (1991): 693.

191   *The press began referring to him:* Peter Aldhous, "Hadley Quits Two OSI Investigations," *Nature* 352 (1991): 268.

     "It is not the business of the subcommittee": Quoted in Christopher Anderson, "Black Eye for NIH," *Nature* 350 (1991): 100.

     Furious about the leak: Philip J. Hilts, "FBI Pursues Leak of Documents in Science Misconduct Inquiries," *New York Times,* March 13, 1992; Barbara Culliton, "NIH Need Clear Definition of Fraud," *Nature* 352 (1991): 563

     "There is a lesson for science": Quoted in "Healy Ready to Take on NIH," *Nature* 350 (1991): 178.

192   *He immediately called for a hearing:* Aldhous, "Hadley Quits Two OSI Investigations"; Peter Aldhous, "Healy and Dingell Lock Horns," *Nature* 352 (1991): 461.

     The continuous "public blood-letting": Beardsley, "Troubled Homecoming."

     "What I was hearing from faculty people": Interview with Jim Darnell; subsequent quotations are also from this interview.

193   *. . . indicting Baltimore for his "egregious departure":* Paul Doty, "Responsibility and Weaver *et al.*," *Nature* 352 (1991): 183–184.

     Baltimore wrote that "the data have proved more durable": David Baltimore, "Open Letter to Paul Doty," *Nature* 353 (1991): 9.

     Indeed, scientists such as Alan Stall: David Hamilton, "Verdict in Sight in the 'Baltimore Case,'" *Science* 251 (1991): 1168–1172.

     "Many of those who were not opposed": Quoted in Beardsley, "Troubled Homecoming."

     Science magazine claimed that "it was at this point": Quoted in Hall, "David Baltimore's Final Days."

194   *"He really found that very difficult":* Interview with Paul Berg.

194 *"Paul's right, I suppose":* Interview with Jim Darnell

  "David and I talked": Ibid.; subsequent quotations from Darnell are also from this interview.

195 *"It is in the best interest of the University":* Letter from Jim Darnell to Richard Furlaud, November 27, 1991.

  "One, the continuing ball-in-play": Quoted in Hall, "David Baltimore's Final Days."

  "I was really outraged": Interview with Paul Berg;

  "I was a threat": Interview with David Baltimore, January 13, 1995.

196 *"I would have come":* Interview with David Baltimore, March 23, 1994.

  "Well, that was probably": Interview with David Baltimore, April 25, 1994.

  "The fact that David": Interview with Jim Darnell.

  Shortly after Baltimore's resignation: Interview with Maurice Fox, January 2, 2000; see also Daniel Kevles, *The Baltimore Case* (New York: Norton, 1998), 287.

197 *On July 14, 1992, because of Lyter's conclusions:* Malcolm Gladwell, "Prosecutors Halt Scientific Fraud Probe," *Washington Post,* July 14, 1992; David P. Hamilton, "U.S. Attorney Decides Not to Prosecute Imanishi-Kari," *Science* 257 (1992): 318.

  "So far as I can tell": Quoted in Hamilton, "U.S. Attorney Decides Not to Prosecute."

  He would wait until things calmed down: Gladwell, "Prosecutors Halt Scientific Fraud Probe"; Richard Stone and Eliot Marshall, "Imanishi-Kari Case: ORI Finds Fraud," *Science* 266 (1994): 1468–1469.

  The manuscript remained incomplete: "Dr. Bernard Davis, 78, Professor and Leader in Genetics Research," obituary, *New York Times,* February 5, 1994. Davis's thoughts on scientific conduct, taken from his incomplete book, were recently published as "The Scientist's World," *Microbiology and Molecular Biology Reviews* 64 (2000): 1–12.

198 *"Howard's death at such a young age":* David Baltimore, "In Memoriam: Howard Temin, the Fierce Scholar," *Cell* 76 (1994): 967–968.

  "The group that he had at the Rockefeller": Interview with Irving Weissman, August 13, 1997.

TEN: HOMECOMING

199 *"I don't know that I relax much":* Interview with David Baltimore, January 13, 1995.

200 *"She said she never wanted":* Ibid.

  "The essential reason the office": Quoted in Philip Hilts, "Institutes of Health Close Fraud Investigation Unit," *New York Times,* May 5, 1993.

  He declared victory: Eliot Marshall, "Fraudbuster Ends Hunger Strike," *Science* 260 (1993): 1715; Bernard Davis, "The New Inquisitors," *Wall Street Journal,* April 26, 1993.

201 *The appeals process was expected:* Jock Friedly, "Trial and Error," *Boston Magazine,*

January 1997; Gina Kolata, "Inquiry Lacking Due Process," *New York Times,* June 25, 1996.

201 *Several other authors published studies:* Kolata, "Inquiry Lacking Due Process." Papers from Imanishi-Kari's lab included Iacomini et al., "Endogenous Immunoglobulin Expression in μ Transgenic Mice," *International Immunology* 3 (1991): 185–196, and T. Imanishi-Kari, C. A. Huang, J. Iacomini, and N. Yannoutsos, " Endogenous Ig Production in μ Transgenic Mice, II: Anti-Ig Reactivity and Apparent Double Allotype Expression," *Journal of Immunology* (IFB) 150 (1993): 3327–3346. Confirming results from other labs included Durdik et al., "Isotype Switching by a Microinjected μ Ig Heavy Chain Gene in Transgenic Mice," *PNAS* 86 (1989): 2345–2350; Rath et al., "Quantitative Analysis of Idiotypic Mimicry and Allelic Exclusion in Mice with a μ Ig Transgene," *Journal of Immunology* 143 (1989): 2074–2080; and A. Stall, F. Kroese, F. Gadus, D. Sieckmann, L. Herzenberg, and L. Herzenberg, "Rearrangement and Expression of Endogenous Immunoglobulin Genes Occur in Many Murine B Cells Expressing Transgenic Membrane IgM," *PNAS* 85 (1988): 3546–3560. See a detailed explanation of the Herzenberg data in Daniel Kevles, *The Baltimore Case* (New York: Norton, 1998), 128–133.

The panel amassed over 6,500 pages: Department of Health and Human Services, Research Integrity Adjudications Panel, "Decision No. 1582," June 21, 1996, 1.

"The Panel found that much": Ibid., 11, 12, and 14–15.

202 *"For example, the 'January Fusion' controversy":* Ibid., 12–13, 14, and 115.

203 *The appeals panel concluded that the matches:* Ibid., 37–49.

Secret Service agent Hargett admitted, "[We] didn't know": Ibid., 31.

The appeals panel became even more skeptical: Ibid., 31.

Ironically, the panel also noted: On the data selection techniques, see ibid., 106, 61, and 80–84.

204 *The panel dealt yet again with the disagreement over BET-1:* Ibid., 58, 123, and 92.

She claimed at the hearings: Ibid., 35.

"After hearing Dr. O'Toole": Ibid., 93, 167–168.

"As long as I stay": Quoted in Daniel Kevles, "The Assault on David Baltimore," *New Yorker,* May 27, 1996, 95; see also Judy Sarasohn, *Science on Trial* (New York: St. Martin's Press, 1993).

205 *"I don't get upset":* Interview with Thereza Imanishi-Kari, May 18, 1998.

Donald Kennedy . . . "the end of the sorriest chapter": Quoted in Kolata, "Inquiry Lacking Due Process."

"It's a sad fact that his exoneration": Quoted in Rick Weiss, "Researcher Absolved of Data Fraud," *Washington Post,* June 22, 1996.

"There was a lot of cruelty": Quoted in Kolata, "Inquiry Lacking Due Process."

"What could David have done": Interview with Irving Weissman, August 14, 1997.

205　*"I think that would be destructive":* Interview with David Baltimore, January 13, 1995.

206　*Dingell's aides "went after 'The Big Story'":* Interview with confidential congressional source, January 1996. This view is supported by both Suzanne Garment (author of *Scandal: The Culture of Mistrust in American Politics*) and Judy Sarasohn (author of *Science on Trial*).

　　The NIH investigations proved that point: House Committee on Science and Technology, Subcommittee on Investigations on Oversight, "Fraud in Biomedical Research," March 31 and April 1, 1981.

　　"While scientists may be very good": Quoted in Kolata, "Inquiry Lacking Due Process."

　　"It had become obvious": Quoted in ibid.

　　"Sadly and inexplicably, the scientific community": Maxine Singer, "Assault on Science," *Washington Post,* June 26, 1996; Kevles, *Baltimore Case,* 256–258.

　　He sweepingly declared: Bernadine Healy, "The Dangers of Trial by Dingell," *New York Times,* July 3, 1996; Kevles, *Baltimore Case,* 258; interview with Bernadine Healy, June 23, 2000.

207　*"Watson was vicious":* Interview with Paul Berg, June 24, 1997.

　　"There was no reason for this": Interview with confidential source.

　　"There were scientists on the East Coast": Interview with Irving Weissman.

　　Mark Ptashne, Walter Gilbert, John Edsall, and Paul Doty: Interviews with confidential sources; Sarasohn, *Science on Trial,* 165; Friedly, "Trial and Error."

　　Ptashne wrote letters: Ptashne letter in *Nature* 352 (1991): 101. Ptashne found O'Toole a job at the biotech company Genetics Institute, in Cambridge (Sarasohn, *Science on Trial,* 166). Rockefeller story from Kevles, *Baltimore Case,* 258.

　　Gilbert, a man whom: Friedly, "Trial and Error"; see also Kevles, "Assault on David Baltimore."

　　She considered the appeals board hearings a "great human experience": Interview with Thereza Imanishi-Kari, May 18, 1998.

208　*"The self-serving reason":* Singer, "Assault on Science."

　　"Simply at the mundane level of money": John Cairns, "To an Officer of the National Academy of Sciences, 28 June 1991," *Nature* 352 (1991): 101.

　　"Publicly Mark said it was": Interview with confidential source, 1998.

209　*Gilbert proclaimed that "the total human sequence":* "Proposal to Sequence the Human Genome Stirs Debate," *Science* 232 (1986): 1598–1600; see also David Baltimore, "Genome Sequencing: A Small Science Approach," *Issues in Science and Technology* 3 (1987): 48–50; Walter Gilbert, "Genome Sequencing: Creating a New Biology for the 21st Century," *Issues in Science and Technology* 3 (1987): 26–35.

　　But, in a replay of his position on the War on Cancer: Interview with David Baltimore, September 16, 1997; *Issues in Science and Technology.* spring 1987.

　　"The most benevolent thing": Interview with Paul Berg.

209 *"Everyone could have walked away"*: Quoted in David Hamilton, "Verdict in Sight in the 'Baltimore Case,'" *Science* 251 (1991): 1168–1172.

Gilbert said elsewhere that "this case": Sarasohn, *Science on Trial*, 265.

210 *"The late Richard Feynman captured"*: Paul Doty, "Responsibility and Weaver *et al.*," *Nature* 352 (1991): 183.

"We've learned from experience": Richard Feynman, *Surely You're Joking, Mr. Feynman!* (New York: Norton, 1985).

"The test you will face": House Committee on Energy and Commerce, Scientific Fraud Hearings, May 4 and 9, 1989, serial no. 101–64, 101.

Doty's words, "leave to others the responsibility": Doty, "Responsibility"; Ptashne's sentiments are noted in Sarasohn, *Science on Trial*, 237.

"I think that the . . . ": Interview with David Baltimore, January 13, 1995.

"What do I think?": Interview with Irving Weissman. His observation implies the putative connection between idiotype networks and immune response.

211 *"Baltimore is the premier"*: Comments quoted in MIT *Tech Talk*, June 5, 1995.

212 *Yelling commands to Alice and Paul:* Interview with Paul Berg, June 27, 1997.

AIDS fatalities continued to rise: UNAIDS, *Report on the Global HIV/AIDS Epidemic* (Geneva: UNAIDS, 2000).

In Zimbabwe, HIV: International AIDS Vaccine Initiative Newsletter, Spring 1999.

Baltimore's name "kept coming up no matter where you looked": This and subsequent comments quoted in Friedly, "Trial and Error."

213 *"We spent a shitload of money"*: Interview with Irving Weissman.

214 *Since then, it has been shown that Hilleman's hepatitis B vaccine:* Francis Mahoney and Mark Kane, "Hepatitis B Vaccine," in *Vaccines*, ed. Stanley Plotkin and Walter Orenstein, 3rd ed. (Philadelphia: W. B. Saunders, 1999).

215 *Their sacrifice led to a poliovirus vaccine:* Monkey data from Jane Smith, *Patenting the Sun* (New York: Anchor Books, 1990), 352. Most of these monkeys were ordered for vaccine production purposes, as the Salk vaccine had just been licensed. Polio deaths estimated in American Society of Hospital Pharmacists, *Drug Information 1997* (Bethesda: American Society of Health System Pharmacists, 1997).

Companies cited surveys that suggested: Jon Cohen, "Bumps on the Vaccine Road," *Science* 265 (1994): 1371–1373. See also Jon Cohen, "Are Researchers Racing towards Success, or Crawling?" *Science* 265 (1994): 1373-1375.

216 *Most important, no one in AIDS-ravaged third world countries:* World Health Organization, *World Health Report 2000* (Geneva: WHO, 2000).

"Even if we hit something really good": Interview with Irving Weissman.

The most important result to come: On the protection of monkeys from AIDS using antibodies, see T. W. Baba, V. Liska, R. Hofmann-Lehmann, J. Vlasak, W. Xu, S. Ayehunie, L. A. Cavacini, M. R. Posner, H. Katinger, G. Stiegler, B. J. Bernacky, T. A.

Rizvi, R. Schmidt, L. R. Hill, M. E. Keeling, Y. Lu, J. E. Wright, T. C. Chou, and R. M. Ruprecht, "Human Neutralizing Monoclonal Antibodies of the IgG1 Subtype Protect against Mucosal Simian-Human Immunodeficiency Virus Infection," *Nature Medicine* 6 (2000): 200–206; and J. R. Mascola, G. Stiegler, T. C. VanCott, H. Katinger, C. B. Carpenter, C. E. Hanson, H. Beary, D. Hayes, S. S. Frankel, D. L. Birx, and M. G. Lewis, "Protection of Macaques against Vaginal Transmission of a Pathogenic HIV-1/SIV Chimeric Virus by Passive Infusion of Neutralizing Antibodies," *Nature Medicine* 6 (2000): 207-210.

On non-antibody-dependent protection of monkeys from AIDS, see I. Ourmanov, C. R. Brown, B. Moss, M. Carroll, L. Wyatt, L. Pletneva, S. Goldstein, D. Venzon, and V. M. Hirsch, "Comparative Efficacy of Recombinant Modified Vaccinia Virus Ankara Expressing Simian Immunodeficiency Virus (SIV) Gag-Pol and/or Env in Macaques Challenged with Pathogenic SIV," *Journal of Virology* 74 (2000): 2740–2751; A. Cafaro, A. Caputo, C. Fracasso, F. Titti, and B. Ensoli, "Control of SHIV-89.6P Infection of Cynomolgus Monkeys by HIV-1 Tat Protein Vaccine," *Nature Medicine* 5 (1999): 643–650.

217 *It remains a substantial challenge to integrate:* On the feasibility of an AIDS vaccine, see A. Schultz, "Encouraging Vaccine Results from Primate Models of HIV Type 1 Infection," *Aids Research and Human Retroviruses* 14 (1998): S261–263; J. Stott, S. L. Hu, et al., "Candidate Vaccines Protect Macaques against Primate Immunodeficiency Viruses," *AIDS Research and Human Retroviruses* 14 (1998): S265–270; A. McMichael and T. Hanke, "Is an HIV Vaccine Possible?" *Nature Medicine* 5 (1999): 612–614.

When these and related vectors were tested: On viral vaccine vectors, see A. Schultz, "Using Recombinant Vectors as HIV Vaccines," *International AIDS Vaccine Initiative (IAVI) Report 3* (1998), 1–4, and R. W. Ellis, "New Technologies for Making Vaccines," in Plotkin and Orenstein, *Vaccines*. On viral vectors providing protection against SIV in monkeys and (in the McMichael paper) demonstration of immunogenicity, see N. Davis, I. J. Caley, K. W. Brown, M. R. Betts, D. M. Irlbeck, K. M. McGrath, M. J. Connell, D. C. Montefiori, J. A. Frelinger, R. Swanstrom, P. R. Johnson, and R. E. Johnston, "Vaccination of Macaques against Pathogenic Simian Immunodeficiency Virus with Venezuelan Equine Encephalitis Virus Replicon Particles," *Journal of Virology* 74 (2000): 371–378; Ourmanov, Brown, et al., "Comparative Efficacy"; J. Benson, C. Chougnct, M. Robert-Guroff, D. Montefiori, P. Markham, G. Shearer, R. C. Gallo, M. Cranage, E. Paoletti, K. Limbach, D. Venzon, J. Tartaglia, and G. Franchini, "Recombinant Vaccine-Induced Protection against the Highly Pathogenic Simian Immunodeficiency Virus SIV(mac251): Dependence on Route of Challenge Exposure," *Journal of Virology* 72 (1998): 4170–4182; T. Hanke, R. V. Samuel, T. Blanchard., V. Neumann, T. Allen, J. Boyson, S. Sharpe, N. Cook, G. Smith, D. Watkins, M. Cranage, and A. J. McMichael, "Effective Induction of Simian Immunodeficiency Virus-Specific Cytotoxic T Lymphocytes in Macaques by Using a Multiepitope Gene and DNA Prime-Modified Vaccinia Virus Ankara Boost Vaccination Regimen," *Journal of Virology* 73 (1999): 7524–7532.

217 *Only time will tell:* Progress of AIDS vaccine trials in humans is reported on the in-

ternet sites of the International AIDS Vaccine Initiative (www.iavi.org), the United Nations AIDS Division (www.UNAIDS.org), and Americans for AIDS Research (www.amfar.org).

ELEVEN: CALTECH

218 *"I was sure he was not going to take it"*: Interview with Paul Berg, June 24, 1997.

"If it was not a challenge": Quoted in Robert Lee Hotz, "Reversal of Fortune," *Los Angeles Times,* September 28, 1997.

"It can't not have influenced him": Interview with Paul Berg, June 24, 1997.

219 *"I have said a lot about what I have learned"*: David Baltimore, Caltech inauguration speech, March 8, 1998.

Alice said lovingly, "He has aged well": Conversation with Alice Huang, September 16, 1997.

INDEX

199–200; and Nobel Prize, 115, 116, 120; VSV research of, 66, 73, 76

Huber, Brigitte, 153, 155, 186

Human Genome Project, 208–9

human immunodeficiency virus. *See* HIV

human T-cell lymphotrophic virus type I (HTLV-I), 143

human T-cell lymphotrophic virus type III (HTLV-III), 142. *See also* HIV

Hunter, Tony, 144

Huntington's disease, 127

Hurwitz, Jerry, 61–63

hybridomas, 150

Imanishi-Kari, Thereza, 4, 6, 147–53, 155–59, 165–76, 192, 196–97, 209–11, 233–34n, 245n, 246n, 253n; congressional hearings fraud charges against on, 166–76, 191, 200, 206; exoneration of, 201–5; and "Harvard Cabal," 207; MIT review of, 156–57, 167, 186–90; NIH investigation of, 157–59, 165–72, 177, 182–92, 197–98, 200, 205, 206; ORI investigation of, 197–98, 200–204, 206, 207; O'Toole's initial allegations against, 153, 155; Secret Service investigation of, 169, 171–74, 182, 187, 201–3; Tufts review of, 155–57, 167, 189, 204;

immunology, 5, 23, 131, 146–47, 143, 149–52, 178, 198; allegations of fraud in, 153–59, 165–78, 182–98, 200–207; cell types and, 12. *See also* AIDS

imprecise joining, 148

Indiana University, 25

infertility, 127

influenza virus, 44, 50, 76, 162, 163, 233n

Ingram, Vernon, 30

Institute of Genetics, 147

Interagency Commission on Recombinant DNA, 123, 124

International Conference on Recombinant DNA. *See* Asilomar conference

introns, 92–93

Jackson, Roscoe B., Memorial Laboratory, 9–13, 21, 23, 76, 78, 130

Jacobson, Michael, 66, 67

Jerne, Niels, 102, 150

Johns Hopkins University, 66

Johnston, Robert, 217

Journal of Immunology, 201

Journal of Virology, 3, 75

junk DNA, 93

Kaposi's sarcoma, 142

Karolinska Institute, 120

Kendrew, John, 31

Kennedy, Donald, 191, 205

Kennedy, Edward M., 108, 123–25

Kent State University, 78

Khorana, Gobind, 85

Killian, James, 35

Kim, Peter, 142

King, Jonathan, 113, 124

King, Martin Luther, Jr., 73

Kirkegaard, Karla, 5

Koch, Robert, 3

Korean War, 16

Kornberg, Arthur, 31, 87–88, 100

Koshland, Marian, 147

Kramer, Larry, 212

Kyoto University, 149

L-cells, 45–47, 49, 56

Ledeen, Bob, 20, 29

Leder, Phil, 236n

Lederberg, Joshua, 22, 27, 30, 91, 105–6, 179

leukemia, 80, 81, 130

Leukemia Society, 115

Levinthal, Cyrus, 31, 35, 36, 38–40, 45, 140

Lewis, Hermann, 94, 99, 102, 237n

Lewis, Sinclair, 43–44

Lincoln, Abraham, 200

Lipmann, Fritz, 42, 54

Loeb, Tim, 53

Long, John, 153, 155, 165

lupus, 149, 153

Luria, Salvador, 27, 37; in antiwar movement, 68; Dulbecco and, 50, 63; at MIT, 31, 35, 40, 41, 70, 72, 140; Nobel Prize of, 26, 85; phage research of, 25, 28, 30, 39, 45

lymphadenopathy-associated virus (LAV), 142. *See also* HIV

Lyter, Albert, 197

MacLeod, Colin, 25
macrophages, 12
Maddox, John, 156, 170, 186
Madwoman of Chaillot, The (Giraudoux), 13
Manhattan Project, 82, 113, 163–64, 216
Maplethorpe, Charles, 158, 203, 204
Marburg incident, 95
Marcus, Philip, 40
Massachusetts, University of, Medical School, 155
Massachusetts General Hospital, 2, 155
Massachusetts Institute of Technology (MIT), 67, 68, 70–72, 92, 94, 114, 116, 117, 159, 196–98, 199, 218, 230n; antiwar movement at, 73–75, 77–78; Center for Cancer Research (CCR), 85–86, 116, 140, 148, 170, 199, 219; Darnell's lab at, 40–42, 51, 58–61; graduate program in biology at, 32–33; and Imanishi-Kari affair, 147, 149, 156–57, 167, 169, 186–90, 197; institute professors at, 211; Luria at, 31, 35, 40, 41, 70, 72, 140; Medical Center, 153; military research at, 35–36; Nobel laureates at, 85, 170, 211; presidency of, 178, 179; Radiation Lab, 35; in recombinant DNA safety controversy, 97, 113, 122, 125; virology course taught by Baltimore at, 76–77; Whitehead Institute's affiliation with, 4, 140–42
mathematics, 8
McCarty, MacLyn, 25
McMichael, Andrew, 217
measles vaccine, 213n
Medawar, Peter, 33, 37, 39
Mendel, Gregor, 23
mengovirus, 44–50, 55, 56, 58
Merck Pharmaceuticals, 213, 214n
Mertz, Janet, 90, 236n
Meselson, Matthew, 31, 235n
messenger RNA, 93
military research, 35–36
Millikan, Robert, 219
Molecular Cell Biology (Baltimore and Darnell), 166
Moloney mouse leukemia virus, 130

monoclonal antibodies, 245n, 247n. *See also* BET-I
mononucleosis, 95
Montaigne, Luc, 161
Morgan, Thomas Hunt, 23–24, 40
Morrison, Philip, 113
Morrow, John, 98, 99
Mt. Sinai Hospital, 20
mumps vaccine, 213n

Nathans, Dan, 54, 67, 98
National Academy of Sciences (NAS), 97, 114, 122, 125, 128, 239n; Asilomar conference funded by, 104; Committee on a National Strategy for AIDS, 160–65; Institute of Medicine (IOM), 1–2, 159, 160; *Proceedings* of, 100; Recombinant DNA Molecules Committee, 100–102; and scientific fraud allegations, 166, 171, 207–8
National Cancer Institute, 80, 81, 85, 95, 154, 161
National Commission on AIDS, 164
National Defense Education Act, 16
National Institute of Diabetes and Digestive and Kidney Diseases, 200
National Institutes of Health (NIH), 130, 154, 165, 200, 220; AIDS Vaccine Research Committee, 212; allocation of funds to, 83; and discovery of reverse transcriptase, 81; Imanishi-Kari affair investigated by, 157–59, 165–72, 177, 182–92, 197–98, 205, 206; in recombinant DNA safety controversy, 111, 113, 123–25, 126, 127, 239n; and tumor virus research, 76
National Science Foundation (NSF), 29, 94, 99
NATO, 93
Natural Resources Defense Council, 112, 124
Nature (journal), 78–79, 81, 100, 142, 156, 158, 170, 183–90, 193, 207–10, 234n, 253–54n
network theory, 150–51, 210–11
Neurospora, 22
neutrophils, 12
Newcastle disease virus, 44, 50, 76

Design: Nola Burger
Composition: Integrated Composition Systems
Text: 12/14.5 Adobe Garamond
Display: Perpetua and Adobe Garamond
Printing: Data Reproductions
Index: Ruth Elwell